Forbidden Drugs 3E

For Renée, Harry and Sophie

That humanity at large will
ever be able to dispense
with Artificial Paradises
seems very unlikely.
Aldous Huxley

The best of life
is but intoxication.
Lord Byron

Every form of addiction
is bad, no matter whether
the narcotic be alcohol
or morphine or idealism.
C.G.Jung

Diseases are
the tax on pleasures.
John Ray

I was teetotal
until prohibition.
Groucho Marx

Preface to Third Edition

"It is rare to come across anybody who feels neutral or unconcerned about the issues surrounding the forbidden drugs." This statement seems as true today as when I wrote it in the preface to the first edition of this book in 1994. Everyone is touched in some way by the use of drugs taken for pleasure whether as consumer, purveyor, parent, teacher, treatment provider, policy maker, or victim of a drug-related crime.

The aim of the book is to provide a readable, authoritative and at times entertaining account of every substance consumed for enjoyment or self-enlightenment throughout the world. It begins with an analysis of why people choose to consume psychoactive drugs, and then goes on to consider the likely consequences. Next follows an account of each individual drug or drug class covering the historical background, preparation and distribution, pharmacology, medicinal uses (if any), subjective effects, pattern of recreational use, unwanted effects and risks. Chapters then deal with the nature of addiction and therapeutic approaches for people whose drug use has become problematic. The book ends with a comparison and critical analysis of drug policies in various countries, leading to some proposals for future strategies.

Recreational drug use is a world-wide phenomenon, and in this new edition I have adopted a more international approach to its epidemiology and politics. The structure of the book remains the same as that of the second edition, but every chapter has been thoroughly revised and updated. The book is based, as before, upon a critical analysis of the relevant scientific literature and the extensive clinical and research experience of the author. Conclusions are dispassionate and evidence-based, and sometimes surprising. Whilst containing enough detailed information to be of value to clinicians, researchers and policy makers, the primary target of the book is to provide a comprehensive and intelligible account of every aspect of the subject for the interested general reader.

In order to strengthen the international perspective, I have invited contributions from three North Americans pre-eminent in their respective fields. Professor Ethan Russo has collaborated as co-author on the two chapters dealing with cannabis and the hallucinogens. In the final chapter, Dr Robert DuPont and Dr Ethan Nadelmann provide contrasting perspectives of present and future US drug policy as part of a critical appraisal of international drug control. Biographical sketches can be found on page xvii, and I am most grateful for this invaluable input.

For the first time I have a commercial interest to declare. In 2000 I left the NHS and until 2005 took on the role of Medical Director at GW Pharmaceuticals plc whilst retaining a Senior Research Fellowship within the Oxford University Department of Psychiatry. GW is a pioneering public company founded in 1998 to research and develop plant-derived cannabinoid prescription medicines. In my judgement, this approach offered the best prospect of harnessing valuable therapeutic benefits of cannabis in serious diseases whilst minimising unwanted effects. It has now generated standardised formulations which are convenient for patients and acceptable to international regulatory authorities. In the light of my long-term interest in the medicinal potential of cannabis the opportunity to be a part of such an innovative venture was irresistible. From 2005 to the present date I have retained a part-time input into GW as Medical Director of the Cannabinoid Research Institute within the company. I would like to emphasise that the opinions expressed in this book are entirely my own and should not be taken to represent the views or position of GW Pharmaceuticals.

It has been a pleasure, as always, to enter into a project with Oxford University Press. I would like to thank in particular my editor Nicola Ulyatt, whose cheerful and positive approach from start to finish has been much appreciated.

Oxford   P.R.

May, 2009

Preface to Second Edition

A request from a publisher for a second edition, like the ingestion of a recreational drug, is bound to result in a mixture of pleasure and pain. Pleasure, because of the implication that the initial offering was not entirely devoid of merit; pain in contemplating the mountain of unforeseen work that is suddenly conjured up.

The subject matter of the book certainly remains topical. The controversy and concern generated globally by 'the drugs problem' show no sign of abating as we approach the millennium. The British Prime Minister must have echoed the thoughts of many world leaders when he stated in 1998 that this country would be a better place to live ' . . . if we could break once and for all the vicious cycle of drugs and crime which wrecks lives and threatens communities'.

The book is based primarily upon a critical analysis of the relevant scientific literature. It is also shaped by the research I have been involved in over the years exploring various aspects of the human response to drugs, both prescribed and recreational, and by my daily contact with patients and their often anguished families at the drug dependency unit in Oxford. But I was conscious of a wider personal perspective as I wrote the new edition: as a parent of teenage children; as one whose contact with certain friends and acquaintances has ensured of familiarity with most forms of recreational drug use in the real world outside the clinic and the laboratory; and as one whose formative student years were spent in the patchouli-laden atmosphere of swinging London during the psychedelic Sixties.

In preparing this second edition I have taken note of the comments of friends, patients, and reviewers, and paid heed to sagacious voices from within Oxford University Press. My purpose remains unchanged: to provide a readable and informative appraisal of recreational drugs and the issues which surround their use, and to blow away some of the cobwebs of myth, prejudice, and hyperbole which envelop them.

The first part of the book explores the reasons why people take drugs and the likely consequences of this; the second examines the nature of the drugs themselves; and in the final section there is a discussion of the meaning of addiction, a review of the various ways of helping people cope with drug-related problems, and an analysis of contemporary drug policy in various countries. The most obvious change is the addition of three new chapter on tobacco, alcohol, and anabolic steroids. I always regretted not including these in the first edition, not least because their omission might perpetuate the illusion that there is some logic in setting them apart from other, less socially acceptable recreational drugs. Nor can they be sensibly excluded on account of the book's title: all three have been forbidden at some time or place.

All the other chapters have been fully revised and updated, and the layout has been improved by the introduction of subtitles throughout. The fairly detailed historical accounts of the various drugs met with some approval, so these have been retained and in some cases slightly expanded. Sections dealing with scientific matters are written in plain English and with no expectation of prior knowledge.

No author could wish for a more agreeable and constructive relationship with a publisher than I have experienced with Oxford University Press. In particular, I would like to thank Alison Langton, without whom the book would never have been conceived; Susan Harrison, who always looks for new angles; Martin Baum, a feisty new editor for the second edition; and, above all, John Harrison, whose amiable and undeviating support, encouragement and wise advice sustained me through both editions.

Oxford   P.R.

April, 1999

Preface to First Edition

I try my best never to talk about drugs at social gatherings. This is because I have learnt from hard experience that if I do forget my golden rule and get drawn on the subject and my wife is not on hand to turn the conversation to safer matters, the discussion invariably becomes heated. On one memorable occasion in Australia, I would undoubtedly have been knocked unconscious had it not been for the diplomatic skills of our hostess.

It is rare to come across anybody who feels neutral or unconcerned about the issues surrounding the forbidden drugs. This is because you don't have to be a user to be profoundly affected by them on a personal level. Parents concerned about what their children are up to; teachers, doctors, lawyers, and other professionals who come into contact with drug use in the course of their work; victims of the spiralling levels of drug-related crime; policy makers, social activists, and libertarians; and almost anyone who ever opens a newspaper.

This sense of personal involvement introduces an emotional tone into any debate which can lead to bombast and speculation taking the place of a calm appraisal of the various dilemmas. 'Stamp out reality' was a typically provocative slogan of the hallucinatory sixties, but it would also seem an apt motto for some of the modern rhetoricians and gurus who support or oppose the 'war on drugs'.

Recent opinion polls have indicated that many North Americans think that illegal drugs represent the nation's number one problem, with the related nightmares of AIDS and crime close behind. We don't yet seem quite so concerned in the United Kingdom, possibly because organized crime is less high-profile, and many of us still do not connect the soaring levels of muggings, car crime, and burglaries with someone's need to feed a drug habit. The bald truth is that tens of thousands of people in Britain are faced with the challenge of raising £100 or so every day of their lives to maintain their supply of heroin or cocaine, with no legal income except a social security cheque worth about £40 a week.

Discovering that they are addicted is sometimes the first inkling that people have of the potency of the drugs they have been ingesting. Only the other day, this account was published in the letters section of a national newspaper:

'I made the decision to stop ... in my quest for a healthier lifestyle, and [had my last dose] ... last Thursday morning. By evening I had a mild headache. On Friday morning I had a fierce headache and felt dizzy and sick. I could not go to work. Friday evening I was physically sick and the headache was worse,

with shooting pains in my neck and shoulders. Saturday I still had a bad headache, but I wasn't feeling sick and pain relief was possible.

Today, Sunday, I have a mild headache but I still feel very drowsy. I hope I
shall continue to feel better tomorrow.'

This writer was describing the consequences of breaking her addiction to
coffee and tea. Many people today would either not classify caffeine as a real
drug at all or would see it as being of negligible potency. My 11-year-old
daughter enjoys a cup of tea most days and nobody reports me to Social
Services, yet in 17th-century Britain coffee was regarded very much as cannabis is nowadays: a potent mind-altering chemical which should be treated with
respect. Since one only becomes aware of being addicted to something when it
ceases to be available, most people remain blissfully unaware that they are
indeed hooked – just as many 19th-century Britons and North Americans
remained unaware that they were hooked on opium or cocaine since these too
were freely available at that time.

Cultural conditioning is very powerful and accounts for much of the glaring
inconsistency in attitudes towards familiar and unfamiliar drugs, and it is fascinating to look back and see how these cultural attitudes have fluctuated over
the decades. The public perception of cocaine is a case in point: from a harmless tonic and constituent of that refreshing beverage Coca-Cola in the 19th
century to a terrifyingly addictive narcotic fit only for debauchees and criminals between the world wars, to being *de rigueur* for everyone who aspired to a
Porsche or even just a mobile phone in the Thatcher/Reagan years. The properties of cocaine, although significantly influenced by the way it is used, have
remained constant, but the way they are interpreted by 'experts' and the public
at large continually changes.

My aim in writing this book has been to set out for the interested reader with
no special experience or scientific knowledge what is known about the drugs
themselves and why people take them, the meaning of addiction and the treatments that are available for it, and the natural history of drug use. I have also
described the current policy on drugs in Britain, and discussed some ideas for
reducing drug-related problems in the future. I have not tried too hard to resist
expressing some personal opinions along the way and I hope these are consistent with the known facts. This will be for the reader to judge and react appropriately with assent or outrage; the only response that would disappoint would
be indifference.

Oxford   P. R.

June 1994

Contents

Contributors

Chapters 5 and 7

Dr Ethan Russo
Neurologist, Ethnobotanist and acknowledged expert on psychoactive herbs.

Ethan Russo, MD, has held faculty appointments at the universities of Montana and Washington. He is currently Senior Medical Adviser to GW Pharmaceuticals, visiting professor at the Chinese Academy of Sciences, Secretary of the International Cannabinoid Research Society, and board member of the International Association for Cannabis as Medicine.

Dr Russo is author of *Handbook of Psychotropic Herbs* and *The Last Sorcerer: Echoes of the Rainforest,* and co-editor of *Cannabis and Cannabinoids: Pharmacology, Toxicology and Therapeutic Potential.* He was founding editor of *Journal of Cannabis Therapeutics,* selections of which were published as books: *Cannabis Therapeutics in HIV/AIDS, Women and Cannabis: Medicine, Science and Sociology, Cannabis: From Pariah to Prescription,* and *Handbook of Cannabis Therapeutics: From Bench to Bedside.* Dr Russo has published numerous other book chapters and articles concerning neurology, pain management, cannabis, and ethnobotany.

Chapter 15

Robert L. DuPont
President, Institute for Behavior and Health, Inc.

Robert L. DuPont, MD is President of the non-profit Institute for Behavior and Health which uses the power of new ideas to reduce the use of illegal drugs. He is Clinical Professor of Psychiatry at Georgetown Medical School and Vice President of Bensinger DuPont and Associates providing employee assistance services and working to reduce the nonmedical use of prescription drugs.

Dr. DuPont was the first Director of the National Institute on Drug Abuse (NIDA), under three presidents (Nixon, Ford and Carter).

The second White House Drug Czar, he has written more than 300 professional articles and chapters and 18 books and monographs including *The Selfish Brain – Learning From Addiction* published by Hazelden Information & Educational Services in 2000.

Ethan Nadelmann
Founder and Executive Director, Drug Policy Alliance.

Ethan Nadelmann received his BA, JD, and PhD from Harvard, and a master's degree in international relations from the London School of Economics. He then taught politics and public affairs at Princeton University where his speaking and writings on drug policy attracted international attention. In 1994, Dr Nadelmann founded the Lindesmith Center, a drug policy institute created with the philanthropic support of George Soros. In 2000, this merged with another organization to form the Drug Policy Alliance, which advocates for drug policies grounded in science, compassion, health and human rights. A new book, co-authored with Peter Andreas and entitled *Policing the Globe: Criminalization and Crime Control in International Relations*, was published by Oxford University Press in 2006.

Described by *Rolling Stone* as "the point man" for drug policy reform efforts, Ethan Nadelmann is widely regarded as the most prominent proponent of drug policy reform.

Chapter 1

Why use drugs?

We live in an age of unprecedented reliance upon drugs. Whether it is a prescription medicine, an 'over-the-counter' pharmaceutical or a herbal remedy, pills and potions are seen by many as a quick and easy solution to problems which have little or nothing to do with medical disorders. Family doctors are besieged by distressed and demanding people who would much rather walk out of the surgery with a prescription than set about the more demanding task of finding practical solutions to their economic, social, and interpersonal difficulties. In this context it is hardly surprising that there is an equally unprecedented appetite for 'recreational' psychoactive drugs.

According to the Oxford Shorter English Dictionary a drug is 'any substance that affects the physical or mental functioning of a living organism', and psychoactive or psychotropic means 'affecting a person's mental state'. The most widely consumed psychoactive drug in the world is caffeine in the form of tea, coffee, soft drinks, energy supplements, and chocolate, Most regular daily consumers of coffee or cola would not see themselves as drug dependent, but the reality is that caffeine is a highly addictive stimulant associated with both physical and psychological withdrawal symptoms following abrupt termination of intake. Caffeine also has numerous toxic effects, and overdoses are a relatively common cause for emergency room treatment in countries such as the US. It currently enjoys world-wide acceptance of unrestricted use for all age groups yet in previous centuries many governments tried unsuccessfully to ban or control it. For example, in 17th century Britain coffee was generally viewed as a substance with powerful (and sometimes highly undesirable) psychoactive effects, and its regular users were often looked upon with disapproval; rather similar, in fact, to the way cannabis is seen today. Caffeine is now disregarded as a bland nonentity whilst cannabis, almost entirely unregulated prior to the 20th century, is a global pariah.

Around 208 million people (4.9% of the world's adult population) have used an illegal drug at least once during the past year and more than one in three adults will do so during their lifetime. Recreational or 'non-medical' drug use is a global phenomenon, but there are considerable national and regional variations in both patterns of use and choice of drug. Despite having exceptionally stringent drug control laws and an unusually high minimum age for alcohol consumption, the US tops the league for drinking and illegal drug use. A high disposable income is an important factor influencing prevalence, due not only to the ability of the consumer to bear the cost but also to the motivational effect on black market suppliers in the selection of their national targets. Accurate quantification is hampered by the unreliability of prevalence data. Epidemiogical studies, surveys, seizure statistics from police and customs, databases, and official audits all have their shortcomings. Readers should take the figures throughout this book as approximations rather than hard facts. In developing countries these inaccuracies are likely to be even more pronounced, and certain drugs (e.g. solvents; home-cultivated marijuana) may be very difficult to monitor.

Initiation into both legal and illegal recreational drug use peaks in the mid to late teenage years, the former marginally earlier than the latter. Range of initiation remains wide, however, especially for illegal drugs. Young people aged between 16 and 30 account for three quarters of all illegal drug use, but in 2007 it was noted that consumption among individuals in their fifties and sixties has been increasing steadily, suggesting that many babyboomers who grew up in the 1960s and 1970s are carrying the habits of their youth into their retirement years. Children who begin taking drugs in their early teens or even sooner have usually experienced personal or family disadvantage which predates this. Males are more likely to use drugs and in larger amount than females in all age groups, but there are some interesting exceptions. For example, in the UK among 15-year-olds significantly more girls smoke tobacco than boys, and in the past decade the number of young women drinking more than twice the recommended weekly limit has doubled. Multiple drug use is not uncommon amongst 16 to 24-year-olds, and one survey discovered that a quarter of young people were in the habit of taking two or three drugs other than tobacco or alcohol. Easy availability of both legal and illegal drugs aggravates this tendency to excess.

Despite ratification by 130 countries of international treaties under the auspices of the World Health Organization (WHO), regulations aimed at denying children access to alcohol and tobacco are usually not rigorously enforced. The most powerful predictor for taking up smoking is having a sibling or parents who smoke. The habit is more common among children with only one parent, living in a poor neighbourhood, or with lower educational attainments. A small proportion of medical students and a larger group of nurses still puff away in defiance of the mute testimony of the specimen jars and pathology slides that surround them. Alcohol consumption peaks in the late teens and early twenties. Among university students there are large variations between the different courses, with the highest consumption among male students of biological sciences who average 40 units per week. Overall, around a half of male and a quarter of female students drink more than the recommended safe drinking levels. Only 6% of white students are non-drinkers, in contrast to 50% of non-whites.

The majority of children are offered illegal drugs at some point in their school career, and obtaining them is not perceived as difficult by most pupils. The starting point is experimentation with cigarettes, wine, beer, or solvents. Frequency of drunken episodes correlates with future intake of cigarettes and illegal drugs, the first of which is almost always either solvents or cannabis. The greater the consumption of cannabis, the more the chance that other drugs will be tried. Stimulants, 'party drugs', and hallucinogens might follow, and heroin or crack cocaine are the end-points for a tiny minority. There is no convincing evidence that this is a causative sequence. The argument that cannabis inexorably leads to harder drug use is confounded by the observation that a majority of users never touch any other illegal drug, and only a very small proportion will progress to heroin or cocaine.

Three-quarters of those who ever try an illegal drug will have done so by the age of 18, with peak use occurring in the late teens and early twenties. Thereafter a steady decline correlates with progressive involvement in the structures of society as work, relationships, and parenthood take their toll. Married people use less drugs than those who are single or divorced, but the highest rates of all occur in men living with women to whom they are not married. In later life women are higher consumers of prescribed psychoactive drugs, while men rely more on alcohol to soothe, or inflame, their nerves. Drug use is also related to employment status, educational achievements, and geographical location.

Only 3% of the drug-using population ever injects a drug. Heroin and crack cocaine remain minority interests, with only 1% of those under 30 years of age admitting ever having tried either, but people who try heroin find it hard to use sparingly. In one large survey, the number of adolescents who had tried heroin was only 1.7% of the total sample. But of those who had used it once, 65% used it again, and of these two-thirds were using it weekly and 15% daily. Only tobacco carries a higher risk of addiction for the casual user.

A recent survey in the US indicated that at some point in their lives 92% of the adult population had drunk alcohol, 74% had smoked tobacco, 43% had taken cannabis and 16% had used cocaine. Tobacco and cannabis were marginally down from levels 10 years previously (76% and 46% respectively), alcohol and cocaine remained constant. In 2007, nearly 20 million Americans were current illegal drug users, representing 8% of the population aged 12 and above. More encouragingly, overall use of both legal and illegal recreational drugs seems to have declined over recent years. Use of an illicit drug within the past month among 12 to 17-year-olds decreased from 11.6% to 9.5%, with cannabis down from 8.2% to 6.7%, alcohol from 17.6% to to 15.9% and cigarettes from 13% to 9.8% (figures from US Substance Abuse and Mental Health Services Administration (SAMHSA)). Cocaine and methamphetamine have also declined in this age group.

In the UK, a worrying development among young people is a marked increase in problems related to excessive alcohol consumption. Only Ireland, Denmark, and the Isle of Man have higher levels of drunken episodes out of 35 European countries. Smoking has declined amongst young males but not females, who are also binge-drinking more than ever before. However, the prevalence of illegal drugs among all age groups is at its lowest level since the mid-1990s, mainly reflecting a steady decline in cannabis smoking. In the 16 to 24 age group in 2008, 21.3% used an illegal drug in the past year compared to 31.8% in 1998.

There is marked variation in patterns of drug use across Europe. The top five countries for alcohol consumption are Luxembourg, Czech Republic, Hungary, Estonia, and Germany. Tobacco smoking is exceptionally high in Spain, Switzerland, Slovakia, Hungary, Bulgaria, Greece, and Belarus. Cannabis smoking is most prevalent in the Czech Republic, Switzerland, Ireland, France, and the UK.

A growing concern in many countries, and particularly the US, is non-medical use of prescription medicines. Prescription rates for the opioids hydrocodone and oxycodone have increased fourfold and ninefold respectively in the US over the past decade, and this has been paralleled by a dramatic rise in opioid overdoses presenting to hospital emergency rooms. Figures from SAMHSA show that almost 7 million Americans abused prescription medicines in 2007, up 80% from 2000 and more than all the consumers of cocaine, heroin, hallucinogens, ecstasy, and inhalants combined. This has resulted in a four-fold increase in the number or Americans requiring treatment for dependence upon pharmaceuticals. Deaths from overdose of diverted prescription opioids have gone up 160% in five years and now outnumber all the deaths resulting from heroin and cocaine. The illicit trade in prescription drugs is worth billions of dollars annually, and they are now the most popular intoxicants for pre-teen children.

Despite the modest decline over the past decade in the overall use of illegal drugs in the US and Europe it is evident that the appetite for mind-altering drugs, both legal and illegal, remains a universal attraction. Not content with just alcohol and cigarettes, millions of ordinary people are prepared to flout the law and face considerable risk and inconvenience in order to consume forbidden drugs. Why do they do it?

This question can be approached on two levels: first, by contemplating the attraction or function of intoxication, and secondly by a more utilitarian search for human or environmental characteristics which make initial experimentation or persistence with drugs more likely.

The search for 'altered consciousness'

Some writers interested in psychoactive drugs have come to the conclusion that a desire or need for 'altered consciousness' has always represented more to mankind than mere hedonistic self-indulgence. Andrew Weil (*The Natural Mind*, 1973) has argued that it is a basic human appetite, recognizable throughout history from the most primitive beginnings. Of interest here is the observation that some animals in their natural habitat seem interested in intoxication, seeking to experience it repeatedly. Dogs have been observed snuffling the fumes from rotting vegetation to the point of incoordination, and I knew of a cat which confounded its carnivorous nature by gobbling up any marijuana its owner inadvertently left lying around.

Weil argues that drug-induced mental changes are part of a whole range of natural 'altered states' which fulfill an important revitalizing or insight-producing function. Psychoactive plants and drugs are only one way to reach this endpoint. Religious or spiritual practices achieve it for millions, as do meditation, fasting, sleep deprivation, music, exercise, yoga, or hypnosis. Twilight states between sleep and waking, daydreams, trances, and even delirium can also serve a restorative function. Weil sees evidence of the in-built attraction and need for these states in the antics of children making themselves dizzy, faint, or even unconscious by whirling or breath-holding. He quotes a more famous writer, Aldous Huxley: '. . . *the urge to escape, the longing to transcend themselves if only for a few minutes, is and always has been one of the principal appetites of the soul. Art and religion, carnivals and saturnalia, dancing and listening to oratory—all these have served, in H. G. Wells's phrase, as Doors in the Wall*'.

The writings of Weil and others challenge the assumption that consciousness alteration is undesirable, dangerous, or 'wrong'. Does 'reality', he asks, only equate to ordinary waking consciousness? Huxley certainly did not think so, and modern brain research has supported his conception of the brain as a sort of filter or reducing-valve, diverting from conscious awareness information that has no immediate survival value. He felt that the inhabitants of a modern, materialistic society progressively stripped of a spiritual dimension had more need than ever to transport themselves beyond such sterile boundaries. Street graffiti in the late 1960s called on people to 'stamp out reality'.

This is a controversial line to pursue because it suggests that at least some of those who use mind-altering drugs, who take the chance of freeing themselves from a perceptual strait-jacket, may reap significant benefits from the experience. At the very least, they may gain insight into the robotic, stereotyped nature of much human behaviour. This can be a profoundly unsettling realization, and none of these writers suggest that it is an undertaking without risk. Weil concedes that drugs can '... *hurt your body, hurt your mind, impede your development*'. But the possibility does arise that these might be risks worth taking.

Practical reasons for experimenting with drugs

If you ask teenagers why they use drugs, most will simply tell you that they are pleasurable or exciting. Other reasons include getting rid of unpleasant feelings of shyness, anxiety, boredom or lack of confidence, boosting energy and diminishing the need for sleep, improving concentration or performance, fitting in with their friends, or because it makes them feel sophisticated or pleasantly rebellious and independent. Scientists have tried to refine these simple explanations or attach numbers to them. One investigator found that fun and curiosity accounted for half, peer pressure a third, and self-medication a fifth of the stated motivation. This pattern held true for all drug types except the stimulants; here, fun and curiosity was the prime mover for 40%, with the other two categories 30% each. Among Oxford undergraduates the main reason for using recreational drugs was pleasure, with stress relief the principal benefit for around a fifth of the students. Social pressure was slightly more influential in encouraging alcohol use than for other drugs. Enhanced recreational drug use at university is more likely because of emergence from the controls of family and school life, the excitement of a new environment and circle of friends, social and academic pressure, and enhanced availability of legal and illegal substances. Expectations of positive consequences vastly outweigh the anticipation of problems, but most people are well aware of possible negative outcomes. Drinkers in one survey listed 'awful effects' (89%), cost (76%), health hazards (74%), risk of accidents (66%), and fear of losing control (51%). Another survey showed that the main dislikes for illegal drug use were health risk (13%), cost (7%), breaking the law (7%), hangovers (6%), and fear of addiction (6%). However, the main reason for stopping was insufficient pleasure rather than a fear of adverse consequences. Young people say they get their information about drugs from the following sources in descending order: media, friends, school teachers, and the police.

What it boils down to is that most people try a drug for one of three main reasons: the expectation of a positive outcome in terms of pleasure, relaxation or a boost in performance, to fit in with their friends, or to medicate themselves for some unpleasant emotion and forget their troubles. But the interesting question remains: what makes one teenager say 'yes please' and another 'no thanks'? To answer this we have to examine some individual and environmental characteristics.

Biological explanations

Gender is a major influence. Males are much less likely to be total abstainers, and tend to consume larger average quantities of drugs and alcohol than females of similar age and social circumstances.

Psychoactive drugs produce their rewarding effects by influencing the release, uptake, and functionality of neurotransmitters (chemical messengers) in various brain circuits (see Chapter 13). Our understanding of how genetics may influence the response to drugs and susceptibility to pleasant or unpleasant effects remains rather rudimentary. Temperament is to some extent genetically determined, and in turn predisposes to particular lifestyles (see below). Adoption studies suggest that certain types of alcoholism can be transmitted genetically in males, and in animals a predisposition to the abuse of morphine or barbiturates can be inbred. Genetic inheritance can influence routes and rates of drug metabolism, and relevant physiological systems; for example, brain electrical reactivity (as measured by an electroencephalogram) to drug administration is in part genetically mediated. It is possible to breed animals which are more or less sensitive to specific drug effects, vulnerable to tolerance, dependence, or withdrawal symptoms, or likely to develop drug-seeking behaviour. Such genetic traits could evolve naturally in humans. There is also some evidence that exposure to a psychoactive drug such as alcohol or nicotine in the uterus through maternal consumption may affect that individual's future response to the drug and even likelihood of becoming dependent upon it.

The balance of the brain's neurotransmitters may vary between individuals. A person who happens to be a bit short of, say, serotonin in a particular brain system may still function normally in most circumstances because other neurotransmitters can compensate. If that person takes a drug which particularly boosts serotonin activity, however, there may be more positive effects than would occur in someone who has a natural sufficiency of serotonin. People differ in the way they metabolize drugs and this can greatly alter the balance of pleasant and unpleasant effects. For example, some Asians are genetically programmed to generate a large build-up of the toxic metabolite acetaldehyde in response to a small amount of alcohol. The cracking headache which results is unrewarding, so these individuals are much less likely to drink regularly if at all. These pharmacological factors are considered in more detail in Chapter 13.

Psychological explanations

A considerable amount of attention has been focused on the personal attributes and early influences which might increase the likelihood of a child or young person experimenting with drugs and going on to develop problems. Unfortunately, much of this work has targeted young people who are already problem drug users and in whom it is impossible to separate cause from effect. For example, problem drug users are often found to have low self-esteem and some investigators have concluded that this is likely to have been a causative factor in the development of harmful drug use. In reality, unless the study can show that the low self-esteem pre-dated any exposure to drugs, an equally likely explanation is that the problem drug use caused the low self-esteem.

Unsuspecting adolescents in university cities throughout the world have been exposed over the years to bulky questionnaires and earnest interviewers in an attempt to give poorly defined personal characteristics a more scientific gloss. The gargantuan Minnesota Multiphasic Personality Inventory alone has formed the centrepiece for well over a hundred papers. Not surprisingly, this effort has generated many apparent associations and predictors of future drug use. For what it is worth, the typical drug-user-to-be is likely to possess at least some of the following characteristics: alienation, rebelliousness, nonconformity to conventional values, and a tolerant attitude towards unusual or deviant behaviour; a relative lack of ambition and commitment to school work or career building; independent mindedness, self-reliance, and a reluctance to abide by rules; impulsivity; a preoccupation with pleasure-seeking and minimal concern for risk; poor problem-solving, coping, and 'refusal' skills; a history of physical or psychological illness; and impaired emotional well-being or consistently low self-esteem. It is calculated that up to 40% of children and adolescents experience at least minor mental health problems at some time, and up to 10% have moderate to severe problems. Such emotional difficulties are reportedly twice as common in urban as opposed to rural areas. The prevalence of depression increases steadily in the teenage years, and eating disorders peak at age 17.

Certain personal attributes, attitudes, and behaviours in early adolescence predict an increased likelihood of experimentation with street drugs at some point in the future. These include minor delinquency, early sexual experience, active participation in political or other 'protest activity' (American studies only!), and a general willingness to get involved in exciting but risky activities. Temperamental characteristics such as feeling persistently bored or irritable, and regular tantrums in very young children, are associated with 'problem behaviours' in adolescence and delinquency in adults. Traits such as high novelty seeking and low harm avoidance in six-year-olds have been shown to predict early onset of substance use. Children who generally have internal rather than external explanations for things that happen (e.g. explaining failure in an exam because 'I didn't work hard enough' as opposed to 'the paper was too hard') are much less susceptible to peer pressure.

A measure which reliably predicts drug experimentation is called the Sensation Seeking Scale. 'Sensation seeking' has been defined as *the need for varied, novel, and complex sensations and experiences and the willingness to take physical and social risks for the sake of such experience* (Zuckerman, 1979). The measure provides a global score and ratings on four sub-scales labelled 'thrill and adventure seeking', 'experience seeking', 'disinhibition', and 'boredom susceptibility'. People who like cigarettes, alcohol, and stimulating foods also score high on this scale, which its author believes provides a measure of 'sensitivity to reinforcement'.

The Sensation Seeking Scale does not have much value as an explanatory tool. It is like trying to account for the consumption of cakes by a measure of liking for sweet things. A person who craves excitement and doesn't dwell too much on the risks is more likely to race motor-bikes or smoke cannabis than someone who lacks these attributes. So what? The majority of people with these same attributes will not do either of these things, but will select any one of a thousand other pursuits which fulfill their requirements but do not happen to be on the investigator's list. The real question to be answered is one step back: what are the biological or existential precursors of a craving for excitement and disdain for risk?

As mentioned above, the importance of low self-esteem in the development of drug-related problems remains uncertain but many of the personal characteristics which have been linked with vulnerability to compulsive drug use are also associated with poor self-esteem: submissiveness, a tendency to depend upon others and constantly crave approval, lack of confidence, a sense of helplessness, anxiety, low expectations for the future, and a readiness to give up if the going gets tough. Having inherently high self-esteem is valuable quite apart from the obvious feel-good factor. People who have it are likely to be more confident and self-determining, better able to handle stress and criticism, more willing to express a controversial opinion and resist pressure to conform, enjoy better relationships, and be less likely to suffer from anxiety and depression. Development of self-esteem is a multifaceted process, but the role of the family is very important. The ideal upbringing is to be on the receiving end of unconditional love and acceptance from a pair of cheerful and reliable adults whose own relationship is warm and supportive, and who evolve clearly defined rules and boundaries for the child's behaviour with plenty of latitude for individual decisions and actions within those boundaries.

Family and cultural explanations

It is not surprising that the personal relationships which envelop every individual are extremely important in shaping attitudes and behaviour, and it makes sense to look first at the influence of the family. Inconsistent family practices (mealtimes, bedtimes, television or computer access, homework rules, parental reliability, discipline, rewards for good behaviour), poor maternal interaction at an early age, and low expectations by the parents of future success for their offspring are all associated with increased likelihood of regular smoking, drinking, and drug use. Familial religious beliefs will have a powerful influence, and in some circumstances will result in complete abstinence (e.g. the forbidding of alcohol in Islam). Ethnic influences are also important, and may result from cultural or biological mechanisms. The children of an alcoholic father or a mother receiving prescribed psychoactive drugs are more likely to use an illicit drug other than cannabis, and perhaps this is because they have learnt from their parents that psychological stress requires a chemical solution. The presence of one smoking adult in the family doubles the risk that the children will take up regular smoking. This influence is more powerful in girls who are also more successful in keeping their smoking secret from their parents. The risk of becoming a smoker increases fourfold if an older brother or sister smokes. Three quarters of school students who do not drink alcohol abstain in respect of their parents' wishes. Consumption of illicit drugs is higher in teenagers who lack one or both of their natural parents, who come from families with high levels of stress and conflict, whose parents themselves use illegal drugs, or who have a close relative who is 'antisocial' or 'alcoholic'. It is lower in families with pronounced religious beliefs, or a warm, trusting, and conflict-free parent-adolescent relationship—a state which may exist more frequently in the pages of psychology textbooks than in the real world. Cannabis use was found to be six times less common in families where disapproval of its use had been firmly expressed. Influences in families cut both ways: a difficult baby may result in weary and exasperated parents who unleash their frustrations in later childhood and heighten teenage alienation. One good parent-child relationship can provide an effective buttress against quite disturbed behaviour in siblings or the other parent.

The more time children spend unsupervised by an adult outside school hours, especially outside the family home, the more likely they are to huff solvents, drink alcohol excessively and smoke cigarettes or cannabis, feel depressed, indulge in more generally risky activities, and do less well in school.

Drug taking by young people may simply reflect rejection of mainstream ideas or values by the adult members of the family. Conventional, conservative families operating along more authoritarian lines are likely to produce children who also conform to rules and have less inclination to challenge external authority. Each style has its advantages and disadvantages. Most of us have come across eccentrics and risk-takers who, whether successful or disaster-prone, have a life-enhancing effect on those who come into contact with them. The family also seems to play a vital role in determining an individual's self-esteem as described above.

Not surprisingly, members of friendship groups tend to share attitudes and beliefs, but it is uncertain whether this is mainly due to like selecting like ('assortative pairing') or one person influencing another. In other words, do similar people simply cluster together, or do certain individuals produce conformity by inducing changes in others? Whichever explanation is true, people certainly do congregate with others of similar attitudes and habits, and this certainly holds true in the case of drug use. This is illustrated by a study which identified the source of a drug on the occasion of a person's first exposure. Most commonly (40%) this was within a group of friends who all shared the same supply, followed by a gift from an older friend (26%) or other aquaintance (12%), bought from a friend (10%), given by an older sibling (5%), bought from a stranger (5%), or given by a stranger (2%).

The effect of this immediate circle of friends and acquaintances outweighs any conflicting pressure emanating from society at large and, temporarily, from the family. Becoming warmly acquainted with established aficionados of any particular drug, be they beery medical students or ecstasy-popping clubbers, is by far the strongest predictor that you will try that particular substance yourself.

Influence can be direct through persuasion or role-modelling, or indirect by a subtler inculcation of beliefs and values, and that of friends and associates interacts in a complicated way with that of the family. It seems that the influence of siblings fades with age, presumably as that of peers increases, but the power of one peer group declines rapidly as the person moves to a fresh milieu or social circle. Indirect influence is much longer lasting, and is the characteristic effect which the family exerts. Parental influence, although it may be swamped by succeeding peer groups from time to time, constantly re-emerges. Whilst immediate and overtly-stated parental rules may seem totally ineffective in curbing adolescent excesses, the subtler modelling of attitudes and behaviour results in psychological structures or mind-sets which remain active for a lifetime. Unfortunately, they may not result in the outcome anticipated or intended by the parents. A father preoccupied with hard work and long hours might expect his progeny to be impressed by the money and prestige this is producing: instead, the child may be more influenced by awareness of the loneliness and lack of support experienced by the mother.

Interrupted schooling, academic failure, socio-economic disadvantage and truancy are each associated with a greater prevalence of drug use. Truants aged 14–16 are twice as likely to smoke regularly, three times more likely to abuse solvents or smoke cannabis, and four times more likely to try 'hard' drugs than non-truants. They are more likely to come from large or broken families, to have smoking parents and unemployed fathers, and to engage in heavy drinking, fighting, and vandalism. Pre-teen drug use is almost always associated with disadvantage, either personal (bereavement; bullying or being bullied; low IQ; personality disorder; delinquency) or familial (socio-economic deprivation; parental drug use or criminality; family breakdown; single parent or step-parent).

Observation of adult behaviour outside family and peer groups also influences young people. For example, in schools which permitted teachers to smoke on the premises, twice as many 16-year-olds became regular smokers. Active promotion, availability, and cost have a significant influence on most forms of drug use, but the law does not seem to be a major deterrent. In a survey of university students, users said that the law had not been a significant factor in weighing up the decision to try a drug. Very few non-users said they would try a currently illegal drug if it was legalized. Geographical variations in the patterns of drug use may be explained by either cultural variations or differences in drug availability.

Risk taking

Risk taking is part of the normal process of developing independence and individual identity during the progression from childhood through adolescence into adulthood. Society deems some risks acceptable and some not, often with little justification to teenage eyes. There are many hidden variables which can subtly alter risk profiles. Putting a small child into a safety restraint when you drive to the supermarket is obviously sensible, but research suggests that mothers who do this drive faster than those whose children are just rolling around in the back, and are therefore at increased risk of having an accident.

Adolescents approach risk assessment differently to adults. It is rather unlikely that they will sit down and consider fully the pros and cons of any particular adventure. They may lack knowledge or tune out the possibility of danger. Powers of introspection tend to be undeveloped, they may well be impulsive and impatient, and most young people have a sense of invulnerability if thoughts of mortality or serious damage even cross their minds. External influences also impinge on risk awareness and judgement; for example, adolescents from intact families take less risks than those with divorced or separated parents.

Risks cluster together: the young person overtaking you at 120 m.p.h. on his motor-bike probably smokes, drinks, and fornicates far more than would be deemed advisable by the Health and Safety Executive. Smokers are much more likely to drink heavily than non-smokers.

Most people confronted with a possible course of action which seems attractive but also risky carry out some sort of rapid mental cost-benefit analysis which is subject to all sorts of idiosyncratic biases. The key calculation is the likely balance of positive and negative outcomes, and the expected intensity of those outcomes. Rewards are often immediate while possible harms are deferred, leading to an underestimate of both the likelihood and severity of the latter. The majority of young smokers remember risks being discussed within the family and can repeat the message from health awareness sessions at school. There is no doubt that awareness of the dangers of smoking among children has increased greatly over the last 10 years, but this has not been mirrored by proportional reductions in the numbers taking up the habit.

Even if a decision to avoid risk is taken, this may be thwarted at the last moment as other factors intrude. For example, there is a large discrepancy between initial intention to wear a condom and actually using one. Spiralling lust, too much alcohol, or embarrassment may overwhelm earlier decisions. Having indulged in risky behaviour and apparently got away with it unscathed is in itself extremely rewarding and encourages further exposure.

Is experimenting with drugs 'abnormal'?

Many of the normal psychological changes associated with adolescence present challenges both to the young people experiencing them and to concerned adults looking on. This is a time of learning to exert control over emotion in the face of stress, becoming an individual separate from the family and clarifying a sense of self, developing the ability to consider alternative outcomes and make rational decisions about competing choices, and beginning to plan beyond the immediate. Experimentation in many aspects of living is an essential part of the developmental process. In an era when legal and illegal drugs are part of the environment in every school, can we automatically assume that trying out illicit drugs (which include cigarettes and alcohol for those legally classified as children) is automatically pathological or even abnormal? One US study, controversial but scientifically impressive, would suggest not.

The investigators selected 100 three-year-old children and followed them up regularly until they were 18. At regular intervals they were interviewed and subjected to psychological testing. Quality of parenting was assessed when they were five, and feedback from teachers was obtained from time to time. At the end of the study, the subjects mostly fell into three categories with regard to their use of recreational drugs: 29 total abstainers, 36 experimenters (cannabis once a month or less and no more than one other drug), and 19 regular users (cannabis at least once weekly plus at least one other drug). Sixteen subjects could not be classified. There were significant psychological differences between the three groups and those with the healthiest psychological profile turned out to be the experimenters. These differences were discernible in the children's earliest assessments, and those who were destined to become regular users showed 'interpersonal difficulties, poor impulse control, and emotional distress from an early age'. Quality of parenting was significantly better in the families of those who evolved into experimenters than in either of the other groups.

So it is clear that experimenting with illicit drugs is certainly not an automatic sign of an alienated or unhappy young person. On the contrary, it may be the product of psychological traits which are associated with many positive outcomes in life.

Selected references

Advisory Council on the Misuse of Drugs (2006). *Pathways to Problems*. HMSO, London.

Anstey, K. J., Christensen, H., Low, L-. F. (2006). Prevalence, risk factors and treatment for substance abuse in older adults. *Curr Opin Psychiatry* **19**(6), 587–92.

Brook, J. S., Whiteman, M., Gordon, A. S. (1983). Stages of drug use in adolescence: personality, peer, and family correlates. *Development Psychology*, **19**, 269–77.

Brook, D. W., Brook, J. S. (1990). The etiology and consequences of adolescent drug use. In: *Drug and alcohol abuse prevention* (ed. R. R. Watson). The Humana Press, Inc., New York.

Brown, G. L., Linnoila, M. I. (1990). CSF serotonin metabolite studies in depression, impulsivity, and violence. *Journal of Clinical Psychiatry*, **51** (Suppl.), 31–43.

Coopersmith, S. (1967). *The antecedents of self-esteem*. W. H. Freeman, San Francisco.

Degenhardt L, Chiu W-T, Sampson N et al. (2007). Epidemiological patterns of extra-medical drug use in the United States: Evidence from the National Comorbidity Survey Replication, 2001–3. *Drug & Alcohol Dependence* **90**, 210–23.

Degenhardt L, Chiu W-T, Sampson N et al. (2008). Towards a global view of alcohol, tobacco, cannabis, and cocaine use: findings from the WHO world mental health surveys. *PLoS Medicine*, **5**, e141, 0001–0015.

Dembo, R., Shern, D. (1982). Relative deviance and the process(es) of drug involvement among inner-city youths. *International Journal of the Addictions*, **17**, 1373–99.

Galizio, M., Rosenthal, D., Stein, F. A. (1983). Sensation seeking, reinforcement, and student drug use. *Addictive Behaviours*, **8**, 243–52.

Gorsuch, R. L., Butler, M. C. (1976). Initial drug abuse: a review of predisposing social psychological factors. *Psychological Bulletin*, **83**, 120–37.

Hawkins, J. D., Catalano, R. F., Miller, J. Y. (1992). Risk and protective factors for alcohol and other drug problems in adolescence and early adulthood: implications for substance abuse prevention. *Psychological Bulletin*, **112**, 64–105.

Jaffe, L. T., Archer, R. P. (1987). The prediction of drug use among college students from MMPI, MCMI, and sensation-seeking scales. *Journal of Personality Assessment*, **51**, 243–53.

Jessor, R. (1976). Predicting time of onset of marijuana use: a developmental study of high school youth. *Journal of Consulting and Clinical Psychology*, **44**, 125–34.

Joffe A, Yancy WS (2004). Legalization of marijuana: potential impact on youth. *Pediatrics* **113**, e632-e638.

Kandel, D. B. (1980). Drug and drinking behaviour among youth. *Annual Review Sociology*, **6**, 235–85.

Kandel, D. B., Kessler, R. C., Margulies, R. Z. (1978). Antecedents of adolescent initiation into stages of drug use: a developmental analysis. *Journal of Youth and Adolescence*, **7**, 13–40.

Kandel, D. B., Davies, M. (1996). High-school students who use crack and other drugs. *Archives of General Psychiatry*, **53**, 71–9.

Kershaw, C., Nicholas, S., Walker, A. (2008). *Crime in England and Wales 2007/08*. Home Office Statistical Bulletin July 2008; ISBN 978-1-84726-753-5.

Malhotra, M. K. (1983). Familial and personal correlates (risk factors) of drug consumption among German youth. *Acta Paedopsychiatrica*, **49**, 199–209.

Measham, F., Newcombe, R., Parker, H. (1993). The post-heroin generation. *Druglink*, **May/June**, 16–17.

Measham, F., Newcombe, R., Parker, H. (1994). The normalisation of recreational drug use among young people in North West England. *British Journal of Sociology*, **45**, 287–312.

Moore, S., Gullone, E. (1996). Predicting adolescent risk behaviour using a personalized cost–benefit analysis. *Journal of Youth and Adolescence*, **25**, 343–59.

Morgen, C. S., Bove, K. B., Larsen, K. S et al. (2008). Association between smoking and the risk of heavy drinking among young women: a prospective study. *Alcohol & Alcoholism* **43**, 371–5.

Novacek, J., Raskin, R., Hogan, R. (1991). Why do adolescents use drugs? Age, sex, and user differences. *Journal of Youth and Adolescence*, **20**, 475–92.

Pritchard, C., Cotton, A., Cox, M. (1992). Truancy, illegal drug use, and knowledge of HIV infection in 932 14–16 year-old adolescents. *Journal of Adolescence*, **15**, 1–17.

Richardson, J. L., Radziszewska, B., Dent, C.D., Flay, B. R. (1993). Relationship between after-school care of adolescents and substance use, risk taking, depressed mood, and academic achievement. *Pediatrics*, **92**, 32–8.

Robson, P. (1988). Self-esteem—a psychiatrist's view. *British Journal of Psychiatry*, **153**, 6–15.

Robson, P. (1996). Young people and illegal drugs. In: *Adolescent medicine* (ed. A. Macfarlane). Royal College of Physicians, London.

Sadava, S. W., Forsyth, R. (1977). Person – environment interaction and college-student drug use: a multivariate longitudinal study. *Genetic Psychology Monographs*, **96**, 211–45.

Sell, L., Robson, P. (1998). Perceptions of college life, emotional well-being, and patterns of drug and alcohol use among Oxford undergraduates. *Oxford Review of Education*, **24**, 235–43.

Shedler, J., Block, J. (1990). Adolescent drug use and psychological health: a longitudinal survey. *American Psychologist*, **45**, 612–30.

Smith, G. M. (1974). Teenage drug use: a search for causes and consequences. *Personality and Social Psychology Bulletin*, **1**, 426–9.

Sutherland, I., Willner, P. (1998). Patterns of alcohol, cigarette, and illicit drug use in English adolescents. *Addiction*, **93**, 1199–208.

Teichman, M., Barnea, Z., Ravav, G. (1989). Personality and substance use among adolescents: a longitudinal study. *British Journal of Addiction*, **84**, 181–90.

Trad, P. V. (1994). Developmental vicissitudes that promote drug abuse in adolescents. *American Journal of Drug and Alcohol Abuse*, **20**, 459–81.

Webb, E., Ashton, H., Kelly, P., Kamali, F. (1997). Patterns of alcohol consumption, smoking, and illicit drug use in British university students: interfaculty comparisons. *Drug and Alcohol Dependence*, **47**, 145–53.

Zuckerman, M. (1979). *Sensation seeking: beyond the optimal level of arousal*. Wiley, New York.

Chapter 2

The consequences of drug use

An individual's reaction to a drug is shaped by many factors: the pharmacology of the drug including its potential to induce dependence, its purity and the presence or absence of contaminants or adulerants, the route by which it is taken, the way it is metabolized and stored in the body, and possibly by the person's unique pre-existing biological make-up; the individual's personality and experience, mood, and expectations when the drug is taken; and the physical and social environment in which the experience happens. The existence of so many variables explains the unpredictability of drug effects, and why a particular drug may affect a person differently from one occasion to another. This will be discussed further in Chapter 13.

The relative risk posed by individual recreational drugs has received considerable attention recently. The United Nations (UN) position is to code illicit drugs on four dimensions: treatment demand per 1,000 users; prevalence of injecting use; toxicity (ratio of recreational to lethal dose); and drug deaths per 1,000 users. This approach would put opioids and cocaine at the top of the tree. An alternative approach encompassing both legal and illegal drugs was published by Professor David Nutt and colleagues in a 2007 *Lancet* paper. This calculated risk on the basis of three factors, each with three subdivisions: the potential physical harm (acute/chronic/intravenous); the tendency to induce dependence (intensity of pleasure/psychological dependence/physical dependence); and effects on families, communities, and society (intoxication/other social harms/health care costs). Comparing 20 recreational drugs on this basis, the two drugs with the highest harm ratings were again heroin and cocaine. More thought provoking was the high harm ranking for alcohol (5), well above tobacco (9) and cannabis (11). Ecstasy, a Class A/Schedule 1 drug, was way down the ranking at 18. As the authors note, the fact that all nine components are given equal weighting leads to some anomalies, notably a ranking for tobacco which does not do justice to the unique lethality of its delivery mechanism in long-term use. Nevertheless, the ranking certainly calls into question the logic of current legal classifications.

'Visible' and 'invisible' drug users

The great majority of people who use drugs never come to the attention of doctors (tobacco excepted), lawyers, or policemen. They are invisible to research unless briefly flushed out of cover by population surveys, and so do not feature in the statistics of the prevalence or outcome literature. The problem that this presents to those with an interest in understanding the consequences of drug use beyond the boundaries of the addiction clinics can be illustrated by reference to the recent cocaine epidemic in North America. Population surveys indicated that over 25 million US citizens had tried the drug in one particular year in the 1980s. Animal experiments, emergency room surveys, and the pronouncements of experts suggest that cocaine is one of the most toxic and addictive of street drugs, yet only a tiny proportion of these people presented for treatment or help of any kind, or were ever prosecuted. The rest remained completely invisible, and we have no idea how things turned out for them. Did they just snort the stuff a few times, enjoy it or not as the case may be, then simply drop it as new priorities took shape? Similarly in the case of heroin, of the 1% or even 2% of the general adult population who tell researchers that they have tried it at least once, relatively few go on to contribute to the casualty statistics.

The discrepancy between the numbers who admit to having at some time smoked cannabis, or swallowed LSD, ecstasy, or amphetamine, and those who ever present for help with drug-related problems is even more enormous. The assumption must be that the vast majority use these drugs only briefly or in small amounts, or that they prove pretty well harmless to most people.

'Experts' in drug misuse and addiction, whether they be doctors, psychologists, social workers, or members of any other learned profession, never see these invisible users and so base their expertise on observations of visible users who either become addicted, ill, or arrested. Consequently, they tend to have an unduly pessimistic view of both the toxicity and addictive potential of recreational drugs. Most are no more knowledgable about non-problematic drug use than the average person on the street, and some a good deal less so.

Since so little is known about the natural history of this invisible population of relatively problem-free users, the few studies that have been carried out are particularly interesting. Every heroin or cocaine user in treatment can tell you about friends or aquaintances who seem able to limit their use of these drugs to weekends or special occasions, but subjective and anecdotal opinions do not carry much authority. Besides, who can be sure that these apparently controlled users are not simply in transit to addiction?

A handful of studies do give limited support to the idea that relatively stable, controlled use of both opiates and cocaine is possible. Such users develop rituals and routines which ensure that the drug remains just a part of their lives, rather than its epicentre. We shall see in Chapter 13 that environmental and social context is all-important to the formation and maintenance of addictive behaviour. It seems that if the drug taking can be ritualized and compartmentalized, then it can be more easily contained. The social drinker limits her consumption of alcohol to particular times and places, sanctioned and reinforced by society's rules. Studies among opiate 'chippers' suggest that many are successful in creating a similar structure around their heroin use. Such people are very likely to have stable accommodation and employment, non drug-using friends and good family relationships, clear plans for the future, and a sense of being in control of their lives. They are wary of tolerance, the need for bigger doses to achieve the same effect that results from too-regular consumption, recognizing that this is the hook which can draw them into dependency.

Many chippers do give a history of episodes of addiction, but usually seem to have been able to overcome these without professional help. Some oscillate between drug and 'straight' cultures, while others lead completely conventional lives apart from this one discrepancy. Intermittent users are much more likely to prefer snorting or smoking heroin to injecting it.

In one large sample of young men selected because they had tried heroin at least once, only a third had ever reached the point of using it almost every day. Two-thirds of those who had taken it as often as once a month also reported periods of daily use. This suggests that it is difficult to avoid becoming dependent unless you rigorously restrict yourself to very infrequent indulgence, and is mirrored by observations of US soldiers who used heroin in Vietnam. Although the majority of these did not become addicted, three-quarters of those who tried it more than five times did become dependent. This group also demonstrated that a period of addiction does not inevitably mean that any future dabbling is bound to give rise to re-addiction as a third of the once-addicted sample did use heroin again in an infrequent, controlled manner on their return to the US.

Invisible cocaine use has been examined using the 'snowballing' technique. Cocaine users identified through advertisements, personal contacts, or fieldworkers were invited to introduce the investigator to similarly inclined friends and acquaintances, who in turn were asked to do the same thing. This uncovers a sample which does not have as its common denominator a connection with treatment services, and which should therefore be more representative of drug users in general. In groups of cocaine users discovered in this way dependence was found to be the exception rather than the rule. Episodes of progression to heavy use followed by spontaneously regained control or abstinence were not uncommon but many people were able to cope with regular or irregular intake without losing control over lengthy periods. Long-term prospective studies are rare and involve only small numbers but, for what they are worth, also suggest that dependency on cocaine requiring professional help is quite unusual. Most individuals who are able to take cocaine in a controlled manner over many years do so rather sparingly, no more than once or twice a month. If a period of heavy use does supervene, most people can respond to the writing on the wall: in one sample, only 20% of those who had escalated to daily use were still taking cocaine one year later. On the other hand, many years of controlled use can lead to an unwarranted sense of invulnerability, since loss of control after a decade or more of problem-free experience is also well recognized. All of this research focuses upon snorted or, much more occasionally, injected cocaine and less is known about the consequences of flirting with crack, except that certain populations seem particularly vulnerable to compulsive patterns of use (see Chapter 13).

One study showed strikingly different population characteristics between visible and invisible users of cocaine, amphetamine, and heroin. In sharp contrast to the visible group, most invisible users expressed little or no concern about their drug use and no wish for help or advice. They were much more likely to use stimulants only, less likely to inject anything or if they did so to share equipment, and less likely to use drugs on a daily basis. The invisible group showed a much lower propensity to compulsive or dependent use of any of the three drugs. The similarity in age, gender ratio, and duration of drug history argues against the alternative explanation that the two groups are simply at different stages of their drug 'careers'.

These studies indicate that addiction to heroin and cocaine requiring treatment occurs in only a minority of those who try them. Since addiction usually has devastating consequences for those who do fall within its grip, it is unfortunate that it remains so difficult to predict with any confidence who will be so afflicted.

Short-term consequences

All drug use, legal or illegal and no matter how fleeting, carries some immediate risk. Alcohol is by far the most dangerous recreational drug in terms of accidents, violence, and immediate social impact. It is a factor in a high proportion of fatal road accidents (e.g. 17,000 US deaths in 2006) and a third of other accidental deaths, and in up to half of all head injuries reaching hospital. It is involved in more than half of all visits to hospital accident and emergency departments. The 2007/8 British Crime Survey (BCS) revealed that almost half of all violent incidents were fuelled by alcohol, especially those perpetrated by a stranger (58%). Reliable data on the contribution of intoxication from other drugs (prescribed or recreational) to road traffic statistics and other incidents is less reliable, but US surveys show that between 10–22% of drivers involved in crashes have psychoactive drugs other than alcohol detectable in blood tests. The BCS suggests that drugs other than alcohol are a factor in 19% of violent incidents. Young people who took an illegal drug in the previous year are twice as likely as those who did not to commit a criminal offence. In the US more than half of those arrested for major crimes test positive for drugs on arrest. A third of all adolescent suicides are intoxicated at the time. Heavy drinkers and regular drug users often have poor employment records, and in the US alcohol or drug misuse by parents is a factor in more than three quarters of incidents leading to children being taken into foster care.

Illegal drugs have an added dimension of immediate risks because they are manufactured, distributed, and sold by criminals who do not put quality control high on their list of priorities. Purity is hugely variable, making accidental overdose an ever-present possibility. For example, analysis of street heroin shows that the diamorphine content can vary between 0% and 80%. The number of drug-related deaths has doubled in both the US and UK over the past twenty years, and escalating prescriptions of opioid analgesics and sedative hypnotics have contributed to this rise. A government sponsored team analyses deaths in the UK related to illegal drugs on an annual basis. The 2008 report revealed that there were 1,900 drug-related deaths during the previous year of which 63% were the result of accidental overdose. Opioids were a factor in three quarters of these, and 38% of fatal cases had also consumed alcohol. Mortality rates associated with acute reactions to opioids or cocaine are much higher in men than women, and are at their peak in the mid to late twenties age group. Interactions as a result of poly-drug use are no doubt an important contributory factor.

Street drugs can also contain toxic solvents, accidental by-product of manufacture, adulterants, or bulking agents. They may be contaminated with pesticides, fungi, or bacteria. The intensity of the psychological effects of stimulants, hallucinogens, or unusually potent forms of cannabis may prove overwhelming. Solvents can produce a fatal cardiac dysrhythmia in naive and experienced users alike. Young people are particularly at risk from the lifestyle consequences of the street drug scene, such as violence and sexual exploitation.

Legal and illegal recreational drugs, both 'hard' and 'soft', can interfere with many aspects of ordinary living. Effects on energy, concentration, mood, or physical health can cause tension and disruption within families, and confrontations or disappointments at school or in the workplace. Some employers operate drug (and alcohol) policies which involve regular urine screens for illicit drugs. Positive tests can result in dismissal even if there has been no discernible effect on performance.

Countries vary in their approach to drugs and driving. In Britain the Road Traffic Act requires applicants or licence holders to inform the Driver and Vehicle Licensing Agency (DVLA) of any 'prescribed or prospective disability' which could pose 'a source of danger to the public'. Such disability includes 'addiction/use or dependency on illicit drugs' or 'chronic solvent misuse or dependency'. If the DVLA receives evidence of 'persistent use or dependency' on cannabis, amphetamine, ecstasy or 'other psychoactive substances' the driving licence will be revoked until a minimum period of six months' (one year for public service vehicle drivers) abstinence has been demonstrated. Persistent use of opioids, cocaine or methamphetamine results in more pro-longed licence withdrawal and stringent requirements for rehabilitation. The 2008 pre-Christmas blitz on drugged driving in the UK incorporated a return to the use of roadside tests of coordination to test for effects of drugs other than alcohol. Consultant-supervised maintenance on oral methadone or buprenorphine (see Chapter 14) is no bar to retaining a driving licence, but if injectable prescriptions of controlled drugs are provided it must be surren-dered. Covert drug use revealed in testing following an accident may invalidate insurance cover. In the US, regulations concerning drugged driving vary widely across the nation. In some states it is illegal to drive a vehicle if you have even a trace of illegal recreational drugs or their metabolites detectable in your blood. President Bush declared December 2008 as National Drunk and Drugged Driving Prevention Month, in the hope of encouraging '. . . *all Americans to help keep our Nation's roads safe by making responsible choices and taking appropriate measures to prevent drunk and drugged driving'*.

Approximately a third of all US drug users are women of child-bearing age, and more than half a million unborn babies are exposed to illicit drugs each year. Damage to the foetus, though theoretically possible with most drug types, is extremely rare when the mother is an occasional or social user, though some adulterants commonly found in street drugs are potentially very toxic. Drug users overall fall into the 'high normal' range for congenital abnormalities with an incidence of around 3% of live births. Common sense (but not much in the way of hard data) suggests that risks will be greater for addicted mothers who are likely to be consuming more drugs, and may also be suffering from the effects of poor nutrition, chronic infections, lack of family support and antenatal care, and a chaotic lifestyle. It is important to note that *all* drugs taken during pregnancy—legal, illegal, or prescribed—especially during the first three months, represent a potential risk to the foetus and should be avoided if possible. Tobacco is identified as a cause of low birth-weight and premature delivery, whilst a heavy consumption of alcohol has been associated with malformations, growth retardation, and impaired mental capacity.

In the UK the Children Act (2004) requires that in cases where a child appears to be at risk in terms of health or development, it is incumbent upon social workers and other professionals to ensure that the interests and welfare of that child take precedence over all other considerations. Interventions will almost always be aimed at helping the parent or parents to provide the emotional and physical environment that the child requires.

Longer-term consequences

Good quality research into the long-term consequences of teenage smoking, drinking, or drug taking is in short supply, but some broad conclusions can be reached. Modest, controlled consumption of illegal drugs is much more common than regular, heavy, or compulsive use, and many young people seem able to use these substances in the same socially appropriate way as most adults use alcohol. Such transient or experimental use does not seem to be associated with measurable long-term harm.

On the other hand, about 10% of those who experiment with alcohol or illegal drugs will go on to develop problems with them at a later stage. Starting at an unusually early age or rapid escalation in the teens are bad prognostic signs. Other factors which contribute to a higher likelihood of problem drug use include parents who do not impose discipline or smoke and drink to excess themselves; a history of running away from home or truanting from school; living in a children's home or foster care; socio-economic deprivation; or a lack of local amenities (e.g. gym or sports clubs, green space, affordable public transport). Regular or heavy use during adolescence has a strong association with emotional and physical problems then and later, difficult family, social, and sexual relationships, and disruption of education and employment. Problem drug use overlaps with many other undesirable behaviours such as delinquency, teenage pregnancy, and school drop-out and probably shares many causative factors. Drug effects join with these to disrupt the developmental processes involved in progressing from adolescence to adult roles and responsibilities. Such teenagers almost always have poor relationships with those outside their peer group, are less good at practical problem-solving, and become alienated to some degree from families and school life. This disaffection can eat further into an already precarious sense of purpose and ambition, and fuel anxiety, hostility, boredom, and feelings of emptiness. It then becomes tempting to blame the drug directly for these psychological problems, but the drug use may be just one more symptom of a more complicated system of causation, such as a dysfunctional family. There are gender differences in the expression of distress by young people: males tend to manifest it by antisocial behaviour, girls by emotional symptoms. Women are more stigmatized by alcohol or drug problems in most societies.

School students who drink regularly will admit to a range of alcohol-related problems. Most commonly reported in a UK sample are problems with relationships (22%—quarrels with parents, teachers, or friends), personal difficulties (21%—impaired school work, damage to objects or clothing, loss of money or valuables, accident or injury), sexual regrets (15%—engaged in unwanted or unprotected sex), and acts of delinquency (12%—fights, victim of theft, driving while drunk, trouble with the police).

Very little is known about the natural history of young, intermittent users of drugs such as cannabis, amphetamine, cocaine, ecstasy, and hallucinogens or the impact, if any, these may have on their physical or mental health. It is likely that the risk of psychological problems in association with such drugs will be considerably higher in individuals with pre-existing mental health problems or a strong family history of serious psychiatric illness such as schizophrenia. For risks associated with individual drugs see the appropriate chapter.

A number of attempts have been made to follow the progress of opiate users over years rather than months. Addiction is seen in these studies to be a chronic relapsing and remitting process which carries a significant mortality from accidents, illness, suicide, and violence. Despite this, the outcome is not as gloomy as generally thought since up to half the subjects are found to be abstinent after 10 years. In those addicts that survive, the natural history of the condition seems slanted towards slow but steady recovery, which may lead to the beneficial effect of treatment being overestimated. Most addicts become heroin-free by middle age, with a typical addiction 'career' lasting about 10 years. The fluctuating course is marked by longer and longer intermissions of controlled use or abstinence. Notwithstanding this trend, between 5% and 10% of addicts are more than 45 years old. Some may switch dependency to alcohol or other drugs as heroin loses its appeal. Physical problems are mainly related to lifestyle, poor injecting technique, and adulterants in street drugs. Pharmaceutical opiates are remarkably non-toxic and there are well documented examples of doctors and others with access to pure drugs who have injected opiates over decades and still managed to lead stable and productive lives.

If this is the broad pattern of opiate addiction, the details vary considerably from study to study and region to region. For example, mortality among drug injectors in Glasgow was found to be 22 times higher than would be expected in that age group, compared to a ratio of 18 for Stockholm, 11.9 for London, and 10 for Rome. By far the commonest cause of death was overdose, accidental or intentional. Variations in local practices (e.g. simultaneous use of IV benzodiazepines) or treatment availability may account for some of these differences. US follow-up studies usually make for grimmer reading. A quarter of the sample is likely to have died over a 20-year period, and between a quarter and a half remain addicted for the whole time. Nevertheless, a favourable outcome for long-term natural recovery is still discernible for survivors.

Injecting drug use represents a massive, world-wide public health problem because of its role in the spread of several diseases. There are over 16 million intravenous drug users (IDU) globally, almost half of whom live in Asia, South America, Russia, or Eastern Europe. Many share syringes or needles on a regular basis. With the exception of sub-Saharan Africa approximately a third of all infections with the human immunodeficiency virus (HIV) are acquired in this way. This currently equates to around three million HIV positive IDU. Sexual contact with an IDU is an important bridge by which the virus reaches the heterosexual, non drug-using population: a study in New York showed that 80% of cases of heterosexual spread involved an IDU at some point of the chain. The spread of the virus through an injecting population can be terrifyingly rapid: in 1984, the proportion of infected IDU in Edinburgh leapt by 40% within a single year. There are very large national variations in the prevalence of HIV among IDU: in the UK, only 2.3% carry the virus, compared to almost 40% in Russia and Spain, over 40% in Thailand, and almost 50% in Argentina and Brazil.

Other diseases spread in this way include hepatitis B, which is 10 times more infectious than HIV and afflicts between 40% and 60% of regular IDU. An even bigger problem in terms of morbidity and mortality is the more aggressive hepatitis C which is a major cause of serious liver disease globally. The majority of IDU in the US test positive for hepatitis C and up to 80% of the 40,000 new cases each year in the country are acquired in this population. In the UK nearly half of all injectors carry the disease. Sexually transmitted diseases are commoner in this population, as is that ancient and currently re-emerging scourge tuberculosis.

Influences upon the outcome of dependent drug use

Treatment is just one of a number of factors which may impact upon the profile or duration of addiction careers. The common denominator of those treatments which do have some demonstrable impact seems to be their ability to introduce or enhance structure in people's lives. Natural events which achieve the same result, such as a new relationship or job, can be just as beneficial. Factors which most commonly lead people to seek help include health or legal problems, pressure from the family, the expense of the habit, and in the case of illegal drugs the inconvenience and risk of obtaining black market supplies.

Short-term treatment measures, though they may be a necessary preliminary or stepping-stone, have not been shown to exert any effect upon long-term outcome. Detoxification is a case in point, with some people undergoing hundreds of these procedures in the course of their addiction career. In one series, 100 addicts clocked up 770 detoxifications between them, and on only 3% of occasions was this followed by a period of abstinence of a year or more.

When detoxification is linked with some continuing therapy, results are often better than they appear at first glance. Although 71% of heroin addicts in one study used again within six weeks of completing detoxification, many of these did not revert to dependent use and the abstinence rate increased steadily over time. At six months, 45% were off drugs and living in the community, whilst a further 14% were using only on an occasional basis. The greatest number of lapses happened in the first week after detoxification, and the results from other studies show that 80–90% of full-scale relapses will have occurred within the first few weeks or months. Reasons given for relapse include re-exposure to the drug culture and drug-using friends, recurrent craving, interpersonal conflicts, unpleasant mood states or environmental conditions, and reduction of staff support.

Long-term outcome relates quite consistently to the length of time spent in treatment, and if that duration is less than three months it is unlikely to be more effective than detoxification alone or no treatment at all. Of relevance to this observation is the finding that methadone or buprenorphine maintenance programmes retain clients better than drug-free outpatient programmes or therapeutic communities.

Predicting outcome for the individual addict is very difficult. Having a serious pre-existing psychiatric illness is a definite disadvantage, and there are some other relatively weak indicators of an unfavourable prognosis: poor pre-addiction social stability, employment history, or educational attainment; heavy involvement in the drug culture, or having a drug-using partner; history of serious criminal activity; heavy alcohol use before or during treatment; an inability to maintain long-term relationships; and being raised in a culture different to that of the parents. Interestingly, the severity of the addiction in terms of frequency of use or quantity consumed has little or no bearing on the likelihood of successful rehabilitation.

Two factors stand out above all the others in determining a successful outcome. These are achieving a structured and rewarding lifestyle and changing location after becoming abstinent.

Addicts who are successful in beating their habit are usually those who are able to find alternative sources of interest and gratification which lead to new routines and preoccupations. These may be achieved by a new relationship, a job, or even an alternative less damaging dependence. The latter could take the form of religious involvement or regular attendance at a self-help group. There is no doubt that membership of Alcoholics Anonymous (AA) is associated with prevention of relapse into alcoholism, and it likely that the same is true of Narcotics Anonymous (NA). At the very least, AA and NA are very effective at breaking an unhealthy self-focus through their emphasis on helping others, and provide an inspiring model of attainable abstinence to those who have begun to abandon hope.

An occupation or career fulfills many functions beyond the obvious one of generating a supply of money. It provides a sense of belonging and purpose, contributes to self-esteem and confidence, permits an escape from the humdrum tasks of day-to-day living even though it may itself be quite routine and dull, introduces the worker to another circle of acquaintance, and adds shape and structure to life.

The other quite striking predictor of a good outcome is a change of domicile after coming off drugs. According to the published opinions of ex-addicts themselves, this seems to have played the decisive role in maintaining abstinence in at least a quarter of cases. One investigation followed a group of 171 heroin addicts over a period of two decades. Abstinence occurred for 54% of the time spent away from the home city and for only 12% of the time spent living in it. Abstinence lasting a year or more was three times more likely to be achieved away from home, and 81% of abstinent addicts relapsed within one month of returning to their home city. Presumably, this can be explained by re-exposure to a familiar and welcoming drug scene, alongside a resurgence of family pressures and conflicts.

Selected references

Arasteh, K, Des Jarlais, D. C. (2008). Injecting drug use, HIV, and what to do about it. *Lancet*, **372**, 1709–10.

Blackwell, J. S. (1983). Drifting, controlling, and overcoming: opiate users who avoid becoming chronically dependent. *Journal of Drug Issues*, **13**, 219–35.

Bradley, B. P., Phillips, G., Green, L., Gossop, M. (1989). Circumstances surrounding the initial lapse to opiate use following detoxification. *British Journal of Psychiatry*, **154**, 354–9.

Cottrell, D., Childs-Clarke, A., Ghodse, A. H. (1985). British opiate addicts: an 11-year follow-up. *British Journal of Psychiatry*, **146**, 448–50.

Dawson D. A., Goldstein R. B., Patricia Chou S. et al. (2008). Age at first drink and the first incidence of adult-onset DSM-IV alcohol use disorders. *Alcoholism: Clinical & Experimental Research* **32**, 2149–60.

Driver and Vehicle Licencing Agency (2008). *At a glance guide to the current medical standards for fitness to drive.* Drivers Medical Group, DVLA, Swansea.

Edwards, J. G., Goldie, A. (1987). A ten-year follow-up study of Southampton opiate addicts. *British Journal of Psychiatry*, **151**, 679–83.

Frischer, M., Goldberg, D., Rahman, M., Berney, L. (1997). Mortality and survival among a cohort of drug injectors in Glasgow, 1982–1994. *Addiction*, **92**, 419–27.

Gossop, M., Green, L., Phillips, G., Bradley, B. (1987). What happens to opiate addicts immediately after treatment: a prospective follow-up study. *British Medical Journal*, **294**, 1377–80.

Gossop, M., Green, L., Phillips, G., Bradley, B. (1989). Lapse, relapse, and survival among opiate addicts after treatment. *British Journal of Psychiatry*, **154**, 348–53.

Judson, B. A., Goldstein, A. (1982). Prediction of long-term outcome for heroin addicts admitted to a methadone maintenance programme. *Drug and Alcohol Dependence*, **10**, 383–91.

McLellan, A. T., Luborsky, L., Woody, G. E., O'Brien, C. P., Druley, K. A. (1983). Predicting response to alcohol and drug abuse treatments. *Archives of General Psychiatry*, **40**, 620–5.

McLellan, A. T., Luborsky, L., O'Brien, C. P., Woody, G. E., Druley, K. A. (1982). Is treatment for substance abuse effective? *Journal of the American Medical Association*, **247**, 1423–8.

Maddux, J. F., Desmond, D. P. (1982). Residence relocation inhibits opioid dependence. *Archives of General Psychiatry*, **39**, 1313–17.

Marshall, E. J., Edwards, G., Taylor C. (1994). Mortality in men with drinking problems: a 20 year follow-up. *Addiction*, **89**, 1293–1298.

Mathers BM, Degenhardt L, Phillips B et al. (2008). Global epidemiology of injecting drug use and HIV among people who inject drugs: a systematic review. *Lancet* **372**, 1733–45.

Milby, J. B. (1988). Methadone maintenance to abstinence: how many make it? *Journal of Nervous and Mental Diseases*, **176**, 409–22.

Mulleady, G., Sherr, L. (1989). Lifestyle factors for drug users in relation to risks for HIV. *AIDS Care*, **1**, 45–50.

Newcomb, M. D., Scheier, L. M., Bentler, P. M. (1993). Effects of adolescent drug use on adult mental health: a prospective study of a community sample. *Experimental and Clinical Psychopharmacology*, **1**, 215–41.

Roberts, I., Barker, M., Li, L. (1997). Analysis of trends in deaths from accidental drug poisoning in teenagers. *British Medical Journal*, **315**, 289.

Robins, L. H. (1979). Addict careers. In: *Handbook on drug abuse* (ed. R. L. Dupont, A. Goldstein, J. O'Donnell), pp. 325–36. N.I.D.A., Washington.

Robson, P. (1996). Young people and illegal drugs. In: *Adolescent medicine* (ed. A. Macfarlane). Royal College of Physicians, London.

Robson, P., Bruce, M. (1997). A comparison of 'visible' and 'invisible' users of amphetamine, cocaine, and heroin: two distinct populations? *Addiction*, **92**, 1729–36.

Segest, E., Mygind, O., Bay, H. (1989). The allocation of drug addicts to different types of treatment. An evaluation and a two-year follow-up. *American Journal of Drug and Alcohol Abuse*, **15**, 41–53.

Simpson, D. D. (1979). The relation of time spent in drug abuse treatment to post-treatment outcome. *American Journal of Psychiatry*, **136**, 1449–53.

Simpson, D. D., Savage, J., Lloyd, M. R. (1979). Follow-up evaluation of treatment of drug abuse during 1969 to 1972. *Archives of General Psychiatry*, **36**, 772–80.

Stimson, G. V., Oppenheimer, E., Thorley, A. (1978). Seven-year follow-up of heroin addicts: drug use and outcome. *British Medical Journal*, **1**, 1190–2.

Thorley, A. (1981). Longitudinal studies of drug dependence. In: *Drug problems in Britain: a review of ten years* (ed. G. Edwards, C. Busch). Academic Press, London.

Torralba, L., Brugal, M. T.,Villalbi, J. R., Tortosa, A., Toribio, A., Valverda, J. L. (1996). Mortality due to adverse drug reactions: opiates and cocaine in Barcelona, 1989–93. *Addiction*, **91**, 419–26.

Warburton H, Turnbull PJ, Hough M (2005). *Occasional and controlled heroin use: not a problem?* Report prepared for Joseph Rowntree Foundation, York ISBN 1 85935 425 4

Vaillant, G. E. (1988). What can long-term follow-up teach us about relapse and prevention of relapse in addiction? *British Journal of Addiction*, **83**, 1147–57.

White, N. J. (1989). Prescribing in pregnancy. In: *Oxford textbook of medicine* (ed. D. J. Weatherall, J. G. G. Ledingham, D. A. Warrell). Oxford University Press, Oxford.

Zinberg, N. E., Jacobson, R. C. (1976). The natural history of 'chipping' (controlled use of opiates). *American Journal of Psychiatry*, **133**, 37–40.

Chapter 3

Alcohol

Historical background

It is impossible to say just how long ago it was that humans first learnt to ferment sugars into alcohol, but the founders of the Babylonian Empire were brewing beer 4,000 years before the birth of Christ. An Egyptian papyrus dating from around 3,500 BC describes wine-making techniques, and knowledge of the process had reached the Atlantic coast of Europe by 2,500 BC. Alcohol partially displaced the ritual and medical roles of cannabis and opium which were being cultivated by Stone Age farmers. From that time onwards alcohol has been produced wherever humans have settled.

In polytheistic Ancient Greece, Dionysus, son of Zeus and Semele, may have been a minor god but as patron of wine and dance he was certainly a popular one. Drunken revelries were held by his acolytes every spring and winter. The symposium evolved as a ritual-laden gathering at which men could indulge in bibulous conversation and riotous entertainment, with vast amounts of food and drink being consumed. Public drunkenness outside of these special occasions was unusual even though a love of alcohol was certainly not confined to the ruling classes. The Greeks invented the tavern and were the first to organize the mass production and systematic export of wine. Mead (derived from fermented honey) was also very popular among ordinary people. Plato and Socrates drew attention to the darker side of alcohol, including its association with public disorder and violence, failure to fulfill a useful role within the family, difficulties in work and productivity, and accidents. And for high-profile casualties one need look no further than Alexander III ('the Great'), dead at 32 after one too many alcoholic binges.

Dionysus evolved into Bacchus, and Pliny the Elder reviled wine as 'a thing that perverts the mind and produces madness'. The small Roman vineyards that sprang up around 700 BC were insufficient for home consumption, so trade routes for importation developed rapidly. As the empire expanded both importation and home production soared and prices plummeted. By AD 20 heavy daily drinking had become the norm and was associated with much violence and debauchery. Alcohol was free to the plebs on public holidays, which eventually amounted to around 160 days each year under Nero, and which helped to fuel the growing atmosphere of savagery and decay.

The Hebrews took enthusiastically to wine during the Egyptian captivity. According to the Book of Genesis, Noah planted a vineyard, made full use of its provenance, and 'lay uncovered in his tent'. The Bible veers from condemnation to endorsement, but generally there has been a tendency down the ages for Christian theologians to be indulgent towards over-imbibers. After the decline of the Roman empire it fell to the Christian monasteries in many countries to safeguard the traditions of brewing and viticulture, and it was an ingenious monk who invented the cork and opened the way to bottle ageing and secondary fermentation. Around the same period, approximately AD 616, the adherents of Islam were forbidden alcohol by the law laid down in the sacred Koran (or Qur'an) by the prophet Mohammed.

In the British Isles, ale had been the endemic tipple of the native population since pre-Roman times, and taverns appeared early in the 12th century. In medieval Britain, beer was often safer to drink than water from the local river or well, and was also seen as an important source of energy and nutrition. Ales were relatively low in alcohol content (around 3% by volume), contained useful amounts of B vitamins, calcium, and magnesium, and supplied up to 10% of dietary energy. The addition of hops to prolong storage time and enhance taste probably caught on about 200 years later. This also permitted extended fermentation time so the resulting beer was much more alcoholic.

With the increasing dominance of the 'patriarchal nuclear family' a drunken husband or father came to be seen as failing in his role as an ally of the Government in maintaining social order. The drunkard became socially unacceptable because his incapacity obliged his neighbours to care for his dependants, and no excuse was accepted for what was seen as selfish gluttony or simple greed. Alcohol-induced violence within the family was deplored, but induced little in the way of a practical response because of the low status of women and the expendability of young children. Surviving documents from this period demonstrate contemporary concern about the role of alcohol in fermenting violence, causing accidents, and undermining moral behaviour.

From the 15th century onwards alcohol consumption became increasingly located outside the family home, and the alehouse or tavern evolved as the convivial centre of the working man's social life. It also served as a labour exchange, a staging post for journeys, and a setting for such entertainments las bear-baiting, cockfights, and prizefights. This shift considerably reduced women's access to alcohol, and raised concern among the ruling classes about possible disruption of the availability and reliability of labourers.

The popular belief that alcohol was generally beneficial was endorsed by 17th-century doctors who recommended it for a wide range of conditions as disparate as depression, venereal disease, and gout. It was a staple ingredient of tonics and dietary supplements. Consumption increased steadily through the century, and the Government cashed in on this by imposing the first ever beer duty in 1643. Beer consumption reached an all-time high in 1689 with an average intake for the year of 832 pints for every man, woman, and child in the land. Considerable amounts of home-produced wine were drunk in Britain in the Middle Ages, but the dissolution of the monasteries by Henry VIII resulted in the destruction of virtually all British vineyards. Subsequent patterns of wine consumption were determined almost entirely by shifting treaties and taxes. When relations with the French deteriorated at the beginning of the 18th century the Methuen Treaty was signed with Portugal, turning the wealthier English citizens from claret to port drinkers almost overnight. For the next 80 years only 3.6% of all the wine drunk in England came from France. Smuggling of French wine became vastly profitable until commercial channels were reopened by a new treaty in 1783. Around this time, the vineyards which formed the starting point for the future New World wine tradition were being planted by Franciscan monks newly embarked in California. There were notable peaks of consumption in the middle of the 18th century and the late 1900s, but the industry in Britain went into a steady decline to an all-time low in the 1940s and 1950s. Since then, however, the taste for wine has caught on again in a big way and consumption per capita is far greater now than at any time in the past.

The process of distillation was developed in the Middle East around the 12th century AD with medicinal applications in mind, but consumption of 'acqua vitae' was widespread in Europe by the beginning of the 16th century. Until around 1700, restrictive practices ensured that consumption of distilled drinks in Britain was almost entirely confined to the wealthy. The cancellation of the monopoly hitherto enjoyed by the Worshipful Company of Distillers led to the infamous 'gin craze' among the poor which peaked between 1720 and 1750. Gin was first created in 17th-century Holland by the addition of juniper berries to grain alcohol. When William III restricted importation of French wine and brandy the deregulated home gin industry went into overdrive, and in London alone 8,000 'dram shops' sprang up in which one could become 'drunk for a penny, dead drunk for tuppence'.

The debauchery and squalor associated with this crisis was a shock to the respectable citizenry, but alcohol in all its forms was still central to the everyday life of polite society. Drinking among men tended to be heavy and competitive and public figures such as William Pitt and Richard Sheridan were certainly not ashamed of their reputations as 'six-bottle men'. Gin may have plummeted downmarket but the respectable image of brandy ('bernenwijn' evolving to 'branntwein' or 'burnt wine') remained untarnished.

Whisky ('usquebaugh') was hugely popular in Scotland and Ireland. In the US, despite the prominence and influence of the Puritans, the early colonists adopted similar habits to their countries of origin. The local cider industry developed rapidly along with production of mead and fruit wines, and distillation became widespread early in the 18th century. Alcohol consumption per capita in 1790 was at least twice that of 1990 levels.

The eighteenth century saw the zenith of both British and American drinking, but it was also the period when organized opposition to the habit began to strengthen and doctors began to refer to drunkenness as a disease. As early as 1724 George Cheyne wrote about the eroding power of 'craving' and the physical risks inherent in sudden abstinence after regular, heavy imbibing. This 'medicalization' of alcohol abuse was accelerated by the writings of such physicians as Benjamin Rush (1790) in the US and Thomas Trotter in Britain, who declared in 1804 that the 'habit of drunkenness is a disease of the mind'. The acute withdrawal syndrome was named 'delirium tremens' in 1813, and the term 'alcoholism' coined in 1849 by the Swedish physician Magnus Huss who defined it as follows: '*Those disease manifestations which without any direct connection with organic disease of the nervous system take on a chronic form in persons who, over long periods, have partaken of large quantities of brandy*'. The appropriation of the new syndrome by doctors was part of a wider professional expansionism. This included the birth of the new specialism of 'psychiatry' which sought to redefine abnormal behaviour according to moral and medical principles.

The earliest pioneers of the Temperance Movement promoted the concept of moderation rather than abstinence. They were more concerned about punch, rum, and whisky than beer, wine, or cider, but as the alcoholic increasingly came to be seen as ill and needy rather than immoral or degenerate so the argument for complete abstinence moved to centre stage. The fervour of reformers escalated alongside the growing power of psychiatrists and the increasing use of asylums. Restrictions on alehouse opening hours were introduced in 1828 and tightened further in 1848 and 1854, by which time US temperance associations could boast over a million members. Paradoxically, at around the same time the number of public houses shot up as a result of the Beer House Act which made it much easier to obtain a liquor licence. Wine, too, enjoyed an impressive peak of consumption in the last quarter of the century.

In the American West, the first saloons appeared in the aftermath of the Civil War and were soon to be found in every one-horse town. Cheap whisky, heavily-armed customers brutalized by war and deprivation, and rudimentary enforcement of law and order created an alarming environment which attracted the concerns of the temperance campaigners back East. An 'Antisaloon League' was influential in persuading some states to tackle the problem by going 'dry'.

In 1913 the League joined the political movement calling for national prohibition, which was duly enacted in 1919. Initially this had wide support, but demand for bootleg liquor shot up in the 1920s, and a host of private drinking clubs ('speakeasies') sprang up in every city. Organized criminals took full advantage of this windfall opportunity. Quality control was poor and there were many casualties from impurities in the 'moonshine'. A combination of pressure from voters and a desperate need by the Federal government for taxation income lead to the repeal of the prohibition in 1933 during the Roosevelt era. Control over alcohol retail and distribution was turned over to administration by individual states. Today there are still more than 500 counties in the US where sale of alcohol is forbidden.

Consumption of beers, wines, and spirits fell steadily in Britain from the beginning of the 20th century to the start of the 1950s. Popularity of wine and spirits has increased markedly since then, particularly the former whose consumption per capita now easily eclipses the previous all-time high in the 1740s. Beer showed a much more modest recovery until the mid-seventies, but has declined again more recently. In the England of 1750, 94% of all alcohol was consumed in the form of beer but in 1980 the proportion had slumped to less than 50%.

Levels of alcohol consumption are determined by a complex interaction of price, availability and promotion, national prosperity, social upheavals and periods of recovery, cultural pressures, and educational or moral campaigns. Price seems to be the most influential factor, and taking account of inflation the real cost of a pint of beer in 1980 was less than half that of 1950. A bottle of whisky would have been one third of the cost. In the case of wine, a determined commercial onslaught on the UK market and the startling impact of New World energy and enterprise within the wine-making industry have changed the drinking habits of a nation.

Attempts to ban juvenile drinking are largely a modern phenomenon. In the Middle Ages, infants received ale as part of their normal diet and a page in the Court of Edward IV could expect to receive an allowance of two quarts daily. Prepubertal children were expected to restrict intake to two or three glasses with meals, but there was no question of abstention. This acceptance of modest consumption alongside stern condemnation of excess continued without any legal enforcement until the 20th century. In 1908 it became illegal for children under 14 to enter bars, and in 1923 sale of alcohol to under-18s was forbidden.

Comparison of alcohol consumption across countries is hampered by differing definitions of a 'standard drink' or 'unit of alcohol', with amounts ranging between 8 g (UK) and 14 g (US).

Preparation and distribution

The alcohols are a group of organic compounds characterized by the presence of one or more hydroxy (OH) groups and having a wide range of industrial applications. Ethyl alcohol (ethanol) forms the basis of intoxicating drinks, and the basic method of its production is the fermentation of glucose by yeast.

Yeast consists of a collection of oval vegetable cells, each of which is a tiny, independent plant. If yeast cells are placed in a solution containing sugar in conditions of low oxygen concentration to encourage anaerobic metabolism, they will split each molecule of glucose into two molecules of ethanol plus carbon dioxide. The chemical equation is as follows:

$$C_6H_{12}O_6 = 2C_2H_5OH + 2CO_2$$

The pay-off for the yeast cells is energy generation but the ethanol is a toxic by-product so they excrete it back into the solution. Once the concentration of ethanol in solution approaches 14 or 15% the yeast cell finds it overwhelming and becomes dormant. This is, therefore, the maximum strength which can be achieved for alcoholic drinks which rely on fermentation alone. Different species of yeasts have been found to lend themselves more efficiently to production of particular types of beer or wine.

Drinks such as wine and cider are manufactured in this single-stage operation by direct fermentation of the sugars in grapes and apples. Allowing secondary fermentation after bottling results in champagne. In the case of beer, fermentation is preceded by the malting process in which grain of one sort or another (usually barley) is allowed to germinate in water, roast-dried, and crushed. The malted barley is then mixed with hops and yeast in hot water for fermentation. The strength of beer and wine ranges between 3–9% and 8–15% alcohol by volume respectively. Fortified wines such as sherry or port are boosted with extra alcohol.

Distillation relies upon the fact that ethanol evaporates at a lower temperature than water. If a fermented solution is heated but kept well below the boiling point of water, collecting the resulting vapour by condensation will generate an ethanol concentration up to a maximum of around 96% by volume. The strength of an alcoholic drink is usually defined by this measure. 'Proof' scales are confusing. The British system, which dates from the 17th century, is centred around the concentration of alcohol required for a solution containing gunpowder to explode—this threshold is taken as 100° proof. Spirits are generally around 40% alcohol by volume, which equates to 70° proof. The American proof value is obtained by doubling the percentage of alcohol by volume.

The taste and character of alcoholic drinks do not depend primarily upon the alcohol content. The flavour of wine is greatly affected not only by the type of grape but also soil, climate, additives, and production techniques (together known as 'terroir'). The character of spirits will be shaped by both the material from which it is derived such as grapes (brandy), grain (whisky), molasses (rum), or juniper berries (gin), and the maturing conditions (e.g. malt whisky stored in sherry barrels). All alcoholic drinks contain widely varying amounts of organic materials, minerals, and other chemicals collectively known as congeners. These greatly influence the colour, aroma, flavour, and hangover potential of each particular drink, and include phenols, sugars, tannins, sulphur, esters, and amino acids. Vodka has the lowest level of congeners, whilst port, brandy, and rum bristle with them.

A dubious marketing initiative occurred with the introduction in Europe in the early 1990s and a few years later in the US of a wide range of 'alcopops' ('spiked sodas'), which are sweet and fizzy drinks containing 5% alcohol or more. In the opinion of the editor of the scientific journal Addiction, *'If there were a gold medal for cynical marketing it would surely be awarded to sections of the alcohol industry for the marketing of alcohol products targeted at young people'*. His own research suggested that by the age of 14 more than half of all teenagers have been drunk at least once, and that white ciders, fruit wines, and alcopops are most closely associated with intoxication in this age group. Among children aged 11 to 16, 27% of girls and 21% of boys had consumed alcopops within the previous month. In Europe, the bulk of alcopops are consumed in the UK, Ireland, Norway, and Denmark, and in these countries their use more than doubled between 1995 and 2003.

Methanol (CH_3OH), known as wood alcohol, is widely used as a solvent but sometimes crops up as a constituent of illicitly manufactured alcohol ('moonshine'). Methanol is highly toxic because it is broken down in the body to formaldehyde. Unfortunately, there is a high concentration of the enzyme responsible for this process in the retina of the eye where the resulting formaldehyde destroys the light receptors and causes blindness.

Scientific information

Ethanol is a small, water-soluble molecule which is absorbed rapidly from the small intestine and rather more slowly from the stomach. Absorption is slowed by fatty or carbohydrate-rich food in the stomach and speeded up by carbon dioxide in champagne or mixers. Absorption of drinks with an alcohol concentration greater than 20% may be slowed because of inhibited movement (peristalsis) of the stomach and partial spasm of the valve (pylorus) between the stomach and small intestine. The timing and height of peak alcohol blood levels will be determined by the dose and rapidity of consumption, the alcohol concentration of the drink, gender, the presence of food, and the time of day (because of the influence of diurnal rhythms on hormone levels). Peak levels normally occur about an hour after consumption. The liver is particularly vulnerable to toxic effects because ethanol reaches it directly from the small intestine via the portal vein.

Over 90% of the absorbed ethanol is oxidized in the liver to acetaldehyde which is then broken down to acetic acid, carbon dioxide, and water. The remainder is excreted unchanged in the breath, urine, and sweat. The enzyme which brings about the first step, alcohol dehydrogenase (ADH), exists in nature to break down the ethanol and other alcohols produced by bacteria in the guts. The quantity of ADH contained in the liver and other body tissues varies greatly between individuals, depending upon liver size, genetic make-up, and the regularity and quantity of alcohol intake. Heavy drinking boosts ADH production and results in tolerance—the need to consume more alcohol to achieve the same level of intoxication. Not only is ADH less efficient in females but women also possess less of it, for example in the walls of the stomach. Unlike men, however, they do not face decreasing ADH activity as the years roll on. Other reasons why women are more susceptible to alcohol include greater rapidity of absorption; higher tissue concentrations of alcohol as a result of smaller blood volume and more subcutaneous fat; hormonal influences on peak blood levels (e.g. higher absorption premenstrually and at ovulation); and greater sensitivity of certain tissues to the damaging effects of ethanol. Drugs such as aspirin interfere with the efficiency of ADH.

Genetics also influence the response to alcohol by regulating other metabolic mechanisms and altering the tone of relevant brain chemicals and systems, including the dopamine-powered 'pleasure pathway'. Almost half of all Asian people produce a relatively inactive form of acetaldehyde dehydrogenase, the enzyme responsible for driving the second stage of ethanol metabolism. The resulting build-up of acetaldehyde in the blood produces headache, flushing, dizziness, nausea, and a pounding heart.

There is enormous individual variation, but the average person is able to metabolize approximately 8 g of alcohol (roughly equivalent to a 'standard drink' in the UK (0.57 drinks in US)) each hour, causing the blood alcohol level to fall in that period by 15 mg per 100 ml of blood (%). The legal limit for driving in Europe ranges between 20 mg% (Sweden) to 80 mg% (several countries including UK), and most US states have now standardized to the latter. With larger amounts or more rapid consumption, the metabolic and elimination processes become overwhelmed, so blood and tissue levels increase much more rapidly. The liver begins to run into difficulties if it is presented with more than about 80 g of alcohol in 24 hours. The risk of liver disease is increased sixfold by levels of consumption averaging more than 40 g daily in men and 20 g in women.

Ethanol produces both stimulant and depressant effects within the brain and interacts with neurotransmitters such as dopamine, serotonin, GABA, and the endorphins. Its main direct effect is probably on the ion channels which permit charged chemicals to pass in and out of nerve cells, blocking or generating impulses. Ethanol inhibits glutamate receptors and this is probably an important cause of impaired coordination and cognition.

Finer judgements, prudence, and self-concern are early casualties of even mild intoxication. Visual and auditory acuity, recovery from glare, colour discrimination, muscle coordination and balance, concentration, decisiveness, and reaction time are all measurably impaired after a single drink. The accident rate for drivers is doubled at the British legal limit of 80 mg%.

Alcohol produces a wide range of physical effects. Skin blood vessels dilate, increasing heat loss, while blood pressure and pulse rate increase. Blood sugar first goes up then drops below normal. A direct effect on hormones controlling fluid balance results in the production of larger amounts of dilute urine and net fluid loss (diuresis leading to dehydration). Alcohol has both pain-killing and sleep-inducing effects, though it upsets the balance between REM and slow-wave sleep and often produces rebound insomnia later in the night. Sexual function is impaired in men, though desire may be enhanced in both sexes. Labour is delayed. Alcohol is directly toxic to the liver and the lining of the stomach. Nausea and vomiting can be induced by a direct effect within the central nervous system. Small doses of alcohol probably give a slight boost to the immune system. A gram of alcohol delivers seven calories.

Possible beneficial effects

Over the centuries, the positive image of alcohol in the public mind has never been dented by the dreadful toll it has exacted on individual and public health, or the pronouncements of temperance campaigners. The folklore of medicinal attributes has survived in one form or another despite little or no evidence to support it, and alcohol is often portrayed in the context of rude good health, virility, courage, and friendship.

Despite the modern obsession with health and safety, most doctors would probably accept that a modest intake is unlikely to be harmful and may indeed do some good. Whilst not conclusive, there is quite a lot of evidence to suggest that one or two drinks daily may offer some protection against diseases of the heart and circulation. Red wine is said to be particularly useful due to the presence of certain phenols such as quercetin and rutin which inhibit blood clotting mechanisms, boost the right sort of fats (high-density lipoproteins) in the plasma, and also have desirable antioxidant activity. It is possible that this is the explanation for the so-called 'French paradox', the observation that despite a diet very rich in saturated fats there is a relatively low prevalence of coronary artery disease in France. Other diseases for which small doses of alcohol may reduce the risk include dementia, gall stones and kidney stones, metabolic syndrome and Type II Diabetes Mellitus, benign prostatic hypertrophy, and osteoporosis in women. Unfortunately, beyond around 20 g alcohol daily, these possible benefits are likely to eclipsed by an increasing risk of liver disease and cancers of the mouth and gastro-intestinal tract.

Recreational use

The World Health Organization (WHO) estimates that around two billion individuals world-wide drink alcohol regularly. The average adult in the European Union (EU) drinks 11 litres of pure alcohol each year, higher than any other region. Since 15% of this population are abstainers, each drinker actually consumes 15 litres annually and in any one year an estimated 23 million Europeans are dependent upon the drug. This compares with consumption of around nine litres annually in the US, Australia and New Zealand. Within the EU there is huge variation between countries, ranging from annual averages of less than five litres in Turkey to 17-plus in the Czech Republic, Lithuania and Hungary. Consumption has been declining steadily throughout most of the EU, but increasing in central Europe. Beer makes up almost half the product consumed (principally in Northern Europe), then roughly a third as wine and a quarter as spirits. Attitudes to drunken behaviour also vary within the region, but it is frowned upon in most Southern EU countries. Overall, around 15% of the adult EU population consumes more than rather arbitrary safety limits of 20 g/week for women and 40 g/week for men.

Annual consumption levels in the UK are around the average EU figure and comparable to Spain, France, and Germany, with 75% men and 60% women having had a drink on at least one day during the previous week. In 1987 the Royal College of Physicians recommended 'sensible limits' for safe drinking of 21 and 14 units weekly for men and women respectively (unit = 8 g alcohol, equal to a half pint of ordinary strength beer, a small glass of wine, or a single measure of spirits). Although these levels are not derived from a firm evidence base, they have been influential in defining at-risk drinking. On this basis, far more UK drinkers exceed safe limits than the EU average (40% men and 23%

women on at least one day during the previous week). Alcohol remains central to most social rituals but is much less acceptable in the workplace than it was a decade ago. The teetotaller is still regarded by many as a social deviant. Some trades and professions carry an awesome reputation for heavy consumption and a high prevalence of alcohol-related problems. Factors which contribute to this are ease of access (bar staff, caterers, restaurateurs, business men with generous expense accounts), hedonistic or sociable working environment (showbusiness, advertising industry, journalism), prolonged separation from family and home environment (seamen, oil-rig workers, servicemen), and stress (doctors, farmers). The number of school pupils who have drunk alcohol in the previous week has declined in recent years, but those who do drink consume more and binge drinking seems to be increasing. United Kingdom pupils report more episodes of drunkenness than any other EU country other than Ireland and Denmark, with one in five admitting having been drunk in the last four weeks. Drinking levels amongst 16 to 24 year-olds in the UK gives rise to concern since currently around a third drink more than twice the recommended safe levels at least once a week. Some believe that this is related to the relaxation of licencing laws in order to permit 24 hour drinking in 2005, and the availability of very cheap supermarket alcohol. In the past decade the number of young women drinking to excess has increased sharply. In Britain it is illegal for those under 18 to buy drinks at a bar. Over-16s can buy beer or cider in a restaurant for consumption with a meal. Despite these restrictions over 80% of under-16s quizzed in a recent survey who tried to buy alcohol in a pub or club and 66% who targeted a shop were successful on their most recent attempt.

In the US there has been a move away from beer towards wine in recent years, with consumption of hard liquor remaining unchanged. Past-year alcohol use among 13 to 14 year-olds has declined steadily, from a high in the mid-nineties of 47% to 32% in 2007. Rates of current alcohol use were around 4% in 12 year-olds increasing to 30% at 16, 52% at 20 and 70% at 21. Almost half of imbibers in their twenties admit to episodes of binge drinking. The percentage of regular drinkers remains around the 70% level into the thirties and forties, then slowly declines. Amongst 80 year-olds, 40% men and 60% women are teetotal.

Unwanted effects

The World Health Organization estimated recently that at any one time around 76 million people will be suffering from an alcohol-related disease. Excessive alcohol consumption is the cause of two million deaths world-wide each year, is the third-leading cause of death in the US (twice the toll of road traffic accidents (RTAs)), and is responsible for 11% of the total disease burden in Europe (rising to 22% in Eastern European males). Around 23 million Europeans and 18 million North Americans are dependent on the drug in any one year. It is a causative factor in over 60 serious diseases, and exerts a major influence in RTAs (as high as one in every three accidents at certain times of the week) and other accidents, homicides, and suicides. The main medical sources of increased mortality are liver damage, respiratory infections, cancers of the respiratory and digestive systems, cardiovascular disease, suicides, and violence. Alcohol-related visits to hospital in the UK have been increasing by 10% yearly, and if both direct and indirect consequences are included this amounted to 800,000 people in the past year at a cost of £2 billion. Alcohol-related absenteeism, and crime and disorder cost the state £6.4 billion and £7.3 billion respectively each year. Alcohol related deaths have risen from 6.9/100,000 in 1991 to 13.4/100,000 in 2006. Young people bear a large brunt of the burden, since alcohol is a causative factor in the deaths of 10% and 25% of young females and males respectively. The relationship of dose to morbidity and mortality is J-shaped because total abstainers have a higher overall mortality than light drinkers. Mortality begins to climb at levels of intake over three units daily for men and two units for women. In a 20-year follow-up of problem drinkers, mortality rate was raised by 364% over the normal for this age group.

Acute effects

Levels of intoxication can be related fairly accurately to blood levels of alcohol, and cognitive deficits become apparent at 30 mg% and above. At 80 mg% the risk of an RTA doubles. At 100 mg% garrulousness, elation, and aggression are likely, along with emotional instability, reduced visual acuity, and impaired coordination and reaction time. Levels above 200 mg% will cause these handicaps to become pronounced along with unsteadiness, slurred speech, potentially life-threatening falls in blood sugar, body temperature, and depression of the heart, and the risk of convulsions. Concentrations of 400 mg% are often fatal as a result of cardiac arrythmia, respiratory depression, or inhalation of vomit. The latter may occur at much lower levels, so an unconscious drunkard should always be placed in the recovery position rather than left snoring on his back. After a huge binge the plummeting blood sugar can be enough to cause brain damage, and the build-up of acidic metabolites (lactic acid, ketones) can bring on kidney failure.

The danger of drunken driving has been recognized since the earliest days of the motor car, and scientific tests in the 1930s clearly quantified the risk.

The introduction of the breathalyser in 1967 reduced road deaths by 15%, but this proved a transient effect. Drunken American drivers killed 26,000 people in 1982, accounting for 60% of all fatal incidents. However, in recent years drunk driving has become increasingly socially unacceptable in many countries, including the US: in 2004, 14.2% Americans questioned in surveys admitted driving under the influence at least once in the previous year, and by 2006 this figure had fallen to 12.4%. Fatal, alcohol-related RTAs declined to 12,998 in 2007, 32% of the total. Similarly in the UK, alcohol-related fatal RTAs have declined from around 1,000 annually in the 1990s to 560 last year, but unfortunately this figure represents a 6% rise from 2001. Alcohol is also a major risk factor for pedestrians and cyclists, and plays an important part in accidents in the home and elsewhere. Drunkenness is closely associated with violence. The 1996 British Crime Survey revealed that 53% of people who attack strangers are drunk at the time, a third of such attacks occur within the immediate vicinity of pubs or other licensed premises, and a further third at or near bus or railway stations. Last year throughout Europe, alcohol was a factor in four out of 10 homicides. Alcohol plays a significant part in nearly half the fights between acquaintances and a third of domestic incidents. The risk of becoming a victim of violence is increased by drinking, since those with robbery or sexual attack in mind often target people made more vulnerable by befuddlement. A study among young Swedish soldiers showed a clear association between alcohol intake and the risk of dying as a result of a violent attack.

Anyone who has ever been drunk is familiar with the price to be paid the morning after. The hangover is made up of some or all of the following: nausea, dry mouth, headache, lethargy, light-headedness, irascibility, reduced tolerance to noise, and general all-round misery. All this is due to a combination of dehydration, build-up of acidic metabolites of alcohol, direct effects of toxic congeners especially in darker coloured drinks, and sleep deprivation.

Alcohol crosses the placenta and is toxic to the developing foetus. The greater the dose, the greater the likelihood of damage, but many paediatricians believe there is no completely safe dose and that abstention during pregnancy is the wisest course. A recent study found that women who had three or more drinks per week and two or more episodes of binge drinking had twice the risk of losing the baby than women who avoided alcohol. Heavier maternal drinking may cause the 'fetal alcohol syndrome' (FAS) which occurs in 0.2% of all births in the UK and US. It is possibly related to peak acetaldehyde levels, so a binge-drinking pattern may be the most harmful. Affected infants are small and floppy with a characteristic facial appearance including a flattened nose and small eyeballs, and variable amounts of brain damage. The foetus is at its most vulnerable during the second and third months of pregnancy, a period of important brain development and limb growth. Three-quarters of children with FAS turn out to be hyperactive, and the average IQ is around 70. Drinking alcohol during pregnancy is the only preventable cause of mental retardation.

Chronic effects

Ethanol is toxic to most tissue, so heavy consumption over a lengthy period can damage almost any body system.

Alcohol can irritate, inflame, and ulcerate the digestive tract all the way from the mouth and pharynx down the oesophagus to the stomach and beyond, and is associated with increased risk of cancer in many sites. Back pressure from distorted blood vessels in the liver causes swelling of veins around the base of the oesophagus (varices) which may burst with disastrous results. Malnutrition results from both this direct effect and the narrowing of dietary intake which is so common among dependent drinkers. The B vitamins, especially thiamine, are particularly affected with potentially dire results, as outlined below. Interference with disposal of urates can lead to gout. The pancreas is especially vulnerable to alcohol, and both acute and chronic pancreatitis are heralded by severe abdominal pain. Long-term damage to pancreatic cells can produce diabetes mellitus because of the loss of insulin production, and further impairment of nutrition because key digestive enzymes are no longer secreted. Chronic pancreatitis is associated with an increased risk of pancreatic cancer. The strong association between alcoholism and tobacco smoking is presumably the cause of the much increased prevalence of lung cancer. Breast, skin, thyroid, and nasopharyngeal cancers are also more prevalent in alcoholics.

Alcohol flows straight from the gut to the liver, so it is the organ first in line for the toxic effect. Susceptibility to liver damage is higher in women and also affected by genetically determined tissue types and general quality of nutrition as well as the quantity of alcohol imbibed. Enlargement of the liver due to fatty infiltration is common in heavy drinkers and is usually fully reversible following abstinence. Alcoholic hepatitis (inflammation of the liver) is much more serious and may even prove fatal. Cirrhosis is a progressive disease which occurs when damaged liver cells are replaced with scar tissue and the organ contracts to a fraction of normal size. When insufficient remains to meet the body's metabolic needs the signs of liver failure appear. Other bodily signs of alcoholism usually evident at this stage include skin blemishes ('spider naevi'), red palms, swelling of the parotid salivary gland, excessive bruising, and clawing of the hands due to tightening of tendons in the palms ('Dupuytren's contracture'). Liver cancer develops in up to 11% of people with cirrhosis.

In the brain, there is loss of nervous tissue which can lead to confusion, memory loss, and deterioration of personality. Associated deficits in Vitamin B_1

(thiamine) can produce Wernicke's encephalopathy with its characteristic combination of confusion, abnormal eye movements, and staggering gait. Untreated, many patients will develop severe and permanent loss of memory and ability to learn new information ('Korsakoff's psychosis'). The cerebellum can be injured, leading to problems with balance and coordination. Damage to nerves outside the brain ('peripheral neuropathy') will cause numbness and muscle weakness. The muscles themselves can be affected, especially those in the upper arm and thigh. Neuropsychiatric disorders, particularly depression, are much more prevalent in heavy drinkers. Common cognitive deficits include impaired concentration, information processing, and visuospatial skills.

A large binge can produce an irregular heartbeat, and heavy long-term consumption is associated with raised blood pressure and greatly increased risk of stroke (cerebrovascular accident). Direct toxicity to the heart can result in an enlarged or flabby organ ('cardiomyopathy') which may eventually prove fatal, and heavy female drinkers have a much increased risk of coronary heart disease. Production of blood cells in the bone marrow is suppressed, leading to various anaemias and further increasing the strain on the heart.

Because of its effects on sex hormones and other related mechanisms, alcoholism is associated with impaired libido and sexual function, osteoporosis, and infertility in both sexes. Male alcoholics may develop impotence, testicular atrophy and enlarged breasts (gynaecomastia), whilst females often experience menstrual abnormalities. Overproduction of the hormone cortisol can lead to obesity and raised blood pressure among other problems.

Alcohol increases the risk of acquiring tuberculosis and other serious respiratory infections in a dose related manner. A recent study revealed an increased likelihood of tuberculosis of around 350% in people drinking more than 40 g alcohol daily long-term. The explanation for this is a combination of social factors and direct toxic effects of alcohol on the immune system.

Approximately 13% of male and 4% of female social drinkers will become dependent upon alcohol. Dependence runs in families, with the close relations of alcoholics five times more likely to develop it due to both genetic and environmental factors ('nature and nurture'). Typologies such as those defined by E.M. Jellineck in the 1950s have been superceded by the concept of the 'alcohol dependence syndrome' which has seven characteristics: 'narrowing of repertoire' as the drinker relies less on social cues and more on the need to maintain a steady intake by an increasingly inflexible routine; making the regular supply of alcohol the main priority in the organization of day-to-day activities; increasing tolerance to the effects of alcohol; repeated withdrawal effects (see below), especially first thing each morning; relief of such symptoms by more drinking; awareness of a growing compulsion to drink; and rapid reinstatement of all these symptoms after a period of abstinence.

When a physically dependent person stops drinking abruptly, withdrawal effects appear after a few hours and reach a peak within a day or two. Initially these consist of tremulousness, nausea, sweating, anxiety, and insomnia. In severe cases this may progress to a full-blown toxic confusional state known as delirium tremens (the 'DTs'). The victim becomes agitated and disorientated, suffers from fleeting delusions and hallucinations, and may develop convulsions which can prove fatal. This syndrome is usually accompanied by other physical disorders, including dehydration, increasing blood pressure, and falling blood sugar. These symptoms gradually subside over a week or two but insomnia, anxiety, and depression sometimes persist for weeks or months.

Alcohol dependence is associated with other psychiatric problems including intermittent auditory hallucinations, pathological jealousy which can result in physical attacks or even murder, and serious depression. There is an association with eating disorders, especially the bingeing/starving condition known as bulimia nervosa. The risk of suicide is greatly increased among alcoholics.

Finally, the dependent drinker is likely to run into problems socially and at work. Families are often wrecked by drunkards with violence directed against the partner or children, neglect of duties of caring or material provision, and diversion of resources to maintain alcohol supplies. The impact upon children is potentially devastating with an increased likelihood of physical and emotional abuse, and a greater prevalence of hyperactivity, truanting, and delinquency. Jobs are lost through poor performance or absenteeism, education and training are disrupted. Social life narrows to the dimensions of the pub, relations with non-drinking friends or neighbours degenerate. Loss of work and family support sometimes ends in financial disaster and homelessness. Alcohol is a lubricant for violence and crime.

Such is the savage impact of our favourite drug on personal and public health. The UK Royal College of Physicians called it 'a great and growing evil' but mostly the rest of us seem remarkably complacent in the face of this array of carnage and suffering.

Selected references

Anderson, P., Cremona, A., Paton, A. et al. (1993). The risk of alcohol. *Addiction*, **88**, 1493–508.

Andreasson, S., Romelsjo, A., Allebeck, P. (1988). Alcohol and mortality among young men: longitudinal study of Swedish conscripts. *British Medical Journal*, **296**, 1021–5.

Babor, T. (1986). *Alcohol: customs and rituals.* Burke Publishing Company Ltd, London.

Braun, S. (1996). *Buzz: the science and lore of alcohol and caffeine.* Oxford University Press, New York.

Edwards, G. (1987). *The treatment of drinking problems*. Blackwell Scientific Publications, Oxford.

Edwards, G., Anderson, P., Babor, T. F. et al. (1994). *Alcohol policy and the public good*. Oxford University Press, Oxford.

Fillmore, K. M., Golding, J. M., Graves, K. L. et al. (1998). Alcohol consumption and mortality. 1. Characteristics of drinking groups. *Addiction*, **93**, 183–97.

Institute of Alcohol Studies (2006). *Alcohol in Europe*. http://ec.europa.eu/health-eu/news_alcoholineurope_en.htm

Leino, E. V., Romelsjo, A., Shoemaker, C. et al. (1998). Alcohol consumption and mortality. II. Studies of male populations. *Addiction*, **93**, 205–18.

Luty J, Carnwath T (2008). Specialised alcohol treatment services are a luxury the NHS cannot afford. *British Journal of Psychiatry* **192**, 245–7.

McKeganey, N. (1998). Alcopops and young people: a suitable case for concern. *Addiction*, **93**, 471–3.

Marshall, E. J., Edwards, G., Taylor, C. (1994). Mortality in men with drinking problems: a 20-year follow-up. *Addiction*, **89**, 1293–8.

Mendelson, J. H., Mello, N. K. (1992). *Medical diagnosis and treatment of alcoholism*. McGraw-Hill, Inc., New York.

Merrick, E. L., Horgan, C. M., Hodgkin, D. et al. (2008). Unhealthy drinking patterns in older adults: prevalence and associated characteristics. *J Am Ger Society*, **56**, 214–23.

National Highway Traffic Safety Administration (2008). *2007 Traffic Safety Annual Assessment* NHTSA National Center for Statistics and Analysis, Washington.

Porter, R. (1985). The drinking man's disease: the 'pre-history' of alcoholism in Georgian England. *British Journal of Addiction*, **80**, 385–96.

Rehm, J. Sempos, C. T. (1995). Alcohol consumption and all-cause mortality. *Addiction*, **90**, 471–80; commentaries 481–8.

Robinson, J. (1988). *The demon drink*. Mitchell Beazley International Ltd, London.

Royal College of Physicians (1987). *A great and growing evil: the medical consequences of alcohol abuse*. Tavistock, London.

Spring, J. A., Buss, D. H. (1977). Three centuries of alcohol in the British diet. *Nature*, **270**, 567–72.

Stephens, R., Ling, J., Heffernan, T. M. et al. (2008). A review of the literature on the cognitive effects of alcohol hangover. *Alcohol & Alcoholism*, **43**, 163–70.

Strandberg-Larsen K, Nielsen NR, Gronbaek M et al. (2008). Binge drinking in pregnancy and risk of fetal death. *Obstetrics & Gynecology* **111**, 602–9.

Vale, J. A., Meredith, T. J., Proudfoot, A. T. (1987). *Poisoning by alcohols and glycols*. In: *Oxford textbook of medicine* (2nd edn.) (ed. D. J. Weatherall, J. G. G. Ledingham, D. A. Warrell). Oxford University Press, Oxford.

Warner, J. (1997). Shifting categories of the social harms associated with alcohol: examples from late medieval and early modern England. *American Journal of Public Health*, **87**, 1788–97.

Warner, J. (1998). Historical perspectives on the shifting boundaries around youth and alcohol. The example of pre-industrial England, 1350–1750. *Addiction*, **93**, 641–57.

Zhang Y, Guo X, Saitz R et al. (2008). Secular trends in alcohol consumption over 50 years: the Framingham Study. *American Journal of Medicine* **121**, 695–701.

Chapter 4

Tobacco

We can only guess at when North American Indians (and Aztecs in central Mexico) first incorporated tobacco into religious rituals and social interactions, but it seems to have been long established by the time Christopher Columbus arrived in the 'New World' towards the end of the 15th century. The dried plant was smoked in pipes or roll-ups made from leaves. The addictive quality of the habit was appreciated quickly by the missionaries who were more successful at converting the Indians to Catholicism than persuading their new recruits to desist from smoking in church. There was much bemusement in Spain when the travellers returned with what was, for a short while at least, the original duty-free supply of tobacco. Its reputation was founded on its use as a medicinal plant rather than for pleasurable effects, and it rapidly became sought after throughout mainland Europe as a treatment for intractable headaches, asthma, gout, tumours, and labour pain.

Tobacco probably reached England around 1550 when some Indians arrived in the custody of Sir John Hawkins, carrying with them supplies for their own consumption. Many of the sailors sampled it during the voyage and liked it so much that it became the custom to plant seeds at various stopping points around world trade routes to ensure a ready supply wherever the call of commerce or military necessity might lead. Sir Walter Ralegh is credited with introducing it to the fashionable world in London towards the end of the 16th century.

The popularity of tobacco soared during the 17th century with demand always exceeding supply, and the first commercial plantation was established in Jamestown, Virginia in 1612. Chewing tobacco and inhaling it as snuff also caught on, and at one point tobacco was literally worth its weight in silver. However, the possibility of harmful effects and the difficulty of consuming it in moderation were appreciated quickly, and it had some influential opponents. King James I published his 'counterblaste to tobacco' in 1604 in which he expressed his view that the 'manifold abuses of this vile custom' were 'loathsome to the eye, hateful to the nose, harmful to the brain, dangerous to the lungs'. The realization that vast tax revenues could easily be exacted from habitués soon overcame such considerations, and James's government became the first beneficiary.

Measures aimed at restricting supplies or introducing punitive taxation merely increased the value of tobacco and the rewards of smuggling. No country has ever been successful in suppressing it once use has become endemic, notwithstanding the proclamations of tyrants, the formal decrees of popes, and the direst of penalties: hand and foot crushing in Turkey, nostril slitting in Russia, total confiscation of assets in Japan, molten lead poured into the throat in Persia. Governments soon recognized that immense revenues could be achieved by sale of monopolies or taxation, and formal tobacco duties were introduced in England in 1660.

The first machine-made cigarettes appeared in Havana in 1853, and factories were established in London in 1856 and the US in 1872. Demand for these grew rapidly towards the end of the century, and by the end of the First World War they dominated the market. Filter cigarettes were introduced in the 1930s but were slow to catch on.

UK cigarette sales increased steadily from 11,000 million in 1905 to 74,000 million in 1939, of which less than 1% were filtered. Up to this point, smoking was more or less exclusively a male habit but became much more popular among women during the Second World War. Consumption soared postwar to more than 113,000 million annually (of which 20% were filtered) and thereafter increased more slowly to an all-time peak of 137,000 million in 1973 (83% filtered). The actual weight of tobacco sold peaked earlier in 1961 at which point 60% of men and 50% of women were smokers, but then fell off because of the rapid increase in popularity of filter tips. The average smoker's daily intake of cigarettes went up steadily from 14 in 1949 to 22 in 1973.

Between 1950 and 2000, around 60 million people died from tobacco-related diseases. During the 1960s cigarettes killed more Americans each year than the total combined casualty list of the First World War, Korea, and Vietnam. Health campaigns and adverse publicity in the UK, notably reports published by the Royal College of Physicians in 1962, 1977, and 1983, were associated with a 25% fall in the number of smokers between the mid-seventies and mid-eighties, by which time women were smoking around 45% of all cigarettes manufactured. By 1987, smokers made up only a third of the adult population as compared to well over half 10 years earlier. This reduction occurred despite the fact that smoking had never been cheaper. Even though UK custom duties went up by 900% between 1939 and 1977, and the proportion of the retail price made up by tax went up by 75% between 1956 and 1989, the real cost of 20 cigarettes actually decreased from 1.1% of the average weekly wage packet in 1960 to 0.6% in 1989. Despite a steady smoking reduction in most developed countries between 1970 and 1985, overall world consumption increased by 7% over this period as a result of large increases in Asia (22%) and Africa (42%).

In the UK and US, reductions in prevalence have been disappointingly slow in recent years. In the former, the percentage of adults who smoke declined gradually from 33% in 1987 to around 26% in the early 1990s, creeping down to around 22% in 2008. Surprisingly, the ban on smoking in public places implemented in July 2007 seems to have had a negligible effect on prevalence. The US saw a reduction from 25% in 1997 to 21% in 2004 and a landmark was achieved in 2008 when the rate fell below 20% for the first time in 80 years.

Preparation and distribution

The solanaceous plant *Nicotinia tabacum* was named after a French ambassador to Portugal, Jean Nicot, who was a strong believer in its medicinal properties. Modern cigarette tobacco consists of a blend of three types of leaf: Virginia, Burley, and Oriental. The latter is more intensely aromatic yet lower in nicotine, and is generally sun-cured. Ready-made cigarettes also contain 'fillers', consisting of other plant components and additives including humectants or moisturizers (glycerol, diethylene glycol), sugars to make the smoke less irritant, and flavourings. Ventilated filters were introduced in the 1970s and now dominate the market.

Approximately 40% of the world's cigarette production emanates today from China's state owned tobacco monopoly. This caters for the 350 million smokers in China, almost all of them men, who make up a third of the world's smoking population. Most of the remaining market share is dominated by a small number of vast, multinational companies such as Altria Group (owner of Philip Morris), British American Tobacco (BAT), Japan Tobacco, Reemsta, Imperial Tobacco, R.J. Reynolds, and Altadis. Astonishingly, the EU continues to pay one billion euros each year in subsidies to European tobacco growers, although a resolution has been adopted to begin to reduce this in 2013.

The global tobacco industry currently produces 5.5 trillion cigarettes each year. Although not the bonanza that was enjoyed in the 1970s and 80s this still provides governments with huge tax revenues: for example, £8,000 million to the UK government in 2006, despite the fact that at least one sixth of all cigarettes smoked in Britain that year were bought tax-free on the black market. Tobacco manufacture still generates around 5,000 jobs in the UK. Taking the effects of inflation and wage rises into account, the real price of cigarettes has fallen consistently since the 1960s in the UK and many other countries. This is unfortunate because smoking is quite responsive to price: an increase of 1% in retail cost can be expected to result in a 0.5% fall in consumption.

Despite attempts to outlaw or strictly limit tobacco advertising in many countries including the US, the EU, and all signatories to the WHO Convention on Tobacco Control the global industry still managed to spend over $8 billion on promotion in 1999. A continuing focus on repressing advertising is justified since according to a UK government study advertising bans can lead to falls in consumption of 5–9%. Smoking in public places has now been banned in many countries throughout the world, most recently in India in 2008.

Recruitment of child smokers remains a global problem. For example, under the terms of the Children and Young Persons (Protection from Tobacco) Act (1991) in the UK, it is illegal to sell tobacco products to children under sixteen, yet 450 children start smoking every day and in 2006 approximately 20% of fifteen year-olds were regular smokers. Prosecution of shopkeepers is a rare event.

Routine surveys of cigarette tar and nicotine content by the Laboratory of the Government Chemist (LGC) were initiated in 1972, and carbon monoxide estimates from 1978. The average tar yield of cigarettes halved between 1960 and 1990 from 30 mg down to 15 mg and manufacturers were required to specify these levels on the packets. Over the same period, carbon monoxide generation reduced less impressively from 19 mg to 14 mg. More recently, some governments have taken steps to institute more formal controls: for example, in 2001 an EU directive specified maximum upper limits on tar (10 mg), nicotine (1 mg), and carbon monoxide (10 mg). Unfortunately, there is little evidence that 'safer' cigarettes are actually any safer: people who switch to low tar brands may just increase the frequency and depth of inhalation. Most countries have now implemented health warnings of varying size and horror on cigarette packets.

Scientific information

The tip of a cigarette achieves temperatures of more than 1,000°C during a puff and this tiny furnace releases more than 4,000 chemicals, one of which is nicotine. This drug, which reaches the brain within seconds of inhalation, resembles in structure the neurotransmitter acetylcholine and has a complicated network of effects. Individual reactions to it vary, and sensitivity to the pleasurable effects may be genetically determined.

Absorption of nicotine through mucous membranes in the mouth will only occur if the smoke is alkaline, as is the case with pipe and cigar tobacco. In these circumstances, the drug remains un-ionized and therefore highly fat soluble. Most cigarettes produce acidic smoke which must be inhaled into the lungs for the nicotine to be absorbed, a highly efficient process that assimilates 90% of the nicotine in the smoke. Nicotine is broken down quickly in the liver and elsewhere to inert substances, so that blood levels halve every two hours or so.

Genetic variation in this metabolic process influences vulnerability to addiction. Cotinine is a stable metabolite which can be used in research as an accurate measure of tobacco intake.

Nicotine binds to cholinergic receptors which are widely distributed in the brain and throughout the body. It can either stimulate or depress various parts of the brain and nervous system depending on the dose, environmental conditions, and the mood and personality of the user. The complexity of its effects relates to this variability, and to its ability to cause the release of many other hormones and neurotransmitters, including noradrenaline (norepinephrine), dopamine, serotonin, GABA, glutamate, endorphins, growth hormone, corticotrophin, and antidiuretic hormone. The result is that the reward experienced by smokers will range from calm relaxation to stimulation and euphoria, depending upon the circumstances. Dopamine release is central to this reinforcing effect. Larger doses have a purer stimulant effect leading to agitation, hyperactivity, vomiting, trembling and shaking, and convulsions.

Nicotine has a wide range of consequences outside the nervous system, including an increase in heart rate and blood pressure; irregularities of the heart beat; constriction of some blood vessels and dilation of others; increased concentration of potentially damaging fats (triglycerides, cholesterol) in the blood and a reduction of protective fats (HDL cholesterol); stimulation of components of the blood-clotting process; and increased general metabolic rate. Tolerance (reduced sensitivity) to many of the effects comes on quickly but is also lost within a few hours. Thus the regular smoker notices dizziness or skin tingling from the first cigarette of each day because tolerance has been lost overnight.

Regular smokers usually become physically dependent on nicotine, and withdrawal is associated with changes in electroencephalogram readings of brain electrical activity, tests of physical and mental functioning, mood (e.g. irritability, depression, poor concentration), appetite, and sleep pattern. This is due to subnormal concentrations of dopamine and other neurotransmitters. The psychological component of the addiction is represented by craving for, and preoccupation with, cigarettes.

The chemical components of tobacco smoke are classified as solids ('particulate phase') or gases. Tars are combustion products of organic materials and are therefore absent from unburnt tobacco, snuff, and chewing tobacco. They are responsible both for the pleasurable taste of cigarettes and much of the damage which ensues. Reducing the tar production of cigarettes causes many smokers to increase the rate and depth of inhalation in an attempt to compensate. Sidestream smoke, which enters the environment without first passing through the smoker, contains more tar than mainstream smoke.

Many tars are polycyclic hydrocarbons or N-nitroso compounds which are known carcinogens. Irritation produced by particulates causes an immediate reduction in the efficiency of the lungs. The tiny hair-like structures (cilia), which swirl rhythmically about on the surface of the larger airways to clear foreign matter out of the lungs, at first work harder to try and counter the sudden surge of incoming toxins but gradually become overwhelmed and inactive.

Tobacco smoke contains up to 5% of carbon monoxide (CO) which combines with haemoglobin to form carboxyhaemoglobin (COHb). This reduces the oxygen-carrying capacity of the blood so the heart has to work harder to maintain a constant supply of oxygen to vital organs. Alongside this increased workload the oxygen supply to the heart is being reduced by the presence of COHb and a nicotine-induced constriction of the coronary arteries. As a final insult, the blood-clotting mechanism is also being stimulated by nicotine. The result, as detailed below, is a huge increase in mortality from heart attacks among smokers. Other poisons within the gaseous phase include ammonia, formaldehyde, and hydrogen cyanide.

Possible beneficial effects

A number of diseases are significantly less prevalent in tobacco smokers. These include Alzheimer's disease, Parkinson's disease, and ulcerative colitis. Smoking also seems to improve some of the symptoms of the neurological condition Tourette's syndrome. These benefits are likely to be related to the pharmacology of nicotine, which could be administered as a conventional pharmaceutical rather than by smoking.

Recreational use

There are an estimated 1.3 billion regular tobacco smokers in the world today, most of whom live in developing countries. In parts of Asia well over half the adult population smokes with a large predominance of males. The Westernized countries are at a later stage in the tobacco epidemic with falling levels overall and relatively higher consumption in lower socioeconomic groups. Average smoking prevalence in Europe is 32% with a wide range, from 18% in Sweden to 42% in Greece.

Current surveys in the UK indicate an adult smoking prevalence of 22% (down from 26% in 2000), with a further one million people smoking pipes or cigars. Highest rates (33% males, 29% females) occur in the 20 to 24 age group, and 80% of these started smoking as teenagers. Three out of four regular smokers say they would like to give up. The proportion of heavy smokers (> 20/day) has decreased steadily and is now well under 10%. Smoking levels vary considerably between socioeconomic and ethnic groups. Manual workers have a much higher prevalence than non-manual occupations (29% vs 19%) and start at a much younger age. Bangladeshi and Pakistani men and people of Irish origin have a higher prevalence than the overall population, and the highest regional rates are in Scotland. Since 2007 the legal age for the purchase of cigarettes has been 18, but the law seems to achieved only a modest inhibition of sale to minors.

In the US, prevalence has declined to just below 20% in 2008 (men 22.3%, women 17.4%) but this still amounts to over 43 million people. As in the UK, the highest levels were recorded among young adults (29% males, 19% females) and lower socioeconomic groups. Native Americans had the highest rates (32%), followed by non-Hispanic blacks and non-Hispanic whites. Nearly half of regular smokers say they have made an effort to quit during the preceding year.

Smokers give various explanations for persisting with a habit which they know is dangerous. Some say it improves their mood or helps them relax, 'calm down', or generally cope better. Smoking can reduce aggression or anxiety, improve tolerance of other people's annoying behaviour, and improve vigilance and task performance. Weight gain following cessation is sometimes a reason to continue smoking.

Most new recruits are under 18, and uptake of smoking among teenagers has declined only slightly despite numerous public health campaigns. Since the mid-1980s girls are more likely to start younger than boys and smoke regularly by the age of 15 ((24% girls, 16% boys). The strongest influences on childhood smoking are parental and sibling habits, advertisements, and smoking in films and on TV. Knowledge of health risk is not a strong deterrant because teenagers exhibit a strong bias towards optimism in the consideration of personal risk. Unpleasant outcomes such as illness are delayed long into the future whereas the rewards in terms of status, peer solidarity, affront to adults, and illusions of maturity are immediate.

Environmental factors are also important. Religious belief (even when no direct restrictions on smoking are made explicit) has an inverse relationship with prevalence. Comparisons between schools in similar neighbourhoods demonstrated that the presence of a smoking teacher can double the prevalence of smoking among older pupils. The average prevalence of smoking among 16-year-olds in a group of schools with no restrictive policy on staff smoking was 32% compared to 20% in those that did have a policy.

A third of women becoming pregnant are regular smokers, and only a quarter of these will stop during the course of the pregnancy. Of these, two out of three resume smoking within a few weeks of the birth. Ninety per cent of women who continue to smoke throughout pregnancy are still smoking five years later.

Unwanted effects

Well over five million people die prematurely each year as a result of tobacco smoking. Last year it was directly responsible for approximately 440,000 deaths in the United States and 114,000 in the UK. Annual health costs in the two countries were $75.5 billion and £1.5 billion respectively. In developed countries, 15% of 35 year-old non-smoking men will die before their 65th birthday: for smokers of up to 14 cigarettes daily the figure is 22%, 15 to 24 cigarettes 25%, and 25 or more cigarettes 40%. Smoking causes more deaths than AIDS, alcohol abuse, cocaine use, heroin use, homicides, suicides, traffic accidents, and fires combined.

Tobacco is the primary cause of at least a third of all cancers, and almost nine out of ten cases of lung cancer. Between 1920 and 1950 the prevalence of this disease in men went up 20-fold, and it is now the most common cancer worldwide, with 1.2 million new cases yearly including over 150,000 from the US alone. Regular smokers are 30 times more likely to contract it than non-smokers, and passive smoking may contribute to a proportion of the 15% of cases which occur in non-smokers. The earlier in life the individual starts smoking, the greater the risk. The prevalence is now decreasing in men but increasing in women. Tumours of the mouth, lip, throat, and oesophagus are up to 10 times more common in smokers, and there is also a proven association with cancers of the stomach, pancreas, kidney, liver, and bladder, and certain types of leukaemia.

Coronary heart disease is the leading cause of death in developed countries, killing more than seven million world wide annually, and smoking is one of the three major risk factors (along with high blood pressure and raised blood cholesterol). The damage is done by starving the heart of oxygen through the formation of COHb, coronary artery atherosclerosis, and increasing the clotting tendency of the blood. The good news is that this risk declines rapidly if the smoker quits, and after four years of abstinence is equivalent to that of a life-long non-smoker.

Smoking damages other parts of the circulatory system. Ninety per cent of people with diseased leg arteries are smokers, who also have an increased risk of high blood pressure, strokes (double the risk in smokers), and ballooning (aneurysm) of the aorta.

The risk of fatal chronic bronchitis and emphysema (chronic obstructive airways disease) is six times greater in smokers and kills 2.8 million globally each year. Smoking is also associated with gastric and intestinal ulcers, Crohn's disease, eye damage (e.g. macular degeneration), tooth and gum disease, and asthma. Smokers are more vulnerable to infections including influenza, pneumonia, and pulmonary tuberculosis. Smoking is a risk factor for diabetes and accelerates its vascular complications, increases the risk of complications following surgery, aggravates heart failure, and is linked to cognitive decline in middle age. Nicotine accelerates the metabolism of several prescribed drugs and greatly increases the cardiovascular risks associated with the contraceptive pill.

Fertility in female smokers is reduced and there is an increased risk of miscarriage, toxaemia of pregnancy, congenital malformations, labour complications, low birth weight, and stillbirth. Paternal smoking also has some negative impact on birthweight, either through a chromosomal mechanism or by passive smoking by the mother.

The spotlight on the damaging effects of passive smoking (inhalation of someone else's fumes) has intensified recently, and in particular the impact on children of smoking parents. Such a child inhales the equivalent of between 60 and 150 cigarettes each year. The smoke inhaled passively is largely sidestream, and this contains much greater quantities of nicotine, carbon monoxide, ammonia, and certain carcinogens than mainstream smoke. Living with a heavy smoker increases the risk of lung cancer by between 10 and 30%, and may also increase the chances of developing bronchitis or heart disease.

Maternal smoking is associated with a five-fold increase in atopic (allergic) symptoms in the child, a greater chance of admission to hospital with a chest infection in the first year of life, and an increased prevalence of the sudden infant death syndrome ('cot death'). This link is dose related: in comparison with a non-smoker, the risk for a mother who smokes less than 10 cigarettes daily is increased by a factor of 1.8, and more than 10 by 2.7. If one parent smokes the annual incidence of pneumonia or bronchitis in the child increases from 7.8% to 11.4%, and if both parents smoke this rises to 17.6%. The risk of the child developing asthma increases by at least a third. Glue ear is much more common, and the child's growth may be stunted if the parents smoke more than 10 a day each. It seems possible that the prevalence of some cancers, including leukaemia, is higher among children in smoking households.

It is now accepted beyond doubt that regular cigarette smokers are in the grip of a genuine addiction. Regular smokers who quit usually experience a predictable pattern of physical and psychological withdrawal effects including irritability, restlessness, anxiety, impaired concentration, increased appetite, constipation, and craving for cigarettes. Over 90% of cigarette smokers fulfill the criteria for dependence defined by the American Psychiatric Association. The likelihood of progression from occasional to regular daily use is greater for tobacco than any other addictive drug, and the long-term damage associated with this particular delivery system is in a class of its own. Of all the risky temptations facing young teenagers that responsible parents may lose sleep about, cigarette smoking should head the list.

Selected references

Action on Smoking and Health (2008). Basic fact-sheets on tobacco and the tobacco industry. ASH, London. http://www.ash.org.uk/ash_4k3664v4.htm.

Benowitz NL (2008). Clinical pharmacology of nicotine: implications for understanding, preventing, and treating tobacco addiction. *Clinical Pharmacology & Therapeutics* **83**, 531–41.

Bonnie R. J., Stratton K., Wallace R. B. (2007). *Ending the tobacco problem: a blueprint for the nation (Executive Summary)* National Academy of Sciences http://www.nap.edu/catalog/11795.html.

Campaign for tobacco free kids (2008). *Toll of tobacco in the United States of America* http://www.tobaccofreekids.org/research/factsheets/pdf/0072.pdf.

Centers for Disease Control and Prevention (2007). *Cigarette smoking among adults – United States, 2006* http://www.cdc.gov/mmwr/preview/mmwrhtml/mm5644a2.htm

Dyer, C. (1998). Confidential tobacco documents enter public domain. *British Medical Journal*, **316**, 1186.

Escobedo, L. G., Reddy, M., Giovino, G. A. (1998). The relationship between depressive symptoms and cigarette smoking. *Addiction*, **93**, 433–40.

Heishman, S. J. (1998). What aspects of human performance are truly enhanced by nicotine? *Addiction*, **93**, 317–20.

Henningfield, J. E. (1985). *Nicotine: an old-fashioned addiction*. Burke Publishing Company Ltd, London.

Klein R., Knudtson M. D., Cruickshanks K. J., Klein B. E. (2008). Further observations on the association between smoking and the long-term incidence and progression of age-related macular degeneration. *Archives of Ophthalmology* **126**, 115–21.

Laurence, D. R., Bennet, P. N. (1992). *Clinical pharmacology* (7th edn). Churchill Livingstone, Edinburgh.

Orson F. M., Kinsey B. M., Singh R. A. et al. (2008). Substance abuse vaccines. *Annals of the New York Academy of Sciences* **1141**, 257–69.

Rock V. J., Malarcher A., Kahende J. W. et al. (2007). Cigarette smoking among adults— United States 2006. *Morbidity and Mortality Weekly Report* **56**, 1157–61.

Sabia S., Marmot M., Dufouil C. et al. (2008). Smoking history and cognitive function in middle age from the Whitehall II study. *Archives of Internal Medicine* **168**, 1165–73.

Shiffman, S. (1989). Tobacco 'chippers' – individual differences in tobacco dependence. *Psychopharmacology*, **97**, 539–47.

Smee, C., Parsonage, M., Anderson, R., Duckworth, S. (1992). The effect of tobacco advertising on tobacco consumption. *Health Trends*, **24**, 111–2.

Chapter 5

Cannabis

Invited Co-author: Ethan Russo

Historical background

A robust but otherwise undistinguished weed now labelled *Cannabis sativa* has provided the world with one of its most remarkable drugs. The psychoactive and medicinal properties of cannabis have been recognized for thousands of years, and it was probably humankind's first non-food crop. The use of cannabis as a medicine was described as long ago as the 16th century BC in the Egyptian Ebers papyrus.

In the modern world, no other forbidden drug has provoked such polarization between its defenders and detractors, with reason frequently swamped by rhetoric.

The first systematic account of the pain-killing, fever-reducing, anti-inflammatory, and anti-emetic properties of cannabis derive from oral tradition in China nearly 5,000 years ago. It was particularly prized for its ability to relieve labour pain, speed up delivery, and reduce post-delivery bleeding. The Assyrians made use of it in the eighth century BC with medical claims from their Sumerian and Akkadian forbears extending perhaps one millennium earlier. The Chinese were certainly cultivating it by the fourth century, and it is described in Indian religious writings as early as the *Atharva Veda* in the second millennium BC. It also found an important place in ancient Greek pharmacopoeias. Ceremonial, recreational, and therapeutic use has continued uninterrupted throughout Asia, Africa, Arabia, and South and Central America down the centuries. Traces of cannabis were identified in the remains of a young girl who died near Jerusalem in the fourth century AD. Scientists have deduced that she was in all probability given the drug to ease the pains of childbirth. The archaeological evidence has recently been bolstered by the finding of a large cache of cannabis in the tomb of a shaman in Xinjiang, China, with subsequent biochemical and genetic analyses proving that the material derived from a potentially psychoactive strain.

The other great asset of the plant, its fibrous stem so useful for rope-making and weaving, was utilized by the Romans who initiated cultivation in Britain.

By Tudor times, this had been expanded on a large scale but still the demand for the fibre could not be satisfied. The early settlers in North America were encouraged to grow hemp early in the 17th century, and this soon developed into a considerable rural industry. Apart from the fibre, the seeds were a source of oil for fuel and other commercial applications, and were found to be nutritious for birds.

This tenacious relative of the nettle and the hop grows wild throughout the world. Its psychoactive product is available in the East in many forms varying in potency, refinement, and expense, and goes under many names, including bhang, charas, ganga, kif, dagga, kabak, and hashish. In these endemic areas it is not only used ceremonially, but also in everyday life to alleviate fatigue and boredom. It was introduced into the Caribbean from Bengal and the population took to it readily. The psychoactive and herbal properties of cannabis were probably first introduced to Europeans in any quantity about 1,000 years ago by the Moors from their base in North Africa during their occupation of Spain and Portugal.

The weed was known in the West as Indian hemp until Linnaeus dubbed it *C. sativa* in 1753 following the lead of Fuchs two centuries earlier, and it began to emerge here as a herbal remedy on any scale in the 18th century. It soon gained a popular reputation as a rival panacea to opium in Britain, Europe, and North America but it was not until the 19th century that Western doctors became aware of its potential as a mainstream medicine. The person who brought it to their attention was the Irish scientist and physician, W.B. O'Shaughnessy. He observed its use in India as a pain-killer, anti-epileptic, antispasmodic, anti-emetic, and cure for insomnia. After carrying out experiments on goats and dogs, O'Shaughnessy began giving it to patients suffering from conditions such as rheumatism, epilepsy, and tetanus, and was impressed with the results. Dissolved in alcohol solution it proved an effective pain-killer. He was also struck by its particular utility as an anti-vomiting agent, a finding that has been replicated in modern research.

When O'Shaughnessy returned to England in 1842 he published an influential account of his findings which sparked off a rapid expansion of its medical use. Other clinicians reported '. . . *the remarkable power of increasing the force of uterine contractions, concomitant with a significant reduction of labour pain*', mirroring French reports of its effectiveness in reducing uterine haemorrhage, and its usefulness in the treatment of chloral and opium addiction. By 1854 it had found its way into the United States Dispensatory. Cannabis was soon available 'over the counter' in pharmacies throughout England and Scotland. Queen Victoria is rumoured to have found it useful in relieving menstrual cramps.

J. Russell Reynolds, 'Physician in Ordinary to Her Majesty's Household', wrote in the *Lancet* of his more than 30 years' clinical experience with cannabis.

In his opinion, '. . . *Indian hemp, when pure and administered carefully, is one of the most valuable medicines we possess*'. He found it incomparable for 'senile insomnia', 'night restlessness', and 'temper disease' in both children and adults, but not helpful in melancholia, 'very uncertain' in alcoholic delirium, and 'worse than useless' in mania. It was very effective in a range of painful conditions including neuralgia, period pains, migraine, 'lightning pain of the ataxic patient', and gout, but useless in sciatica and 'hysteric pains'. He had found it impressive in certain epileptiform convulsions related to brain damage from tumour or trauma, but no good at all in petit mal or 'chronic epilepsy', tetanus, chorea, or paralysis agitans. It effectively relieved nocturnal cramps, asthma, and dysmenorrhoea. Reynolds warned of inconsistency of effect consequent upon 'great variations in strength' of the different preparations since the 'active principle has not been separated', and held that toxic effects only occurred with excessive doses.

Reynolds was writing at a time when the zenith of cannabis as a prescribed medicine and home remedy was already past. Although Sir William Osler was still recommending it for migraine sufferers in 1913, by the First World War it was in steep decline. Reasons for this include variable potency of herbal cannabis preparations, unreliable sources of supply, poor storage stability, unpredictable response by mouth, uncertainty as to optimal dosing regimes, increasing enthusiasm for parenteral medicines, the growing availability of potent synthetic alternatives, commercial pressures, and increasing concern about recreational use, particularly in the US, Egypt, and South Africa.

Recreational use was not widespread in 19th-century Europe and North America, but it became a favourite among artists and intellectuals in the bigger cities. Dr Jacques-Joseph Moreau de Tours was introduced to hashish whilst touring North Africa, and on his return to Paris in the 1840s founded the *Club des Haschishchins* at the Hotel Pimodan with like-minded cronies such as Dumas, Balzac, Flaubert, and Baudelaire. The doses consumed by the members of this club were heroic by modern Western standards, and the resulting 'voluptuous intoxications' have been wonderfully described by Théophile Gautier and other contemporary visitors.

Awareness of the popularity of cannabis among the poor and labouring classes in the British colonies, alongside pressure exerted by a distilling industry increasingly alarmed by this competitive product, led the British government to instigate a comprehensive scientific enquiry into cannabis use and its possible dangers in Asia. The Indian Hemp Commission produced its seven volume report in 1894. This survey revealed no convincing evidence of 'mental or moral injury' from moderate use of cannabis. Excessive use was no more likely to occur than with alcohol, and mainly afflicted those with an established tendency to be idle or dissipated. These findings have been broadly confirmed by the many subsequent reviews that have appeared at regular intervals up to the present day.

Cannabis was outlawed in Britain in 1928 when the Government ratified the 1925 Geneva Convention on the manufacture, sale, and movement of dangerous drugs. It did, however, remain available in pharmacies for use in psychiatric indications until its absolute prohibition under the terms of the Misuse of Drugs Act (1971) (MDA).

In North America, the drug was associated in the earliest years of the 20th century with the poorest sections of the community, and the reefer (marijuana cigarette) was introduced into the country by itinerant Mexican labourers. It soon gained wider popularity, initially among the mainly black jazz musicians and their followers, and started to develop an increasingly negative image in the newspapers of the deep South. Lurid fabricated stories linking it with horrific violence and sexual debauchery induced a truly hysterical reaction to the drug in some quarters. Hatred and fear of the minority groups with which it was associated seem to have played a part in stimulating this response.

On the positive side, a rich folklore and grammatical idiom developed around the use of cannabis, which became known by such names as weed, tea, gage, loco-weed, and Mary-Jane. The reefer or 'joint' was sometimes referred to as a 'mezz' after the white jazz musician Milton Mezzrow who was reputed to have had access to material of particularly fine quality.

By 1930 the steady flow of largely fanciful scare stories had led 16 states to ban cannabis and in the same year the Bureau of Narcotics was formed within the Treasury Department. The first Commissioner was Harry Anslinger, and he devoted the next 30 years to doing everything in his power to blacken the image of cannabis and all who used or defended it with fanatical zeal. In 1937, the Marijuana Tax Act effectively outlawed the drug nationwide despite the opposition of civil libertarians and some doctors and psychiatrists.

Contemporary scientific investigations contradicted Anslinger's propaganda but were ignored and their authors pilloried by the Bureau and the media. The scholarly La Guardia Report (1944) was based upon a detailed appraisal of the medical, psychological, and social aspects of marijuana use in New York City. The review found no evidence to suggest that cannabis induced aggressive or antisocial behaviour, increased sexual crime, or significantly altered the personality of the user. The scientists detected no evidence of addiction or mental or physical deterioration in their subjects. Then, as now, sensational anecdote was preferred to painstaking enquiry.

Contrary to the Bureau's statistics, cannabis was little used in the general population right up to 1960, even though it was growing wild and unrecognized throughout the nation. To most British people it was almost unknown as a fun drug until the 1950s when a surge of immigrants from the Caribbean brought their cannabis with them. Marijuana began to turn up in London folk and jazz clubs, and the first white teenager to be busted found himself in the dock in 1952.

In the 1960s cannabis exploded out of this narrow confinement. It became integral to the developing hippy and psychedelic movements, and also found its way into student life and the homes of otherwise unrebellious and non-deviant people. By 1970, upwards of 25 million Americans had puffed on the weed, and there were ten million regular smokers. In Britain four million had tried it, including a third of all university students.

Prevalence expanded steadily through the 1970s, perhaps reaching its peak toward the end of the decade. The figures from contemporary surveys are rather remarkable: 50% of 18 to 25 year-olds questioned in the US said they had tried it at some time, 43 million Americans had sampled it, and 16 million were regular smokers. Ten per cent of American high-school students were toking daily. In Britain, 20% of employed 20 to 40 year-olds had smoked it within the previous month. These were not criminals or deviants. Millions of ordinary people liked dope and used it regularly, in the context of an ordinary lifestyle. The level of demand had, and still has, enormous economic implications for the countries where cannabis is an important cash crop. In the early 1980s the annual export from the Lebanon alone far exceeded 2,000 tons, a significant contribution to the national economy.

So concerned was the British government that it commissioned Baroness Wootton to head an investigation. Her report (1968) concluded: '*Having reviewed all the material available to us we find ourselves in agreement with the conclusions reached by the Indian Hemp Drugs Commission appointed by the Government of India (1893–1894) and the New York Mayor's Committee on Marijuana (1944) that the long-term consumption of cannabis in moderation has no harmful effects*'. She also found no evidence to support the gateway theory that cannabis is dangerous because it leads inexorably to experimentation with more dangerous drugs. She proposed that cannabis should be made available for research and medicinal use.

Despite its carefully argued, unsensational style, the report was castigated histrionically in the media and ignored by the Callaghan government. Subsequent scientific investigations, such as the Canadian Le Dain Commission (1972), have concurred with the findings of Wootton. The British Royal College of Psychiatrists (1987) stated that '. . . *on any objective reckoning, cannabis must at present get a cleaner bill of health than our legalized "recreational drugs"*'. In February 1998, *New Scientist* revealed that the World Health

Organization had suppressed a report on the harmful effects of cannabis which concluded that on balance cannabis is safer than alcohol or tobacco.

In 2002, the UK Advisory Council on the Misuse of Drugs (ACMD) recommended to the Government that cannabis be reclassified from Class B to Class C under MDA (see Chapter 15), and this advice was implemented in January 2004. Concerns expressed in the media about the increasing potency of the drug, its mental health risks and gateway effects, and supposed confusion amongst young people as to whether the drug had been legalized, led to a request for reconsideration. On re-reviewing the evidence the ACMD confirmed that Class C remained appropriate, and this was again accepted by the Government. However, the subject remained a political hot potato, and in July 2007 a new Home Secretary yet again requested a re-evaluation. For the third time, ACMD reconfirmed its evidence-based reasons for retaining the Class C classification. Despite this, the Government decided to ignore expert advice and proceeded with reclassification to Class B in January 2009.

The British police force has recently adopted the policy of limiting the response to possession by an adult of a small amount of cannabis to a warning and confiscation of the drug instead of arrest, providing there are no 'aggravating factors'. This does not, however, apply to young people who will continue to be arrested and dealt with at a police station.

The situation in North America is even more confusing. Cannabis remains Schedule I and forbidden in the USA. Four surviving patients with proven medical need do receive cannabis directly from the Government via a now defunct federal programme closed to new entrants. Additionally, 12 American states have legalized medicinal cannabis usage either by popular plebiscite or legislation, but patients cultivating or using it are still subject to arrest by the federal authorities. In Canada, judicial rulings allow a limited number of patients access to cannabis if they can successfully negotiate a byzantine process of documentation and medical authorizations.

Calls for decriminalization have arisen from time to time in various countries. In 1972, the American Presidential Commission on Marijuana and Drug Abuse recommended that the possession of a small amount of cannabis for personal use should no longer be a criminal offence, and in 1977 the Carter administration advocated legalizing the possession of up to one ounce of cannabis. In The Netherlands, a *de facto* decriminalization of small amounts of cannabis for personal consumption has been in place since 1976 (see Chapter 15). Public opinion about legalization oscillates from country to country and time to time according to the prevailing media image of the drug. Generally, politicians have concluded that the decriminalization of cannabis has no value as a vote winner.

Preparation and distribution

Whilst there are a number of strains of cannabis, namely *C. sativa*, *C. indica*, and *C. ruderalis*, they are all arguably the same plant genetically, since all are capable of cross-breeding. It is thought to have originated in Central Asia but is now to be found growing wild virtually anywhere in the world save the polar icecaps. Resin content and shape depend upon genetics and ambient conditions. If grown in peaty or heavy soil in a warm, wet climate, tall solid plants ideal for fibre extraction result. Plants grown in sandy soil in hot, dry surroundings are rich in resin, most of which is exuded from the flowering tops of female plants, coating nearby leaves and stalks. The plants are harvested towards the end of the summer. A particularly potent form known in India as *ganja* and in the West *as sinsemilla* (literally, without seeds) is obtained by culling out the male plants before pollination can occur. This results in larger flowering heads in the female plants, and a particularly abundant yield from the glandular trichomes of the resin which contains the principal psychoactive ingredient, delta-9-tetrahydrocannabinol (THC). In order to boost robustness, maturation rate and THC content and generally optimize the 'high', Californian enthusiasts in the early 1970s instigated a breeding programme which crossed carefully selected *sativa* and *indica* plants. The result became known as Skunk #1, the first of many hybrids which have resulted in the very high potency of some modern black market material. Typical current strains include Haze, Northern Lights, New York Diesel, and Dutch Moonshine.

Cannabis is grown in 172 out of the 198 countries about which the UN has collected information, often for local consumption only. Almost half of the world's black market supply originates in the Americas, a quarter from Africa, and around 20% from Asia. Jamaica is the biggest producer in the Caribbean, mainly for local consumption. Most material supplied as resin originates from Morocco, Afghanistan, or Pakistan. Global annual cannabis production is currently estimated at around 41,500 tons. This is somewhat lower than previous years as a result of an intensive US eradication programme which destroyed six million plants in 2006 alone. The area under cannabis cultivation in Afghanistan is increasing rapidly, having doubled between 2005 and 2007. Global resin production has fallen slightly to around 6,000 tons annually, for which Europe is the largest customer. Nearly three quarters of this emanates from Morocco, smuggled in via the Iberian peninsula.

In Europe, the proportion of black market material appearing in herbal form has increased sharply in recent years. In the UK in 2002 it constituted only 30% of police seizures but this had shot up to 80% by 2006, mostly consisting of the more potent 'sinsemilla' variety. This change in customer preference has altered the supply chain considerably, with local production increasing markedly in many countries. In the UK, domestic production started in the early 1990s but has now become a huge cottage industry. Often a small suburban terraced house will be surreptitiously converted into a cannabis factory, with hydroponic cultivation under intensive lighting pirated from the local supply. The quantity of plants seized more than doubled between 2004 and 2005 from 95,103 to 212,971. The figure for the same year in the US was a staggering 223 million plants, but the vast majority of these were 'ditchweed' and virtually irrelevant to the black market trade.

Average street prices have fallen over the last decade in almost all European countries. Typical cost ranges from the equivalent of 4–10 euros/gram. Quality domestically cultivated cannabis may fetch prices of $300–400 per ounce in the USA, and somewhat less in Canada.

Cannabis is usually less adulterated than other street drugs, but may be contaminated with other inactive or active (e.g. datura-containing) plant material, bacteria, and fungi. Imported hashish may contain bulking agents (e.g. wood ash) binders, solvents, or other materials used in manufacture, but when derived from ganja/sinsemilla via sifting or cold-water extraction is often of high quality and purity. Inferior cannabis may be adulterated with various psychoactive substances to increase its potency. In the past tobacco juice was often used and is reputed to enhance the psychoactive effects. Modern adulterants include the dangerous hallucinogen phencyclidine (see Chapter 7), opium, henbane, and datura. Cannabis grown in the US or imported from Mexico or Central America may be contaminated with highly toxic herbicides sprayed from aeroplanes as part of eradication programmes.

Scientific information

More than 400 chemicals have been identified in the resin, including more than 60 aromatic hydrocarbon compounds unique to the plant (cannabinoids). The principal psychoactive ingredient is THC which was isolated in 1964. Cannabis is available on the street in three different forms which vary considerably in their THC content. These are herbal material (often called marijuana or grass), resin compressed into blocks (hash), and a thick oil or tincture usually of very high potency. The herbal form can be subdivided into traditional imported material and the much more potent home-grown sinsemilla or ganja (see section above). From seizures, it appears that most herbal material smoked in Britain is now of the latter variety. This is a cause for concern, since average THC content of sinsemilla has increased steadily from around 6% in 1995 to 16% today. Importantly, this average conceals a very wide range from 4–25%. The consumer is thus exposed to an extraordinary variability in potency. These levels compare to averages for resin of around 5% THC (again with a very wide range) and 9% for imported herbal cannabis. Atmospheric oxidation causes THC concentration to be lower at the outer surface of a block of resin. Another complicating factor in terms of impact is the presence or absence of another cannabinoid, cannabidiol (CBD). This non-psychoactive substance interacts with THC, and appears both to modulate the high and protect against its unwanted psychiatric effects. Historically, cannabis often contained a significant proportion of CBD (more so in Europe than the US), and this remains true of resin available in the UK. However, sinsemilla has generally been found to be almost entirely devoid of CBD and its protective effect.

In the last 20 years fundamental advances have been made in clarifying how cannabis actually produces its effects. Two specific receptors labelled CB_1R and CB_2R have been discovered (and more will surely follow), the former located principally on nerve cells both inside and outside the brain and the latter in immune tissue. Several naturally occuring chemicals (endocannabinoids) which interact with these receptors have been identified, the most important of which are called anandamide and 2-arachidonoyl glycerol (2-AG). These receptors, endogenous ligands, and enzymes for synthesis and degradation are known collectively as the endocannabinoid system (ECS). It has become apparent that ECS plays an important role in normal physiology, modulating amongst other things mood, memory and awareness, sensory perception, movement, coordination, posture and balance, sleep, hormonal regulation, temperature control, appetite, and immune response. ECS plays an important part in maintaining normal mental health, and there is a high density of receptors in key areas such as neocortex, cerebellum, hippocampal formation, amygdala, and basal ganglia. Cannabis produces its psychoactive effects as a result of stimulation of CB_1R in the brain by THC.

The drug is metabolized within the body to both active and inactive metabolites, some of which are absorbed into fat and take a very long time to eliminate, so that urine tests for cannabinoids can remain positive for weeks or even a month or more following abstinence from regular use. THC levels in plasma or urine can be measured accurately but there is no consistent relationship between blood levels and intensity of drug effects. It is theoretically possible for passive inhalers of other peoples' cannabis fumes to test positive if sensitive immunoassay techniques are used, but only after extreme exposure at close quarters. THC freely crosses the placenta into the unborn child and is detectable in breast milk.

Medical uses

Despite the fact that no government currently recognizes cannabis as a legitimate medicine, millions of people throughout the world use it illicitly for this reason. 'Medical marijuana' remains a highly controversial and divisive concept, with activists at each pole characterizing it either as a cruel hoax or a veritable wonder drug. This controversy extends into the legislature, with some countries adopting an ambiguous position on law enforcement. For example, despite its legal status as a Schedule I controlled drug in the US, 12 states have decriminalized its use for medicinal purposes. This has led to high profile conflicts between state and federal legislature, and the persecution of physicians who prescribed or recommended marijuana within state guidelines. Some small, placebo-controlled clinical trials of smoked cannabis have recently demonstrated statistically significant benefits for HIV-related neuropathic pain, loss of appetite, and weight loss. Synthetic versions of THC (nabilone, dronabinol) have been available in many countries for decades with licences usually restricted to the treatment of intractable nausea and vomiting, or cachexia in cancer or HIV. In 2008 the American College of Physicians (ACP) called for '. . . *reclassification into a more appropriate [legal] schedule, given the scientific evidence regarding marijuana's safety and efficacy in some clinical conditions*'. The ACP rejected the suggestion that medical marijuana would represent a catalyst of serious drug abuse, and pointed out that use of vapourization would eliminate most of the risks of smoking.

The discovery of ECS (see above) helped to boost a resurgence of interest in the therapeutic possibilities of non-smoked cannabinoid medicines (CM) in the late 20th century following government sponsored scientific reviews in the UK and US. Although it is still early days for modern, high quality clinical research of CM, there is growing evidence from methodologically sound clinical trials of their efficacy and safety in a range of medical disorders for which standard treatments are either only partially effective or dangerously toxic. These include various types of neuropathic, inflammatory, and cancer pain; muscle spasticity, neurogenic bladder, and other symptoms of multiple sclerosis; AIDS or cancer-related weight loss; intractable nausea and vomiting; glaucoma, and obesity/metabolic syndrome. As is the case with psychoactivity, many of the beneficial effects have been shown to be the result of stimulation of the CB_1R by THC. Paradoxically, trials suggested that blockade of CB_1R might be a strategy for the treatment of obesity and metabolic problems including diabetes, and to help people relinquish smoking, alcohol, and drug abuse. However, in 2008 concern over psychiatric unwanted effects, in particular an increased risk of suicidal ideas, led the FDA to deny a licence to the

CB_1R-blocker rimonabant (Acomplia) in the US, and the European drug regulator subsequently followed suit.

The non-psychoactive CBD is emerging as a fascinating medicine in its own right as an anti-inflammatory, anti-epileptic, anti-psychotic, and neuroprotective agent. Several other cannabinoids also exhibit interesting pharmacological activity. Manipulation of ECS for therapeutic purposes is also of considerable research interest. An endocannabinoid deficiency syndrome in humans has been hypothesized.

Fundamental dissimilarities between smoked cannabis and CM in terms of constituents, pharmacokinetics, pharmacodynamics and the motivation of the user result in very different profiles of effects. CM and recreational cannabis are therefore entirely separate entities, and it is essential that they are considered as such in both a scientific and political context. Professor Robin Murray, a prominent psychiatrist who has repeatedly emphasised the mental health risks of recreational cannabis, has written (2007): *"In a rational world, the introduction of [cannabis-based medicines] would not be influenced by attitudes towards the recreational use of cannabis. Sadly, however, the two tend to become confused in the public mind, and there is a danger that useful medicines might not be licensed because of rising concerns about the recreational use of cannabis."*

Recreational use

Cannabis (puff, spliff, draw, grass, pot, shit, weed, MJ, jane, dope, skunk, chiba, herb, bud, chronic) remains easily the most widely used illicit drug in the world. The UN estimated that approximately 166 million people used cannabis in 2006, amounting to around 4% of the global population aged 15 to 64. Annual prevalence rates in that age group are highest in Oceania (14.5%) followed by the US (10.5%) and Africa (8%). Average European rates are slightly lower though the range is wide, from 1% (Malta) to 11% (Spain). England, France, and the Czech Republic are towards the top end of the scale at around 10%. Surveys in 2007 reveal lifetime use of cannabis by over 100 million North Americans and 70 million Europeans over the age of 12. Two-thirds of all cannabis is consumed by adults aged 16 to 29, although UK statistics from 2005 showed that 12% of school students aged 11 to 15 had smoked it within the previous year. Approximately half the 15 year-olds in the UK had been offered cannabis at some point, and 38% had tried it at least once. Cannabis use is prevalent amongst prisoners in most countries. In the UK, a third of inmates admitted using cannabis regularly during their current confinement.

Cannabis consumption oscillates over the years, and the circumstances which determine these variations are not well understood. Following a period of steady decline between 1979 and 1992, rates of consumption in the US rose again in the mid 1990s such that current use among 12 to 17 year-olds doubled between 1992 and 1994. At that time somewhere in the region of 20 million US citizens were current users, with as many as five million smoking it daily. Similar trends were noted in Europe. In 1996 42% of young people in the UK under the age of 24 had tried it, of whom 16% were regular consumers. However, since 2000 almost all countries (Canada and Mexico are exceptions) have been seeing a steady decline in use. For example, in Europe use in the last year by 16 to 24 year-olds declined from 27% in 2001/2 to 21% in 2007/8, and in the US current use declined from 8% in 2002 to 5.8% (or 14.4 million) in 2007. Interestingly, cannabis consumption, especially by young people, has dropped notably in states with laws permitting medicinal usage. On the other hand, a US survey in late 2008 suggested that this decline may now have levelled out, with eighth graders perceiving the drug as less harmful than their predecessors. In the UK, the 2004 reclassification of cannabis from Class B to C under the Misuse of Drugs Act had no discernable effect on consumption rates. One possible explanation of the decline over the past decade is a halo effect from a less positive attitude towards tobacco smoking amongst young people.

The UK mental health charity Rethink conducted an interesting survey in 2006 which throws further light on patterns of use. Two thirds of participants were aged 16 to 35, and a large majority of the sample had taken cannabis at least once. Of those who had smoked it during the previous year, 40% used it daily, 20% two to three times a week, 9% once a week and 18% once a month. Herbal material was preferred to resin by four fifths of the sample. Only 10% purchased their cannabis from a street dealer, most obtaining it through friends or a regular source. Setting for use varied widely, incorporating use with friends, at home, at parties, or alone. The commonest reasons for smoking it were to aid relaxation (35%), because friends do it (12%), or just to get high (7%). Other more practical reasons included to relieve pain or physical symptoms (8%), to help sleep (5%) or relieve mental health problems (4%), or to increase creativity (3%). For 4%, habit or dependency was the main reason.

Cannabis accounts for at least half of all illegal drug seizures throughout the world. Out of 161,113 drug seizures by the police and customs in the UK in 2005, 114,202 were accounted for by cannabis. Seventy tons of cannabis (of which 70% was resin) and 208,357 plants were taken into custody. The large majority of these seizures were each of less than 500 grams or less than 50 plants. In the same year the US Drug Enforcement Administration (DEA) seized 283,344 kilos (up to 356,472 kg in 2007).

An average marijuana roll-up or 'spliff' contains around 300 mg of herbal material, though 'fatties' or 'blunts' may pack up to 1 g. Purity and smoking technique will profoundly affect the amount of drug absorbed, but even an expert smoker cannot achieve more than 50% absorption and 25% would be a more likely figure. The dose of THC delivered by a single spliff could be as little as 1 mg or as much as 30 mg depending on the quality and type of material. Since the threshold dose for intoxication is around 2 mg, the impact of a single cigarette will be rapidly apparent. The placebo effect is not unimportant in cannabis smoking and is more prominent in naïve smokers or those with suggestible personalities. Vapourizers are increasingly available via the internet as an alternative to smoking for health conscious consumers.

Intoxication will be discernible almost immediately, peak around 15 minutes, and last for three to four hours. By the oral route, onset is delayed for one or two hours depending on the food content of the stomach, but duration is much longer. The main effects are upon mood, attention and memory, perception, and patterns of thinking. These psychological effects are quite variable, and are described below. Heart rate is increased, clumsiness and slurring of speech may be noted, and the eyes become reddened, but the physical effects of the drug are generally mild. Body temperature may be slightly reduced. Fatal overdose due to cannabis alone has never been reported reliably.

Most users in the West smoke the drug in handmade cigarettes ('joints', 'spliffs', or, for those of Churchillian dimensions, 'blunts' or 'fatties') with or without tobacco, or more ostentatiously in clay 'chillums' or water-pipes. Tobacco is reputed to enhance the effects of cannabis, as well as regulating combustion. One risk of cannabis smoking is that it is a gateway into tobacco smoking: 50% of users also smoke tobacco regularly. Marijuana is sometimes brewed up as a tea, or used in cooking. It is more difficult to get the dose right by mouth and severe intoxication may be the result.

There are hundreds of descriptions in print of what it is like to take cannabis. Although these accounts are rather variable, the common theme is the essential lightheartedness of the experience. The typical high it produces has been labelled as 'fatuous euphoria'.

The effect of any drug is greatly influenced by many factors apart from its pharmacology, and this is particularly true of cannabis. The personality, mood, and expectations of the user, the quality of the drug and the amount actually absorbed into the body, the nature of the environment, and the attitude and behaviour of other people who are around at the time will all shape the experience.

Smoking cannabis is usually a sociable activity. A spliff, usually containing a mixture of cannabis and tobacco, is rolled from one or more cigarette papers to achieve the desired dimensions, and then handed round until it is nothing more than a tiny glowing stub (roach), highly prized for its apocryphal potency. This may get so hot and wizened that it requires a special holder (roach-clip). The experienced cannabis smoker inhales deeply and retains the smoke in the lungs for as long as possible to maximize absorption. This sometimes induces a peculiarly strangulated conversational style which non-smokers may find irritating.

After a few minutes of smoking, a sense of calm, contentment, and well-being is noted. A growing feeling of hilarity and sense of the absurd transforms the most mundane observation or witticism into the funniest thing in the world. There is usually a sense of good will, optimism, and well-being. Inhibitions are reduced or dispelled entirely. Participants may be seized with paroxysms of laughter which can be unappealing to the non-intoxicated observer.

In moderate doses, the effect is to enhance perception rather than distort it. Music, food, and sex may seem more pleasurable and intense but the user remains firmly in touch with reality. Time estimation becomes distorted, so that thirty seconds seems like a minute. With larger doses, lethargy may be pronounced ('couch-lock'). Novices who have misjudged the dose may occasionally find themselves physically transfixed. Their thoughts are racing and they may desperately wish to say something or get up and move about, but are effectively frozen to the spot. On the other hand, more experienced users claim to be able to master their intoxication if circumstances demand it.

As time passes, a dry mouth is likely and enhanced appetite may become evident, often with a particular desire for sweet things ('the munchies'). Sudden feelings of depersonalization or unreality sometimes come on in waves, and the degree of intoxication often seems to ebb and flow.

To the aficionado, this sort of intoxication seems valuable and life-enhancing. Musicians may be convinced that their playing is more free-flowing and inspired, talkers that they are more witty and interesting, lovers that their sexual energy and enjoyment are augmented, writers that their imagination is broadened. Sceptics would say that any idea of improved creativity is pure illusion, literally a pipedream. Users, they say, are banal, clumsy, infantile, irritating, illogical, and almost entirely lacking in judgement.

Unwanted effects

The acute toxicity of cannabis is extremely low, and there are no reliable reports of human fatality due solely to overdose. Animal data from the 1940s showed that the ratio of euphoric dose to lethal dose is 40,000. To put this in perspective, the same ratio for alcohol is about 10. However, as with all intoxicants, cannabis increases the risk of accidents or miscalculations. Acute cognitive deficits include impairment of inhibitory control, attention and task accuracy, sensory perception and time estimation, reaction time, physical coordination, depth estimation, recovery from glare, ability to track a moving object, and executive function. Any of these may prove lethal for drivers, pilots, or others performing tasks requiring skill and prudence.

Most unwanted effects caused by cannabis are minor in nature and brief in duration. Transient psychiatric symptoms are not uncommon as part of the intoxication syndrome including disorientation/confusion, anxiety, depression, paranoid ideas, illusions, hallucinations, and delusional beliefs. All of these effects are related to the THC content. They are self limiting, wearing off spontaneously as the drug is metabolized. Panic attacks may result from misinterpreting the rapid heartbeat which usually accompanies use of the drug as evidence of an impending heart attack, or the psychological effects as a precursor to loss of control or madness. Dizziness or depersonalization may similarly be assumed to herald impending catastrophe. Less experienced smokers may be more vulnerable to transient mood disturbances. There may be interactions with other drugs, especially brain depressants.

Morning-after effects from moderate use of cannabis are usually mild. Larger doses may accentuate the sedative potential of the drug, or result in sensory distortion or frank hallucinations. Members of the *Club des Haschishchins* took huge doses by today's standards, and Gautier has left an interesting description of the phenomenon known as synaesthesia, where the senses become interchanged. Describing a vase of flowers, he wrote: *'My hearing became prodigiously acute. I actually listened to the sounds of the colours. From their blues, greens, and yellows there reached me sound waves of perfect distinctness'.*

There are hundreds of published reports of the more serious adverse effects of cannabis, but their scientific validity is often questionable. Methodological problems include reliance on uncorroborated, retrospective, or subjective data; lack of information on physical, psychological, or personality problems antedating drug use; covert continuation of cannabis use or undisclosed use of other drugs currently or in the past; variations in the quality of illicit drugs and the amounts absorbed; lifestyle factors such as poverty and deprivation, or unrecognized physical or mental illness. The prior assumptions of the experimenter may shape the design of the study or the interpretation of the findings.

The current major public health concern surrounding cannabis is its potential impact on mental health. The ability of cannabis in large doses or in a vulnerable recipient to produce a 'toxic psychosis' with confusion, hallucinations, and delusions has been recognized for centuries. This state will wear off spontaneously as the drug is metabolized, although it may take several weeks for this to occur. Cannabis is by no means unique in this effect since several recreational and prescribed drugs can produce a very similar self-limiting toxic reaction. It is also likely that cannabis can precipitate psychosis in people with pre-existing risk factors (e.g. those with an abnormal personality or a family history of schizophrenia), and it can certainly exacerbate symptoms in psychotic patients. Psychotic patients are more likely to use cannabis and the reasons given for doing so include alleviation of boredom, improving sleep, and reducing anxiety and agitation. They are at increased risk of becoming dependent.

In recent years, evidence has accumulated from several epidemiological studies that cannabis smoking in childhood or adolescence may be associated with a 40% increase in risk of a functional (i.e. primary, as opposed to toxic) psychotic outcome in later life. The effect appears to be dose-related, with increased risk in heavy adolescent consumers. A specific genetic vulnerability may heighten this risk markedly in a sub-group of the population. Although these data are sufficiently compelling to raise real concern, it should be noted that the studies do have some methodological shortcomings. It is difficult to distinguish in a single assessment between toxic and functional psychosis as studies rely on self-report to confirm current abstinence rather than a urine screen. Cannabis smoking is not randomly distributed in samples and the potentially confounding variables which shape this choice are currently unknown. Projections of harm are based on a very small proportion of the total population studied (i.e. those who smoke cannabis and develop psychosis). The research has generated considerable controversy in its interpretation and has led to some wildly exaggerated reports in the lay media. The UK ACMD reviewed the evidence (2006) and concluded: '*At worst, the risk to an individual of developing schizophrenia as a result of using cannabis is very small*'. If cannabis smoking is an important risk factor for schizophrenia, the prevalence of the disease would be expected to increase in countries or regions where the prevalence of cannabis smoking has increased sharply and persistently. This has not yet been observed. Reviewing the evidence once again in 2008, the ACMD concluded that '. . . *the evidence points to a probable, but weak, causal link*' between adolescent cannabis smoking and psychosis later in life. This might represent an increase in the lifetime risk of developing schizophrenia in the order of 1%.

An association has also been reported between recreational cannabis smoking and anxiety and depression, although the evidence is less consistent and the direction of causality even more uncertain. The ACMD in 2008 '. . . *remains unconvinced that there is a causal relationship between the use of cannabis and the development of any affective disorder*'.

The effect of cannabis on memory, in particular the ability to learn new information, is another genuine cause for concern. There is no doubt that impaired concentration, learning, and short-term memory is almost inevitable when a person is intoxicated on cannabis, and for many consumers this is the very point of the exercise—a temporary escape from the trials and tribulations of modern society. These effects are likely to persist for several hours after a single exposure before disappearing gradually. Normalization of cognitive function may take days or weeks following abstinence from chronic, heavy use. An important question is whether some of the deficits associated with long-term cannabis use may prove irreversible even after complete abstinence for months or years. This remains an unresolved and controversial issue. Some deficits have been identified using particularly sensitive electronic techniques (event related potentials), but not everyone is convinced by these results that deficits are of any practical significance. Despite intense investigation, evidence of structural brain damage due to heavy cannabis consumption has not been apparent. However, a recent small brain-imaging study comparing heavy daily cannabis smokers to matched controls revealed volume reductions in hippocampus (12%) and amygdala (7.1%), structures concerned with cognitive function and emotional processing. This work will require replication before its significance can be assessed. Most published clinical studies and meta-analyses suggest a lack of permanent neuropsychological sequelae after prolonged abstinence.

Another problem often attributed to cannabis is that it induces a state of chronic apathy, passivity, and indolence which amounts to a change in personality. This reputation was perhaps initiated in the pages of the Hemp Commission report as a cause of concern in 19th-century India. One must bear in mind that the subjects described tended to be marginalized, unhealthy people perhaps suffering from malnutrition and almost entirely lacking in prospects, who were using potent cannabis in very large doses over long periods. There was some indication that people who were 'mentally unstable' to start with were more likely to use cannabis excessively; in other words, that mental abnormality was possibly a cause of drug use rather than a consequence.

'Amotivational syndrome' was a term coined in the 1960s to describe a cluster of symptoms said to occur frequently in regular cannabis users, including apathy, loss of ambition and determination, impaired concentration, and deterioration in school or work performance. There are many possible explanations for these symptoms in young people, including physical illness, psychiatric disorder, sleep disturbance, 'chronic fatigue syndrome', or enforced proximity to uninspiring teachers. Where cannabis was a major factor, chronic intoxication was probably the key. The case to support the concept of amotivational syndrome was built upon the sand of case reports and is not at all convincing. When at last it was subjected to a proper scientific examination in a large sample of subjects in 2006, it was reported that even long-term daily use of cannabis had no effect whatsoever on motivation.

Cannabis is approximately equivalent to alcohol in its ability to produce psychological dependency, according to a systematic expert appraisal published in 2007. Between 4–9% of those who try cannabis find they are unable to stop using it. Heavy or compulsive users may sometimes be self-medicating for emotional or psychiatric disorders, or using other illicit drugs such as amphetamines, cocaine, or hallucinogens. A physical dependency syndrome may occur in heavy, long-term users, with abrupt withdrawal resulting in irritability, anxiety, gastrointestinal upsets, and disturbed sleep for a week or so. Europe has seen a trebling of cannabis treatment demands between 1999 and 2005. In the US and UK it now represents the primary drug problem for around 15% and 7% respectively of all those admitted to drug dependency programmes, and 75% of young people under the age of 18 seeking treatment for drug-related problems in Britain are concerned primarily about marijuana. Such treatment programmes are only modestly successful, with abstinence rates between 20 and 40% at the end of treatment. Admissions to NHS hospitals for psychological or behavioural problems due to cannabis oscillated between 581–946 per annum between 1998 and 2007.

One concern expressed frequently is that cannabis may act as a 'gateway drug', such that its use may lead either through pharmacological or sociological mechanisms to an escalation to harder drug use and ultimately to heroin addiction. The UK ACMD, the House of Commons Science and Technology Committee, and the RAND Corporation have recently considered separately the evidence for this. All reached the same conclusion, namely that there is little evidence to support the gateway theory despite extensive research.

Cannabis causes the heart to speed up and work harder and blood volume may be increased through salt and water retention. The absorption of carbon monoxide by cannabis smokers reduces the oxygen content of the blood and thus the oxygen supply to the heart muscle. These effects seem of little relevance for healthy individuals, but may add up to trouble for someone with pre-existing cardiovascular disease or high blood pressure.

A cannabis joint delivers a greater burden of tar per unit weight than a tobacco cigarette, assuming a similar smoking profile, although much of this research was performed with low-grade, un-manicured material. In practice, the larger puff volume, increased depth of inhalation, and longer smoke retention by the cannabis smoker can deliver four times as much tar to the lung as would result from a tobacco cigarette. Marijuana tar contains more unpleasant chemicals of known carcinogenicity than tobacco smoke and produces precancerous cell changes in laboratory models. Ammonia, hydrogen cyanide, and aromatic amines are present in much greater quantities in marijuana smoke, whilst polycyclic aromatic hydrocarbons are much less evident. Heavy cannabis consumption over several years is associated with sinusitis, pharyngitis, shortness of breath, chronic cough, and bronchitis. The impact of four NIDA joints daily on the lungs is said to equate to 20 tobacco cigarettes. Inflammatory and precancerous changes have been identified in the airways of chronic smokers and these changes are most marked in those who smoke both tobacco and cannabis. There are anecdotal reports of an increased incidence of tumours of the mouth, larynx, and airways in cannabis smokers. On the other hand, there is no firm epidemiological evidence of an increased prevalence of these cancers or chronic lung disease in countries where large amounts of cannabis are consumed. This may simply be due to lack of systematic investigation, or it is possible that the anti-tumour effects of some cannabinoids observed in laboratory models may be exerting a protective effect. In the absence of definitive research, the consensus among experts is that daily cannabis smoking probably poses all the potential long-term risk to the airways that cigarette smoking does, and that smoking both cannabis and tobacco will maximize this risk. Some cannabinoids are immunosuppressive, so there is a theoretical risk that inhalation may increase the risk of opportunistic infections.

Surveys from various countries suggest that approximately 5% of women have smoked cannabis during pregnancy. Cannabis crosses the placenta and, given to animals in large doses, is damaging to the foetus (teratogenic) and increases lost pregnancies. The picture in humans is much less clear, but the main effects which have been suggested are an association with prematurity and babies of low birth-weight. There is also some evidence of impaired cognitive function, increased incidence of certain childhood cancers, and a greater vulnerability to future dependent drug use amongst offspring of cannabis-smoking mothers. However, regular cannabis use during pregnancy is often associated with low income, social deprivation, poorer education, younger age of conception outside a stable relationship, heavier alcohol and tobacco use, use of other illicit drugs, and poorer maternal nutrition and general health. All of these factors are themselves associated with an increased risk to the foetus. Medications given to the mother, natural birth complications, maternal bonding, feeding practices, and sibling interactions can also confuse the issue. Animal studies show an interaction between exposure to cannabis and a low-protein diet in the induction of stillbirths, postnatal deaths, and delayed developmental milestones. Evidence from children born to Rastafarian mothers in Jamaica using cannabis, but no tobacco or alcohol, during pregnancy seem to support a lack of any attributable complications. Experts continue to differ in their views on whether prenatal exposure puts the unborn child at significant risk. In the absence of certainty it would seem prudent for pregnant and breast-feeding women to avoid this and all other unnecessary drugs.

Laboratory studies suggest cannabis smoking may impair fertility and is not recommended in those wishing to reproduce. It suppresses some immune functions (an attribute of interest for medicinal usage) but this has not been shown to worsen prognosis in chronic infections such as HIV/AIDS. In people with hepatitis C, fatty liver (steatosis) occurs more frequently in daily cannabis users than both infrequent users and non-consumers.

Part of cannabis's folklore is that it provides a stimulus to crime, violent and otherwise. Although its use is highly prevalent in prison communities and among the criminal classes, there is no evidence to suggest that it has a causal role. Cannabis-smoking school students do not commit more crime than non-smokers, for example. Some prison officers believe that prison society would be more violent and disrupted if it ceased to be easily available.

The impact of the increase in potency of herbal material on the physical or mental health of consumers remains uncertain. It is plausible that many will modulate intake according to the perceived effect. Admissions to hospital with cannabis-related toxicity have not increased, but there has been a small but steady rise in numbers seeking treatment for cannabis dependency. On the other hand, increased potency resulting in lower quantities smoked may lessen the pulmonary risks.

In summary, it is evident that cannabis is associated with a large number of unwanted effects, but most of these are minor and transient. Certain groups of people are probably at greater than average risk of more serious consequences and would be well advised to avoid the drug entirely. These include those already anxious, depressed, or psychotic; heavy users of other drugs; pregnant women; some epileptics; patients with existing heart or lung disease; and younger adolescents.

Selected references

Advisory Council on the Misuse of Drugs (2008). *Cannabis: classification and public health*. Home Office, London http://drugs.homeoffice.gov.uk/publication-search/acmd/acmd-cannabis-report-2008?view=Binary.

Barnwell S. S., Earleywine M., Wilcox R. (2006). Cannabis, motivation, and life satisfaction in an internet sample. *Substance Abuse Treatment, Prevention and Policy* 1:2 doi:10.1186/1747-597X-1-2.

Chait, L. D., Perry, J. L. (1992). Factors influencing self-administration of, and subjective response to, placebo marijuana. *Behavioural Pharmacology*, 3, 545–52.

Culver, C. M., King, F. W. (1974). Neuropsychological assessment of undergraduate marijuana and LSD users. *Archives of General Psychiatry*, 31, 707–11.

Deahl, M. (1991). Cannabis and memory loss. *British Journal of Addiction*, **86**, 249–52.

de Fonseca, F. R., Carrera, M. R. A., Navarro, M., Koob, G. F., Weiss, F. (1997). Activation of corticotropin-releasing factor in the limbic system during cannabinoid withdrawal. *Science*, **276**, 2050–3.

Dittrich, A., Battig, K., von Zeppelin, I. (1973). Effects of delta 9 THC on memory, attention, and subjective state. *Psychopharmacologia*, **33**, 369–76.

English, D. R., Hulse, G. K., Milne, E., Holman, C. D. J., Bower, C. I. (1997). Maternal cannabis use and birth weight: a meta-analysis. *Addiction*, **92**, 1553–60.

Erinoff, L. (1990). Neurobiology of drug abuse: learning and memory. *N.I.D.A. Research Monograph 97*.

Feeney, D. M. (1976). Marijuana use among epileptics [letter]. *Journal of the American Medical Association*, **235**, 1105.

Grant, I., Rochford, J., Fleming, T., Stunkard, A. (1973). A neuropsychological assessment of the effects of moderate marijuana use. *Journal of Nervous and Mental Disease*, **156**, 278–80.

Hall, W., Solowij, N., Lemon, J. (ed.) (1994). *The health and psychological consequences of cannabis use*, National Drug Strategy Monograph Series No. 25, Australian Government Publishing Service, Canberra.

Hall W, Room R. (2008). *Beckley Foundation Submission to the ACMD on the classification of cannabis under the Misuse of Drugs Act, 1971*. Beckley Foundation, Oxford. http://www.beckleyfoundation.org/bib/doc/bf/2008_Robin_211352_1.pdf.

Hardwick S, King L (2008). *Home Office Cannabis Potency Study 2008*. Home Office Scientific Development Branch, London

Hezode C., Zafrani E. S., Roudot-Thereval F. et al. (2008). Daily cannabis use: a novel risk factor of steatosis severity in patients with chronic hepatitis C. *Gastroenterology* **134**, 622–5.

Howlett, A. C., Bidaut-Russell, M., Devane, W. A., Melvin, L. S., Johnson, M. R., Herkenham, M. (1990). The cannabinoid receptor: biochemical, anatomical and behavioural characterization. *Trends in Neurosciences*, **13**, 421–3.

Mechoulam, R. (1986). The pharmacohistory of *Cannabis sativa*. In: *Cannabinoids as therapeutic agents* (ed. R. Mechoulam). CRC Press, Boca Raton, FL.

Mendhiratta, S. S., Wig, N. N., Verma, S. K. (1978). Some psychological correlates of long-term heavy cannabis users. *British Journal of Psychiatry*, **132**, 482–6.

Moir D., Rickert W. S., Levasseur G. et al. (2008). A comparison of mainstream and sidestream marijuana cigarette smoke produced under two machine smoking conditions. *Chemical Research in Toxicology* **21**, 494–502.

Moore T. H. M., Zammit S., Lingford-Hughes A. et al. Cannabis use and risk of psychotic or affective mental health outcomes: a systematic review. *Lancet* 2007, **370**: 319–28.

Murray, R. M., Morrison, P. D., Henquet, C., Di Forti, M. (2007). Cannabis, the mind and society: the hash realities. *Nature Reviews (Neuroscience)*, **8**, 885–95.

Nutt D., King L. A., Saulsburg W., Blakemore C. (2007). Development of a national scale to assess the harm of drugs of potential misuse. *Lancet*, **369**, 1047–53.

O'Shaugnessy, W. B. (1843). On the *Cannabis indica* or Indian hemp. *Pharmacology Journal*, **2**, 594.

Pacher P., Batkai S., Kunos G. (2006). The endocannabinoid system as an emerging target of pharmacotherapy. *Pharmacoogyl Reviews*, **58**, 389–462.

Pertwee R.G. Cannabinoid pharmacology: the first 66 years. *British Journal of Pharmacology* **147**: S163–71.

Potter D. J., Clark P., Brown M. B. (2008). Potency of delta-9-THC and other cannabinoids in cannabis in England in 2005: implications for psychoactivity and pharmacology. *Journal of Forensic Science* **53**, 90–4.

Reinarman C., Cohen P. D. A., Kaal H. L. (2004). The limited relevance of drug policy: cannabis in Amsterdam and San Francisco. *American Journal of Public Health* **94**, 836–42.

Rethink (2008). *Cannabis Report*. http://www.rethink.org/how_we_can_help/news_and_media/briefing_notes/educating_reefer.html

Reynolds, J. R. (1890). Therapeutic uses and toxic effects of *Cannabis indica. Lancet.* **1**, 637–8.

Robson, P. (1997). Cannabis. *Archives of Diseases in Childhood,* **77**, 164–6.

Robson, P. (1998). Cannabis as medicine: time for the phoenix to arise? *British Medical Journal,* **316**, 1034–5.

Robson, P. (2005). Human studies of cannabinoids and medicinal cannabis. In: *Handbook of Experimental Pharmacology; Cannabinoids.* (Ed Pertwee R) **168**, 719–56. Springer-Verlag Berlin Heidelberg.

Rochford, J., Grant, I., LaVigne, G. (1977). Medical students and drugs: further neuropsychological and use pattern considerations. *International Journal of the Addictions,* **12**, 1057–65.

Russo, E. B. (2004). Clinical Endocannabinoid Deficiency (CECD): Can this Concept Explain Therapeutic Benefits of Cannabis in Migraine, Fibromyalgia, Irritable Bowel Syndrome and other Treatment-Resistant Conditions? *Neuroendocrinology Letters* **25**(1–2), 31–39.

Russo, E. B., Guy, G. W (2006). A tale of two cannabinoids: the therapeutic rationale for combining tetrahydrocannabinol (THC) and cannabidiol (CBD). *Medical Hypotheses,* **66**, 234–246.

Schofield D, Tennant C, Nash L et al. (2006). Reasons for cannabis use in psychosis. *Australian and New Zealand Journal of Psychiatry* **40**, 570–4.

Schwartz, R. H., Gruenewald, P. J., Klitzner, M., Ferdio, P. (1989). Short-term memory impairment in cannabis-dependent adolescents. *American Journal of Diseases of Childhood,* **143**, 1214–19.

Tashkin, D. P. (1991). Marijuana and lung function. In: *Biochemistry and physiology of substance abuse,* Vol. 3 (ed. R. R. Watson). CRC Press, Boca Raton, FL.

Thomas, H. (1993). Psychiatric symptoms in cannabis users. *British Journal of Psychiatry,* **163**, 141–9.

UK Drug Policy Commission (2008). Submission to the ACMD cannabis classification review 2008. http://www.ukdpc.org.uk/resources/ACMD_Cannabis_Submission_Jan_2008.pdf.

Vandrey R. G., Budney A. J., Hughes J. R. et al. (2008). A within-subject comparison of withdrawal symptoms during abstinence from cannabis, tobacco and both substances. *Drug & Alcohol Dependence* **92**, 48–54.

Varma, V. K., Malhotra, A. K., Dang, R., Das, K., Nehra, R. (1988). Cannabis and cognitive functions: a prospective study. *Drug and Alcohol Dependence,* **21**, 147–52.

Wert, R. C., Raulin, M. L. (1986). The chronic cerebral effects of cannabis use. 1. Methodological issues and neurological findings. *International Journal of the Addictions,* **21**, 605–28.

Yucel M., Solowij N., Respondek C. et al. (2008). Regional brain abnormalities associated with long-term heavy cannabis use. *Archives of General Psychiatry* **65**, 694–701.

Chapter 6

Cocaine, amphetamines, and other stimulants

Cocaine

Historical background

Chewing the leaves of the coca plant (*Erythroxylum* coca) has been part of everyday life in many South American cultures for several thousand years. For millions of people the habit continues to fulfil a comparable role to that of coffee or tobacco elsewhere in the world. A wad of leaves tucked into the cheek for several hours, with perhaps a little woodash mixed in to increase salivation and enhance absorption of the active ingredients, will produce a sense of well-being, reduced hunger, and increased endurance.

Stories about this interesting plant first reached Europe in the 16th century, but it was not until the middle of the 19th century that it became a focus of interest to scientists. An active ingredient was identified in 1855, and this was further purified and named cocaine by the chemist Albert Niemann in 1860. At around the same time the possible medicinal applications of coca were publicized by the writings of an Italian physician who had witnessed its use in Peru. Cocaine soon appeared in an ever-widening array of patent medicines and tonics. A famous example was Vin Mariani, containing the relatively modest dose of 8 mg per glass, which was available in France from the 1860s. This became extremely popular at all levels of European society, and reached the US in 1885. The medical response had at first been muted but interest grew rapidly, with articles by some famous physicians extolling the properties of the drug as little short of miraculous for a variety of ailments. Sigmund Freud was one of the many professionals swept along in the rush. In 1884, his great friend, the scientist Ernst von Fleischl, received morphine for the relief of severe postoperative pain and became addicted. This seemed an excellent opportunity to try out the wonder drug. Freud got hold of some to treat his friend, and was so encouraged by the initial results that he was inspired to write a review article which was, in his own words, '*a song of praise to this magical substance*'. A frequently quoted advertisement of 1885 described coca as '*a drug which through its stimulant properties can supply the place of food, make the coward brave, the silent eloquent, free the victims of alcohol and opium habit from their bondage, and, as an anaesthetic, render the sufferer insensitive to pain . . .'.* Coca-Cola, containing a few milligrams of cocaine in each glassful, was introduced in 1886 and marketed as a refreshing and stimulating alternative to alcohol.

In England, a growing recognition that the miracle drug could have a dark underbelly, reinforced by an element of professional expansionism, resulted in an abrupt restriction of outlets for cocaine alongside the opiates under the Pharmacy Act (1868). In the US, there was a growing preference for sniffing or injecting cocaine rather than imbibing it, and awareness of the risk of addiction began to grow in the last quarter of the 19th century. The outstanding American surgeon, William Halsted, became a compulsive user as a result of his explorations into its local anaesthetic properties. By 1887, even such uncritical adherents as Freud had begun to experience a downturn of enthusiasm. His friend von Fleischl had become pitifully enslaved by the miracle drug, injecting well over a gram of it every day. Commercial acknowledgement of this major shift in public opinion was signposted when caffeine replaced the coca in Coca-Cola in 1903.

Increasing legal restriction in the US stimulated the production of illicit sources of supply. It is interesting that the cost of cocaine on the streets of New York in 1907 was almost identical in real terms to that in 1985. The Harrison Act (1914) limited the use of cocaine to medical prescription nationwide. In 1919, the Supreme Court ruled that maintenance prescribing to addicts was not legitimate medical practice and outlawed it.

The black market in Britain was much less developed, but there were some widely published scandals involving cocaine in the early years of the 20th century. During the First World War, concern grew over the sale of cocaine to soldiers on leave in London, and in 1916 regulation 40 of the Defence of the Realm Act proscribed the supply of cocaine and a number of other drugs to members of the armed forces except on prescription from a doctor. With some additions, this regulation was transferred to the Civil Law in 1920 as the Dangerous Drugs Act.

Cocaine underwent a progressive decline through the second quarter of the 20th century in both Britain and the US, reaching a nadir in the early 1950s. It began a comeback in the middle 1960s, and the public and professional perception of the drug gradually came to resemble that benign and complacent view of a century before. Rapid expansion of use followed in the US, peaking around 1979, at which point 10% of young adults had used cocaine within the last month. By 1986 three million Americans were using it regularly, with a total population prevalence of 3%. The drug's social impact was greatly aggravated by the appearance of smokeable cocaine (crack) in 1985. By 1990 at least 30 million Americans had snorted cocaine at some time in their lives and there were six times as many cocaine addicts presenting to medical centres for treatment as heroin addicts. In the course of 1990, 6.2 million people in the US tried cocaine at least once, half of these went on to use it regularly, and at least 200,000 ingested it daily. The proportion of cocaine consumed in the form of crack in the US and Canada increased very sharply between 1986 and 1990. For example, two-thirds of the cocaine consumed by the youth of Toronto in 1989 was taken in this form.

Europe was much less severely afflicted by the cocaine epidemic, but whilst in recent years US consumption has stabilized some European countries have seen sharp escalations in consumption.

Preparation and distribution

South America currently generates over 900 tons of cocaine each year, which translates into some $60 billion revenue at street level from customers in the US and Europe alone. The slopes of the Andes and the vastness of the Amazon basin play host to the two major species of coca-yielding shrubs. The demand for cocaine emanating from the developed world has created a black economy of stupendous proportions. Peru, Bolivia, and Colombia between them produce 98% of the world's coca leaf, which is estimated to have amounted to 292,430 tons in 2006.

Coca leaf is converted in the country of origin to coca paste, containing up to 80% of the active ingredient. The paste is further purified and refined to produce cocaine hydrochloride, a white, crystalline, water-soluble powder which is very well absorbed by mouth and through the membranes of the nose. The pattern of cocaine use in the source countries has changed markedly as this industry has developed. Paste smoking, virtually unknown before 1970, is now widespread and associated with much physical, psychological, and social harm. Known as bazuco (Colombia), pitillo (Bolivia), or kete (Peru) it is cheap, contaminated with toxic by-products of the manufacturing process such as kerosene and sulphuric acid, and highly addictive. The emergence since 2001 of an epidemic of paste ('paco') smoking in Argentina signals that country's graduation into the big-time of cocaine production.

Cocaine marketing has shifted in recent years as a result of global economic changes and the impact of law enforcement initiatives. These include the destruction of major Colombian cartels and a clampdown on the supply of key chemicals required in manufacture such as potassium permanganate and isopropyl alcohol. Increased demand and better profit margins have led to a new focus on Europe for cocaine marketing. Whilst US supplies continue to gain access via Mexico, cocaine reaches Europe through West African nations such as Guinea-Bissau and thence to the Iberian peninsula or the Netherlands. The effects on society of the titanic criminal organizations which have grown up around this industry are devastating. For example, drug-related violence claimed the lives of 2,682 people in Mexico in the first half of 2008.

Scientific information

Cocaine is an alkaloid which inhibits the reuptake of the brain's neurotransmitters dopamine, norepinephrine (noradrenaline), and serotonin (5-HT), thereby enhancing their effects. It is also a local anaesthetic through its action on fast sodium channels on nerve cells. Average purity at street level ranges between 20–80%.

Cocaine is not very effective if swallowed because the liver destroys most of it before it can reach the brain. If taken orally numbness in the mouth occurs due to its local anaesthetic effect, and this attribute is sometimes used as a measure of purity of street supplies. Absorption is usually rapid when the powder is sniffed ('snorted'), though constriction of nasal blood vessels may cause a delay. By this route, the drug quickly reaches the brain before it passes through the liver. Once absorbed, rapid metabolism in the liver, blood, and elsewhere results in a halving of the blood level every 60 to 90 minutes, so the duration of action is quite short. The powder can also be dissolved in water and injected into a vein. This results in much higher and more rapid peak concentrations in the blood and brain.

Cocaine powder must be heated to over 200°C in order to vapourize it, and at this temperature most of the active ingredient is destroyed. 'Freebase', which consists of cocaine stripped of its hydrochloride salt by a process of alkalinization and chemical extraction, vapourizes at a much lower temperature so that the alkaloid remains mainly intact. Smoking freebase delivers drug to the brain at least as rapidly as would be achieved by injection, albeit at slightly lower peak concentration. A cocaine smoker can be distinguished from a snorter by the presence in the urine of a particular metabolite called methylecgonidine.

Crack is a crude and impure form of freebase, easily prepared from cocaine hydrochloride and bicarbonate of soda in an illicit laboratory or somebody's kitchen, and is so called because of the popping and clicking given off by exploding impurities during smoking. Also known as 'wash', 'stone', or 'rock', it usually takes the form of small, off-white soapy or brittle crystalline lumps costing between £10–20 UK or $10–25 US. It is smoked in a pipe or some form of improvised delivery system, such as a soft-drink can with holes punched in it, or heated on a piece of foil and the fumes inhaled.

Cocaine has a powerful effect upon one particular bundle of dopamine-containing nerves in the brain called the ventral tegmental area (VTA) which is known as the reward or pleasure pathway. These structures mediate the rewarding nature of life's normal gratifications such as food or sex, and appear central to the drug's ability to produce a 'high'. In laboratory models animals will perform any number of tasks to obtain electrical stimulation of this pathway. Most drugs which people use for pleasure have been shown to stimulate these nerves, but none more powerfully than cocaine (or amphetamine). They stimulate the VTA much more intensively than would be the case with normal rewarding events. When animals are given the choice of receiving either cocaine or food they will choose the former, pressing a bar thousands of times to obtain a tiny dose. And given unlimited access, they will continue to dose themselves until they finally die of exhaustion. There is some concern that excessive stimulation of VTA in human cocaine (or amphetamine) users may permanently damage the system so that it remains chronically depleted of dopamine. This might account for the clinical observation that some long-term cocaine users experience a prolonged reduction in their ability to experience reward from the ordinary pleasures of life after giving up the drug.

Cocaine also stimulates the sympathetic nervous system, which is responsible for the so-called 'fight or flight' mechanism. This produces an increase in heart rate and blood pressure, widening of blood vessels to muscles and narrowing of those to skin, a toning-up of the body's chemical and hormonal systems generally, and an increase in the amount of oxygen entering through the lungs. The body is prepared for action.

Frequent use by any route results quickly in reduced sensitivity (tolerance) to the euphoric effects of cocaine, but not to all of the unwanted effects (see below).

Simultaneous use of cocaine and alcohol results in the formation of cocaethylene, which adds to the euphoric effect but also increases the risk of damage to the heart or liver.

Medical uses

Cocaine was used as a local anaesthetic for decades, but has now been superceded by safer alternatives such as lignocaine and bupivacaine. Its use in analgesic elixirs for terminal care is also obsolete. Apart from very occasional use in otolaryngeal procedures, no other medical indications remain.

Recreational use

Cocaine (coke; snow; charlie; blow; 'C'; flake; toot; aunt; bernie; cecil; scottie; lady; nose candy) is the second most trafficked illicit drug in the world after cannabis.

The US has the highest prevalence of use, with 16% of citizens over the age of 18 having taken it at least once, and 2.4 million having used it in the previous month. There are also around 700,000 regular crack users. This compares with current lifetime prevalence rates of 11% in Canada, 4% in Colombia and Mexico, and negligible rates in the Middle East, Asia, and Africa. However, since 2002 US consumption of both powder cocaine and crack appears to have stabilized at levels considerably below the peak in the 1980s, and the proportion of the workforce testing positive for the drug has declined by 36% since 1998. Nevertheless, there are still nearly a million new initiates each year.

The overall European lifetime prevalence is only 4%, but this masks large variations in individual countries and the number of current users has risen sharply in recent years to around two million in 2007. Out of 26 countries providing data, 11 had prevalence figures for use by adults in the last year less than 0.5%. The ranges are from 0.1% (Greece) to 2.7% (Spain) with the UK second highest at 2.4%, up from 1.2% in 1998. Peak usage is between the ages of 18 to 25, and in the UK 6% in this age bracket have used cocaine within the previous year. Males users outnumber females by two to one. Crack use remains relatively uncommon throughout Europe except among injecting heroin addicts.

Prices in the US increased by as much as 40% in 2007 as a result of the dollar's weakness and the average street price in that year was $122/gram, up from $75 in 2003. Street prices vary widely across Europe, ranging between €45–120/gram, but average prices have declined steadily since 2000. In the UK in late 2008 costs as low as £25/gram have been recorded. Purity at street level ranges widely, but averages between 40 and 70% in US and UK.

In many countries, regular cocaine use is the domain of two disparate social groupings who also have very different profiles of use. On the one hand, there are young professionals, typically unmarried males in their twenties, who use cocaine by the nasal route relatively infrequently and in the context of their work or social lives. It is quite unusual for such people to present to doctors or drug services with cocaine-related problems. Women are less likely to use cocaine in large amounts or over long periods.

Then there is the hard drug scene, peopled by men and women of low socio-economic status, unemployed and often homeless, who prefer to inject cocaine or smoke it in the form of crack. They are likely also to be injecting heroin, involved in criminal activities or prostitution to support their drug habits, and experiencing a lot of high-profile, drug-related problems. Crack is very commonly used by heroin addicts, as many as 70% in one recent UK study.

Although it can be taken by mouth or, at the other extreme, dissolved in water and injected into a vein, most users arrange the powder into a 'line' on a hard surface and snort it into the nose through a tightly rolled piece of paper such as a banknote, ideally of high denomination. Some people achieve the same result with a tiny silver spoon or other equipment specially designed for the purpose. An average line delivers around 25 mg cocaine.

As with all psychoactive drugs, the effects are shaped to an important extent by the user's expectations, and the setting in which it is taken. In the case of street drugs, purity and the nature of contaminants are also important factors. Usually, a sense of well-being appears promptly and grows rapidly. Confidence, optimism, energy, self-esteem, and sex drive are all enhanced, and there is an overall feeling of exhilaration and happiness. Most normal pleasures are augmented but not distorted. Sexual desire and performance may be enhanced. The drug often improves social skills, and part of its reinforcing property lies in the positive feedback which may be forthcoming from the user's companions. There is a reduced need for food, rest, and sleep. The heart speeds up, the pupils dilate, and body temperature rises.

Since cocaine is rapidly broken down in the body, the duration of action will tend to be measured in minutes rather than hours. Many people will content themselves with one or two lines, but some will seek to hang on to the high by snorting repeatedly. Once this pattern is established, decreasing sensitivity to the euphoric effects will necessitate rapidly increasing doses at ever briefer intervals. This may get out of control as an all-out binge, ending only when money or drugs run out, or exhaustion supervenes.

One survey found that just under a third of a sample of cocaine users were content to take the drug opportunistically if it happened to be around. About the same proportion bought their own supply but used it in a controlled, infrequent way. A quarter of the sample tended to consume the drug more frequently and regularly, and admitted they devoted a considerable amount of time to cocaine-related friends or activities. The remaining 14% had adopted a compulsive pattern of use and were effectively addicts.

The lungs are a highly efficient absorption system from which the blood carries its cargo directly to the brain without having to swirl round the whole body or pass through the liver, where much of it would be broken down before it could have any effect. For this reason, crack produces sudden euphoria so powerful that words seem to fail people when they are asked to describe it. It delivers a 'rush' or 'high' comparable to that obtained by injecting the drug. Unfortunately, the physical and mental jolt associated with this is also savage. An intense, short-lived euphoria lasting 10 minutes or so is often followed quite rapidly by a very unpleasant down-swing of mood. Regular smokers feel irritable and 'wired', and one unfortunate way of dealing with this is to smoke or inject heroin. Many dealers in crack also sell opiates for this reason, and increases in crack use may therefore be signposted by an upsurge in heroin-related problems. An even more dangerous way to use cocaine is by smoking coca paste, a practice virtually unknown in the US and UK but widely prevalent in South America.

Some people use cocaine in the context of multiple drug use, and they may well choose the intravenous route in order to maximize the intensity of the effect and the 'bang for the buck'. It may be combined in the same syringe with heroin ('speedball') or a benzodiazepine such as temazepam to smooth off the rough edges of the stimulant high. Most people using a number of drugs intravenously, and many crack smokers, are leading the sort of generally chaotic and dangerous lifestyle which will greatly augment the risks to their physical and mental health.

Not surprisingly, injecting or smoking cocaine produces many more casualties than snorting it. When traffickers introduced freebase into the Bahamas in 1984, hospital attendances for problems associated with cocaine abuse increased seven fold. Every year, smugglers (mules) stuff condoms or clingfilm packages with cocaine and swallow them. Should these burst or leak, a fatal outcome is by no means unusual.

Unwanted effects

In estimating the risks associated with cocaine (and amphetamine) it is important to bear in mind that its use may be associated with other risky behaviours such as unsafe sex and driving while intoxicated. Cocaine users often drink a lot of alcohol and smoke both cigarettes and cannabis. Use of opiates, sedatives, and hallucinogens is far higher than in the general population.

Cocaine accounts for more than 100,000 visits to hospital emergency rooms each year in the US, more than any other illicit drug. Chest pain is the commonest presenting complaint. In Europe, over 400 cocaine-related deaths are reported each year and many cases probably go unrecognized since the annual death rate has been estimated at one in every 2,000 users (the figure for cigarette smokers was 12.6/2,000 users). The highest rates of cocaine-related problems occur in men aged between 26 and 34.

Excessive doses are likely to produce sweating, dizziness, high body temperature, dry mouth, trembling hands, and a ringing in the ears. Anxiety and irritability may be evident, as may repetitive skin-picking and involuntary grinding of the teeth. Blood pressure and heart rate go up, occasionally to the point of bursting a blood vessel in the brain. This increased work load on the heart associated with constriction of the coronary blood vessels and effects on the blood clotting mechanism raises the risk of myocardial infarction (heart attack). Cocaethylene, a substance produced when cocaine and alcohol are taken together, augments these risks and also the possibility of liver damage. Convulsions may be caused by constriction or inflammation of the cerebral arteries. Treatment of these events is symptomatic as there is no direct means of neutralizing them. Injectors expose themselves to life-threatening infections and many other hazards.

It is possible that long-term use may irreversibly damage certain nerves or small blood vessels in the brain. More prosaically, narrowing of nasal blood vessels in snorters can lead to a chronic runny nose, ulceration, or collapse of the nasal cartilage with striking effects upon facial architecture. Crack smoking is very hard on the lungs, and is associated with severe chest pain, asthma, bronchitis, emphysema, pulmonary oedema, and fibrosis.

Impulsivity, disinhibition, and impaired judgement may lead to disaster. High doses or a susceptible individual can result in anxiety, panic, irritability, aggression, or confusion. Transient hallucinations or delusions indistinguishable from those seen in schizophrenia sometimes occur. If the delusional beliefs take a persecutory form, there is a risk that dangerously aggressive behaviour may result without warning. Rarely, this loss of contact with reality (psychosis) persists even if no further stimulants are consumed.

Between 10–15% of people who experiment with a snort of cocaine are destined to become compulsive users, usually within two to four years of the first exposure, but it is difficult to predict who will fall victim in this way. Compulsive use is more common among crack smokers than snorters, especially when taken in the context of social deprivation or emotional disturbance. In 2006, 1.7 million people in the US were classified as dependent on cocaine. Requests for treatment of cocaine addiction in Europe have tripled over the past five years.

Compulsive use of both crack and powder cocaine often involves a series of binges lasting hours or days, during which huge amounts may be consumed and ending only when supplies are exhausted or the user has a physical or mental collapse. At the end of such a run three phases of withdrawal have been described. First comes the 'crash'. After a few hours of intense depression, agitation, and desire for more stimulants, the need for sleep becomes irresistable, and this may be induced with depressants such as alcohol, heroin, or benzodiazepines. Intermittent sleep may last as long as two days, followed by a period of low energy and motivation, depression, boredom, and a lack of any sense of pleasure or enjoyment which sometimes goes on for many weeks. This is likely to be accompanied by a powerful desire for cocaine exacerbated by contact with people, places, or things associated in the person's mind with previous drug taking. If this desire is resisted successfully, the third phase consists of a gradual improvement in mood and the ability to find pleasure in ordinary things. The intensity and frequency of the bouts of craving steadily diminish.

Individuals in the grip of compulsive cocaine use, particularly female crack smokers, may become involved in dangerous or humiliating sexual behaviour in the pursuit of supplies.

People with a history of psychiatric illness are more at risk of becoming compulsive users and psychotic or depressive illness may be initiated or exacerbated by stimulants (and many other drugs). In the mid-1980s, one in every five people who committed suicide in New York was found to have cocaine in their bodies at post-mortem. An analysis of 300 psychiatric in-patients showed that 64% could be categorized as 'substance misusers', of whom more than half were cocaine users.

There are important differences between clinical or forensic ('visible') populations and users who remain invisible. Most of the latter are not at all concerned about their drug use and certainly have no desire for help or advice. In studies using well-validated measures, cocaine seems to have a low addictive potential in these people in sharp contrast to 'visible' populations. Heavy intranasal users definitely have higher levels of physical and psychological disorders than abstainers, but light and 'light–heavy' (using up to once a week for no longer than a total of 12 months) do not.

There are reports of impaired hormonal and reproductive function in some long-term users, but of more concern are the effects of cocaine in pregnancy. Cocaine can interfere with the supply of oxygen and nutrients to the foetus through its constricting action on uterine and placental blood vessels, and this can also result in premature labour or stillbirth. The drug causes fetal damage in animal studies, and it is likely this is also possible in humans. Many pregnant women using crack are also seriously undernourished or physically ill, or leading the sort of lifestyles which pose tremendous risks to themselves and the unborn child. Even allowing for these associated factors, low birth-weight is undoubtedly related to cocaine use during pregnancy in a dose-related manner. The effect is more pronounced if the cocaine has been taken in the form of crack, or if other drugs have also been taken. Separation of the placenta during pregnancy, which can kill both mother and baby, is four times more common in cocaine users.

The phenomenon of 'crack babies' has received a lot of publicity. The offspring of crack-addicted mothers may be small for dates, irritable, trembly, poor feeders, and unresponsive to cuddling. These effects usually wear off in the course of a few days. The possibility of longer-term behavioural problems has been raised, but there are so many confounding variables, including social deprivation, poor nutrition, and general health, that this is likely to remain uncertain.

What is clear is that crack-using households are potential breeding grounds for domestic violence and all forms of personal abuse.

Amphetamines

Historical background

The amphetamines lack the glamourous image of cocaine but are used by twice as many people world-wide. Injectable or smokeable methamphetamine is a cyclical international scourge, especially in North America and parts of South East Asia. Despite being second only to cannabis in prevalence in many countries, the amphetamines attract relatively little coverage in either the scientific literature or the lay media.

Plant-extracted ephedrine was an ancient remedy for asthma and bronchial congestion, and synthetic alternatives were required. Amphetamine was synthesized in 1887 and methamphetamine in 1893 (followed by a crystalline formulation in 1919), but they were not tested on humans until the 1920s. Amphetamine sulphate was first licenced as a nasal decongestant in 1932 ('Benzedrine'), and for use in asthma, obesity, pathological somnolence (narcolepsy), and depression soon afterwards. Methamphetamine was marketed in the US as 'Methedrine' in 1940. The unwanted effect of sleeplessness was recognized very quickly, but this did not inhibit their prescription for Parkinson's disease, migraine, addictions, seasickness, mania, schizophrenia, impotence, and apathy in old age. This therapeutic enthusiasm was fuelled by many positive reports in the medical literature.

The utility of the Benzedrine inhaler as a performance enhancer was recognized almost immediately by US students. The first non-medical application of amphetamine was to counter fatigue among soldiers in the Spanish Civil War, and in the ensuing World War this became routine in all armies. In the British Army, it was to be used when the men '. . . *were markedly fatigued physically or mentally and circumstances demanded a particular effort*'. Hitler is said to have received regular injections of methamphetamine (also barbiturates and other drugs) on a daily basis in the closing phases of the war, which must have contributed to his spiralling emotional turmoil and erratic behaviour.

The first recorded outbreak of widespread abuse occurred in Japan immediately after the war when large military stocks of methamphetamine were dumped on to the civilian market. A combination of abundant supplies, low price, heavy advertising, social dislocation, and lack of awareness of the risks fuelled an accelerating epidemic. In 1950 an injectable form appeared, and the epidemic reached its peak in 1954 when there were an estimated half million regular users. Fifty thousand people were treated that year for amphetamine psychosis, and there was a very clear association with crime and violence.

By the 1950s, pill misuse in the US was gaining momentum and the term 'speed freak' was coined. This did not inhibit the continuing expansion of the legal use of amphetamine, with politicians and housewives alike using it as a pick-me-up. The first restrictions on use were introduced in Britain in 1956, but this did little to rein in demand. In the early 1960s, neurasthenia (chronic fatigue) was accounting for a quarter of all amphetamine prescriptions. In 1964, nearly four million prescriptions for amphetamine were issued in Britain, making up 2% of all prescriptions written that year, and in 1971 12 billion tablets were manufactured for medical use in the US. In combination with short-acting barbiturates, amphetamines were found to be a useful aid to interrogation by operatives of various security services.

Pill misuse reached London early in 1960, and a survey among Borstal boys revealed that a third were regular users. A growing black market developed in amphetamine sulphate (Bennies), dexamphetamine (Dexies), methylphenidate (Rit), methamphetamine (Meths, crystal), and Durophet (Black Bombers). A particular favourite among the Mods (a youth cult identified by a particular taste in music and dress) was Drinamyl (Purple Hearts), a potentially lethal combination of amphetamine and barbiturate. In 1964 the law in Britain was tightened, but expansion of the black market sustained the growing epidemic. Injectable methamphetamine prescribing by doctors in the newly formed drug dependency units enjoyed a brief vogue, but several cases of psychosis among recipients caused this to go rapidly out of fashion.

Illicit amphetamine was available in the US from 1962 onwards, but the industry only really took off when the drug was withdrawn from prescription. In the mid-1960s, motorcycle gangs became heavily involved in the manufacture and distribution of methamphetamine ('crank'), a drug whose effects matched closely the violent, high-energy, and high-risk lifestyle they represented. Wide publicity of its damage potential and increased availability of cocaine seemed to limit uptake in the 1970s, but the following decade saw a massive resurgence. Methamphetamine has always been particularly popular in the West and South West of the US, and this has been linked to the particular targeting of cannabis by the authorities in these areas leading to a gap in the market. A similar explanation has been put forward to explain the sudden epidemic of methamphetamine smoking in Hawaii in the late 1980s when socially integrated use of cannabis was vigorously suppressed, leaving the way open to the infinitely more damaging 'ice'.

The risks were well recognized by the streetwise. As Frank Zappa, quoted by Shapiro (1988)) put it: '*I would like to suggest that you don't use speed, and here is why: it will mess up your liver, your kidneys, rot out your mind. In general, this drug will make you just like your parents'.*

Preparation and distribution

Pharmaceutical dexamphetamine sulphate (Dexedrine) and methylphenidate (Ritalin) are often prescribed for narcolepsy and attention deficit hyperactivity disorder (ADHD), and diversion of both drugs to the black market is commonplace. They are also available quite easily via the internet. Modafinil (Provigil) is also used to treat narcolepsy and other causes of excessive daytime sleepiness.

Since the mid-1980s there has been a rapid, world-wide upswing in the illegal manufacture of amphetamines and methcathinone as reflected by the number of illicit laboratories discovered. Vast increases in sales of the chemical precursors (e.g. Ephedrine) have also been noted. Easy availability of the necessary ingredients and the simplicity of the manufacturing process mean that supplies are often produced near the point of consumption and can accurately reflect local demand. Many European, Australian, South American, and African laboratories produce amphetamine sulphate, whereas in the US, Mexico, and much of Asia the emphasis is on methamphetamine.

Methamphetamine production has expanded greatly in recent years and it is now the most commonly produced illegal synthetic drug. It is a major illicit industry in Myanmar (Burma), Thailand, China, North Korea, the Philippines, Mexico, and the US. Alongside the thousands of small, mobile, or transient illegal laboratories are a few hundred 'superlabs' capable of large scale production, and it is estimated that this relatively small number of industrial-scale enterprises account for 80% of the black market supply. Well over 10,000 kg are seized each year in Asia alone. A currently popular route of manufacture is based on diverted pseudoephedrine medicines. The UK is a major consumer of amphetamines, most of which are imported rather than produced locally.

Methcathinone was first synthesized in 1928 and subsequently used as an antidepressant in Soviet Russia up to the end of the 1940s. Its recreational use has in the past been largely restricted to the countries of the former Soviet Union, though it now appears to be gaining wider popularity.

Scientific information

Dexamphetamine sulphate is well absorbed when swallowed or snorted, its effects peak after an hour and last up to eight hours. Methylphenidate has a similar pattern of onset and peak activity, but a shorter duration of action.

Amphetamine bears a close structural relationship to the neurotransmitters noradrenaline (norepinephrine) and dopamine, and its interaction with terminals of catecholaminergic neurones causes their release. A similar effect on noradrenaline neurones outside the brain stimulates the 'fight and flight' mechanism of the sympathetic nervous system. The overall pharmacological effects are similar to those of cocaine, albeit with a much longer duration of action. If this is disguised experimentally, experienced users find it difficult to distinguish the two drugs.

Amphetamine is very potent in animal models of dependency potential. This behaviour is inhibited by the dopamine-blocking drug pimozide, and long-term amphetamine use is associated with depletion of dopamine stores in the dopamine-powered 'reward pathway' (see section on cocaine above). Amphetamine can produce irreversible damage to dopamine nerves in animals, but the significance of this for humans remains unclear. Its impact seems to vary in different parts of the brain, in that receptors in some regions are more responsive to it than others: for example, dopamine D_2 receptors in hippocampus show minimal response.

Methamphetamine is chemically and pharmacologically similar to amphetamine, but the effect on catecholamine neurones is more intense and longer lasting. A greater depletion of dopamine may result in tolerance developing more quickly and a more pronounced withdrawal syndrome. However, the major difference lies in the route of administration, since smoking or injecting a drug vastly increases its impact and potential for damage. The purity of both drugs on the black market varies hugely but currently averages around 50% in the US and UK. Methcathinone is structurally and pharmacologically very similar to methamphetamine.

Potentially dangerous interactions occur with a variety of other drugs, including anaesthetics (heart irregularities), antidepressants (heart irregularities, soaring blood pressure), blood pressure-lowering tablets (antagonizes effect), and 'beta-blockers' (soaring blood pressure).

In overdose, the elimination of amphetamine is much more rapid when the urine is acid. In hospital, this is achieved through the use of ammonium chloride, but the same result can be achieved when medical help is not at hand with large doses of vitamin C.

Medical uses

Use of dexamphetamine, methamphetamine, methylphenidate, and atomoxetine (a noradernergic-specific stimulant) in medicine is now limited to the treatment of severely overactive children, in whom it has a paradoxical calming effect, and narcolepsy (pathological sleepiness). When used in appropriate patients, the risk of dependence or abuse seems very low.

Modafinil (Provigil) is a relatively new drug licenced in several countries to improve wakefulness in narcolepsy patients, obstructive sleep apnoea syndrome, and shift work sleep disorder. The pharmacological mechanism is uncertain but brain dopamine levels are enhanced and modafinil does produce stimulant-like psychoactivity, alterations in mood, perception, and thinking. It also has reinforcing properties in laboratory models and therefore a modest abuse potential.

Recreational use

According to the UN, amphetamines are currently used by around 25 million people world-wide, equivalent to 0.6% of the adult population. This prevalence has been roughly stable since the turn of the century. This overshadows both opiate (15 million) and cocaine use (13 million). Methamphetamine use accounts for 60% of the total, with the remainder shared equally between amphetamine and diverted pharmaceuticals or other synthetics such as methcathinone. Up to two thirds of all stimulant users live in Asia. Apart from those already mentioned, other stimulants available on the black market include fenetylline, phenmetrazine, amfepramone, pemoline, and phentermine.

In the US and Europe there are around 3.7 million and 2.7 million users respectively. In most countries use seems to be slowly declining, but this is offset by sharp increases in a few areas such as North Eastern and South Eastern Europe. This decline is particularly marked in the UK, hitherto Europe's biggest amphetamine market: annual prevalence of overall use declined by 60% between 1996 and 2007 and methamphetamine use remains very unusual. Prevalence in European school students varied widely last year between countries from zero (Greece, Romania, Cyprus) to 7% (Estonia).

Dexedrine (dexamphetamine) is marketed as a small, white 5 mg tablet, while illegally manufactured amphetamine sulphate (speed; whizz; sulphate; billy; bennie; christina; dexies; leapers; sparklers; uppers) is usually sold in wraps or packages of whitish powder (occasionally other colours as a marketing gimmick) costing £10 per gram or less in the UK. The powder can be wrapped in a cigarette paper and swallowed ('bombed', 'Rizla'd'), stirred into a drink, snorted into the nose, or dissolved in water for intravenous injection. Smoking it is less rewarding because the high temperature required to vapourize it destroys most of the active material. When snorted the powder often stings quite unpleasantly, but within a few minutes there is an onset of effects which closely resemble those of cocaine: good cheer, vivacity, and optimism; increased energy and self-confidence; sharpened perception and concentration; reduced appetite for food and sleep. The main differences lie in the much longer duration of action, and the greater relative intensity of peripheral effects such as a racing heart and dry mouth. Decreased sensitivity (tolerance) to the euphoric effects develops rapidly, so that in compulsive users the same binge profile as occurs with cocaine can be anticipated. The intensity of the effects will be limited by the purity of the material, which is likely to be lower than would be usual with cocaine. This difference may have given rise to the false impression that cocaine is a more powerful drug than amphetamine. When injected, a powerful 'rush' or 'flash' is noted within seconds, and both the mental and physical effects are much more pronounced.

Methamphetamine (ice; crystal; glass; tina; christine; crank; crypto; meth) is available as a tablet, powder, oily paste, or in crystalline form. Prices of powder in the US are between $40–120 per gram, and considerably more for crystal which is usually smoked for a particularly intense effect. Yaba is the name (of Thai derivation) for a tablet usually containing a mixture of methamphetamine and caffeine popular amongst clubbers.

Unwanted effects

Community surveys indicate that the majority of amphetamine consumers use the drug quite infrequently in relatively modest doses by the oral route, and in these circumstances the prevalence of problems seems low. Adverse effects correlate quite closely with dose and frequency of use, and are much more common in those who inject or smoke the drug. The likelihood of drug-related problems is unsurprisingly greater in those with pre-existing mental health problems, and inversely related to educational attainment.

As with cocaine, frequent ingestion causes rapidly diminishing sensitivity to the euphoric effects but not to the potentially dangerous effects on the heart. Deaths have been reported from heart attacks and strokes, hyperthermia, and convulsions. High blood pressure and damage to small blood vessels in the eye may occur in chronic users. It seems often to cause rashes, and heavy users may find their teeth rot because of a loss of dentine. Euphoria may be at least partially replaced by depression, paranoia, or aggression ('tweaking').

Amphetamine taken in pregnancy may pose a risk to the healthy development of the baby's heart and bile system, has been linked with cleft palate, and is said to be associated with small-for-dates babies.

Irritability, suspiciousness, heightened aggression, and an unpleasant 'wired' sensation may be prominent, for the relief of which the user may turn to alcohol, sedatives, or opiates. Rapid changes in mood, flight of ideas, and physical tension may culminate in impulsive violence. Methamphetamine has a particular association with aggressive and violent behaviour. As the drug wears off, the user is likely to feel depressed and washed out.

The pattern of immediate and long-term unwanted effects is very similar to that described above for cocaine, except that the time between the escalating doses as the run builds momentum is longer because of the slower rate of metabolism. Binges are followed by a short period of exhaustion and sleep, from which the user emerges into a phase of lethargy and inertia, often accompanied by anxiety or depression which may become intense enough to induce thoughts of suicide or actual self-harm. The temptation to use more amphetamine is tremendous at this stage but, if resisted successfully, a gradual return to normal can be anticipated. Occasionally, anxiety or depression persists for months or even years.

The original description of amphetamine psychosis in 1958 has become a classic paper in psychiatry (Connell, 1958). This alarming condition usually occurs in long-term, high-dose users, but has been recorded after a single ingestion. It comes on a day or two after exposure, and consists of hallucinations (false perceptions which may be visual, auditory, or skin sensation, or any combination of these), disordered thinking, and delusions of persecution. These experiences seem completely real to the sufferer. Pointless, repetitive behaviours sometimes appear, and there may be involuntary picking and scratching at the skin. These symptoms usually disappear gradually after a week or so of abstinence, but occasionally last much longer or become indistinguishable from schizophrenia.

Tolerance (diminishing sensitivity to the drug) causes many regular, long-term users to build their doses up to several grams of street material daily. Emotional lability, poor concentration, insomnia, and fluctuating paranoia are quite common. Heavy consumption of alcohol, benzodiazepines, or opiates may represent an attempt to overcome these effects. A physical withdrawal syndrome is not prominent on giving up amphetamine but depression, fatigue, lack of pleasure in life, extreme craving for drugs, and sleep disturbance are common and may last for weeks or months. Vulnerability to psychological dependence on amphetamines has a strong genetic component, overlapping with increased likelihood of abusing alcohol and other drugs.

In animal models there is consistent evidence that amphetamines are capable of both structural and chemical damage to nerves in parts of the brain which are rich in dopamine and serotonin cells, though the relevance of this finding to human users is unclear. Methcathinone has been associated with an outbreak of Parkinson's disease in Latvia.

Other stimulants

Khat (or Qat)

The stems and leaves of the shrub *Catha edulis* contain a number of psychoactive chemicals, and can be chewed or made into a tea. The most powerful constituent is cathinone, an amphetamine-like stimulant, which is unstable and breaks down spontaneously within days of the plant being picked. Cathinone is prohibited under the Misuse of Drugs Act (1971), whilst Khat itself is not a prohibited substance in the UK, but is illegal in the US.

The shrub is cultivated over large areas of East Africa and the Arabian peninsula, where chewing the leaves has been customary for centuries. Like coca leaves, they induce a sense of energy and well-being, but are also prone to cause stomach upsets, irritability, or sleeplessness. Their use has also been associated with oral cancer and liver disease, but it is difficult to tease out a direct effect from that of detrimental environmental conditions or contaminants. The risk of psychosis and compulsive use is well recognized locally. Unless the leaves are fresh, diarrhoea is likely to be the only consequence noted by the consumer.

Among a group of Somalis living in London, three-quarters of those interviewed had used khat in the past and 86% of these were current users. On average this would happen three times weekly in the evening in a social context. The leaves are sold in bundles costing £5, and the average consumption was seven bundles a month. Adults questioned said they would much prefer their children to use khat rather than alcohol or cigarettes (though 60% of the sample themselves smoked).

Unwanted effects were common but generally mild, and included sleep disturbance, reduced appetite, mood swings, anxiety and panic, depression, and irritability. Dependency upon khat appeared unusual, but many people admitted using more in London than they had in Somalia.

Benzylpiperazine

Benzylpiperazine (BZP, Legal E) was synthesized in 1944 as a potential pharmaceutical, but its amphetamine-like effects have led to its recreational use since the mid-1990s. In many countries (but not the US or UK) it remains technically legal. It is available in powder, tablets of varying colours and capsules, is usually taken orally but sometimes smoked or snorted, and is popular with clubbers as an alternative to amphetamine or MDMA.

Its pharmacology is very similar to that of the amphetamines, but much less potent. Its toxicity profile and dependency-producing potential is probably also comparable with amphetamine sulphate.

Pemoline

Pemoline (round, white, bi-convex tablets marked P9) is a milder alternative to amphetamine in the treatment of overactive children, with a similar duration of action. In addition to the usual amphetamine-like unwanted effect, it some-times proves damaging to the liver and bone marrow and is no longer available on prescription in the UK for this reason.

Appetite suppressants

Some appetite suppressants act by exerting mild amphetamine-like effects, and thus have some modest value on the black market. They include diethyl-propion, mazindol, and phentermine.

Selected references

Advisory Council on the Misuse of Drugs (2005). *Khat (Qat): Assessment of risk to the individual and communities in the UK.* Home Office, London.

Advisory Council on the Misuse of Drugs (2005). *Methylamphetamine review.* Home Office, London.

Bateman, D. A., Ng, S. K. C., Hansen, C. A., Heagarty, M. C. (1993). The effects of intra-uterine cocaine exposure in newborns. *American Journal of Public Health*, **83**, 190–3.

Chen, K., Scheier, L. M., Kandel, D. B. (1996). Effects of chronic cocaine use on physical health: a prospective study in a general population sample. *Drug and Alcohol Dependence*, **43**, 23–7.

Chiarello, R. J., Cole, J. O. (1987). The use of psychostimulants in general psychiatry. *Archives of General Psychiatry*, **44**, 288–95.

Connell, P. H. (1958). Amphetamine psychosis. *Maudsley Monograph No. 5.* Oxford University Press, Oxford.

Gawin, F. H. (1991). Cocaine addiction: psychology and neurophysiology. *Science*, **251**, 1580–6.

Gawin, F. H., Kleber, H. D. (1986). Abstinence symptomatology and psychiatric diagnosis in cocaine abusers. *Archives of General Psychiatry*, **43**, 107–13.

Gawin, F. H., Ellinwood, E. H. (1988). Cocaine and other stimulants. *New England Journal of Medicine*, **318**, 1173–82.

Gawin, F. H., Kleber, H. D., Byck, R., Rounsaville, B. J., Kosten, T. R., Jatlow, P. I., et al. (1989). Desipramine facilitation of initial cocaine abstinence. *Archives of General Psychiatry*, **46**, 117–21.

Glasner-Edwards S, Mooney LJ, Marinelli-Casey P et al. (2008). Identifying methampheta-mine users at risk for major depressive disorder: findings from the methamphetamine treatment project at three year follow-up. *American Journal of Addiction* **17**, 99–102.

Gossop, M., Griffiths, P., Powis, B., Strang, J. (1994). Cocaine: patterns of use, route of administration, and severity of dependence. *British Journal of Psychiatry*, **164**, 660–4.

Gonzales R., Ang A., McCann M. J., Rawson R. (2008). An emerging problem: methamphetamine use among treatment-seeking youth. *Substance Abuse* **29**, 71–80.

Griffin, M. L., Weiss, R. D., Mirin, S. M., Lange, U. (1989). A comparison of male and female cocaine abusers. *Archives of General Psychiatry*, **46**, 122–5.

Griffiths, P., Gossop, M., Wickenden, S., Dunworth, J., Harris, K., Lloyd, C. (1997). A transcultural pattern of drug use: qat (khat) in the UK. British Journal of Psychiatry, **170**, 281–4.

Hall, W., Hando, J., Darke, S., Ross, J. (1996). Psychological morbidity and route of administration among amphetamine users in Sydney, Australia. *Addiction*, **91**, 81–7.

Hando, J., Flaherty, B., Rutter, S. (1997). An Australian profile on the use of cocaine. *Addiction*, **92**, 173–82.

Hulse, G. K., English, D. R., Milne, E., Holman, C. J. D., Bower, C. I. (1997). Maternal cocaine use and low-birth-weight newborns: a meta-analysis. *Addiction*, **92**, 1561–70.

Hulse, G. K., Milne, E., English, D. R., Holman, C. J. D. (1997). Assessing the relationship between maternal cocaine use and abruptio placentae. *Addiction*, **92**, 1547–51.

Iversen, L. (2008). *What are amphetamines and how do they work in the brain?* In: Speed, Ecstasy, Ritalin: the Science of Amphetamines pp. 5–27. Oxford University Press, Oxford.

Kleber, H. D. (1988). Epidemic cocaine abuse: America's present, Britain's future? *British Journal of Addiction*, **83**, 1359–71.

Klee, H. (1997). (ed.) *Amphetamine misuse.* Harwood Academy Publishers, The Netherlands.

McCord J, Jneid H, Hollander JE et al. (2008). Management of cocaine-related chest pain and myocardial infarction. *Circulation* **117**, 1897–1907.

Musto, D. F. (1973). Sherock Holmes and Sigmund Freud: a study in cocaine, *History of Medicine*, **5**, 16–20.

Musto, D. F. (1991). Opium, cocaine, and marijuana in American history. *Scientific American*, **July**, 40–7.

Newcomb, M. D., Bentler, P. M. (1986). Cocaine use among adolescents: longitudinal associations with social context, psychopathology, and use of other substances. *Addictive Behaviours*, **11**, 263–73.

Orson F. M., Kinsey B. M., Singh R. A. et al. (2008). Substance abuse vaccines. *Annals of the New York Academy of Sciences* **1141**, 257–69.

Robson, P., Bruce, M. (1997). A comparison of 'visible' and 'invisible' users of amphetamine, cocaine, and heroin: two distinct populations? *Addiction*, **92**, 1729–36.

Shapiro, H. (1989). Crack: a briefing from the Institute for the Study of Drug Dependence. *Druglink*, Sept/Oct, 8–11.

Sobanski E., Schredl M., Kettler N., Alm.B. (2008). Sleep in adults with attention deficit hyperactivity disorder (ADHD) before and during treatment with methylphenidate: a controlled polysomnographic study. *Sleep* **31**, 375–81.

Stepens A, Logina I, Liguts V et al. (2008). A Parkinsonian syndrome in methcathinone users and the role of manganese. *New England Journal of Medicine* **358**, 1009–17.

Strang, J., Edwards, G. (1989). Cocaine and crack: the drug and the hype are both dangerous. *British Medical Journal*, **299**, 337–8.

Strang, J., Griffiths, P., Gossop, M. (1990). Crack and cocaine use in South London drug addicts: 1987–1989. *British Journal of Addiction*, **85**, 193–6.

Swerdlow, N. R., Hauger, R., Irwin, et al. (1991). Endocrine, immune, and neurochemical changes in rats during withdrawal from chronic amphetamine intoxication. *Neuropsychopharmacology*, **5**, 23–31.

Uhl G. R,. Drgon T., Liu Q. R. et al. (2008). Genome-wide association for methamphetamine dependence: convergent results from 2 samples. *Archives of General Psychiatry* **65**, 345–55.

Volkow N. D., Swanson J. M. (2008). Does childhood treatment of ADHD with stimulant medication affect substance abuse in adulthood? *American Journal of Psychiatry* **165**, 553–5.

Winston A. P., Hardwick E., Jaberi N. (2005). Neuropsychiatric effects of caffeine. *Advances in Psychiatric Treatment* **11**, 432–9.

Chapter 7

Psychedelics and hallucinogens

Invited Co-author: Ethan Russo

The defining characteristic of this group of drugs is their ability to induce profound changes in sensory perception, patterns of thinking, and emotion without at the same time clouding the mind. Terminology is difficult, because it always seems to be judgement-laden; one person's *psychotomimetic* (psychosis mimicker) is another's *psycholytic* (literally mind loosener, and by implication, consciousness expander). *Hallucinogen* is a widely used label derived from the Latin *alucinari* ('to wander in the mind'), which somehow fails to do justice to the complexity of the human response to these substances. The term *true hallucinogen* is perhaps most appropriately applied to crude natural preparations, or to those drugs which disrupt mental functioning to the point of delirium (a mixture of delusions, hallucinations, confusion, disorientation, and memory disturbance) with loss of external frame of reference. For those drugs which have the property of 'blowing the mind' without impairing orientation and consciousness, the word coined in the 1950s by the psychiatrist Humphrey Osmond in the course of his correspondence with Aldous Huxley seems very suitable. '*Psychodelic*' was derived from the Greek words *psyche* (mind) and *delos* (visible). The minor modification, psychedelic, became the noun and adjective of choice.

Historical background

There are hundreds of plants and fungi with hallucinogenic properties which have been used for centuries in a prodigious variety of rituals throughout the Old and New Worlds, but the serendipitous discovery of an immensely potent, synthetic psychedelic in the mid-20th century had a much wider impact upon Western society. It provided the motive force for a counter-culture which developed with great rapidity, ushering in a period of artistic creativity and carrying at its heart a philosophy of life which posed a short-lived but formidable challenge to the existing world order.

Hallucinogenic plants, along with fermented drinks and cannabis, have been used for thousands of years in social and religious rituals, for healing, and as a means of brief escape from a life which might well have been, as in medieval Britain, 'nasty, brutish, and short'. Indeed, it has been proposed that occasional periods of altered consciousness are a necessity for mental health (see Chapter 1).

Solanaceous plants were the source of a number of these hallucinogens, often of peculiar toxicity. Datura, Brugmansia, pituri, mandrake, and henbane are rich in substances which interfere with the action of acetylcholine, one of the brain's important chemical messengers. Traces of black henbane have been discovered at the sites of prehistoric settlements in Britain, and medieval witches were wise in the ways of hallucinogenic potions and unguents, mirroring shamanic activities continents away in the Amazon basin. Apart from alcohol, opium, and cannabis the ingredients of ancient European concoctions might include thorn apple, sweet flag, deadly nightshade, black henbane, and mandrake, bearing their heavy load of the tropane alkaloids scopolamine and atropine.

The Europeans who first settled in North America were fascinated by a local weed which had been a favourite of the native population for centuries. They christened it Jamestown Weed, and as jimsonweed it is still known today. Alkaloids contained in such substances induce a delirious state, but may also produce loss of muscular control, temporary blindness, and paralysis. Many of their less toxic derivatives still find a use in medicine today.

More than 100 psilocybin-containing mushrooms grow freely world-wide. The Aztecs were familiar with the easily recognizable, bright yellow Liberty Cap, which they called the 'flesh of the Gods', but they were also well aware that the safety margin of many other hallucinogenic mushrooms, for example *Amanita muscaria* or 'fly agaric', is dangerously small. These mushrooms produce a similar range of effects to LSD, although less intense and shorter in duration. One should avoid at all costs *Amanita phalloides* ('Death Cap), the cause of the vast majority of mushroom fatalities, or experiments with unidentified small brown mushrooms that may prove much more toxic than psychedelic. Psilocybin is a Schedule 1 controlled drug in the US and possession or sale of hallucinogenic mushrooms was made illegal in the UK in 2005 and the Netherlands in 2008, though they remain legal in some European countries and Canada.

Harmaloid alkaloids, found in the seeds of various shrubs and vines growing in Arabia and Southern and Central America, provided the kick in a whole range of hallucinogenic snuffs and drinks still used ritually today. Empirical indigenous biochemists discovered that combining these materials with dimethyltryptamine (DMT)-donor plants such as Psychotria rendered them orally active and generously psychoactive.

There is an extensive history of psychedelic plant usage in neotropical Native American cultures, most often based upon use of DMT-containing plants. Some evidence suggests that this extremely powerful, if short-acting, psychedelic agent is present in trace amounts in the normal brain, where its function remains unknown. Whilst commonly employed in various psychoactive snuffs, and even eye drops, its most familiar form is as a transendant beverage when combined with *Banisteriopsis caapi*, variously termed *yage, yahe, hoasca,* or *ayahuasca*, the 'vine of the soul'. This usage is widespread in the Amazon Basin, and the associated ritual is an integral part of indigenous culture and cosmology, wherein its employment is considered diagnostic and therapeutic of many maladies, as well as an essential aid to survival in a hostile environment.

Ibogaine, containing similar compounds, retains an important role in ceremonials of certain African societies. It was described by European missionaries in Africa in 1860 and extracted from root material in 1901, and is notably powerful and long-lasting at the expense of enhanced toxicity.

The search throughout the world for new sources of such materials capable of catalyzing entry into the mystic realm left no stone, or creature, unturned; the fact that the skin secretions of certain toads such as the Sonoran Desert toad (*Bufo alvarius*) were rich in a powerful hallucinogen did not escape notice. This produces a psychedelic state awash with intense visual effects of short duration, but with a claimed prolonged 'afterglow'. Pleasure may be somewhat constrained by paroxysmal vomiting or vertiginous dizziness.

Highly toxic mescal beans, psilocybin mushrooms, lysergic acid-containing seeds of the Morning Glory plant, and the mescaline-rich tips of the peyote cactus were used ritually in the Americas thousands of years before the birth of Christ. Partially suppressed for centuries, a formidable peyote cult resurfaced amongst Native Americans towards the end of the 19th century. At that time, peyote enjoyed a brief vogue as a constituent of patent medicines and tonics. As a result of this interest, mescaline was isolated in the 1890s and quickly established a place in Bohemian circles. It also found a niche in psychiatric practice, mainly in the hands of people who were observing and trying to understand psychosis. The use of peyote in the religious practices of the Native American church grew steadily during the 20th century. Four or five cactus tops will produce effects similar in intensity and duration to a modest dose of LSD, though possibly with a greater effect on heart rate and blood pressure.

The pivotal event which was to unleash the phenomenon of psychedelia upon the world occurred in 1943 when Albert Hofmann, a research scientist at the Sandoz pharmaceutical company, accidentally ingested a microscopic amount of a chemical he had isolated five years previously while searching for a new heart stimulant. Feeling restless and dizzy, he lay down and experienced a pleasurable dream-like state lasting a couple of hours. Three days later, he decided to explore its effect further by taking what he thought was a miniscule dose, 250 micrograms, of the new substance which he had labelled lysergic acid diethylamide-25. Bearing in mind that anything over 50 micrograms is enough to produce a hallucinatory effect, the impact of the first recorded 'acid trip' upon Hofmann can readily be imagined. Although at times he feared for his sanity and experienced a cornucopia of the awesome, the inspiring, and the grotesque, he was in no doubt as to the significance and potential benefits of what he later referred to as 'my problem child'.

Hofmann's report of his experience unleashed a flurry of scientific activity. The medical and psychiatric use of LSD expanded rapidly after it was first marketed in 1949 with well over 100,000 patients in the US and Europe receiving it during the 1950s. Indications included depression, anxiety, obsessive-compulsive disorders, alcoholism, neuroses, sociopathy, physical symptoms with no discoverable cause, tiredness, chronic pain, comfort for the dying, and, most frequently of all, as an adjunct to various forms of psychotherapy. Many positive outcomes were reported in the scientific literature, which by the mid-1960s numbered more than 2,000 publications. Outright cures of migraine and psoriasis were claimed after LSD therapy.

The CIA became interested in applications of quite a different nature, since this appeared to be a substance which might facilitate interrogation or the reprogramming of those who had been 'brainwashed'. Field tests included the administration of LSD to agents and others without their knowledge or consent, and on at least one well-documented occasion this had a tragic outcome when an individual in the grip of a prolonged psychotic state after receiving the drug threw himself out of a window. Many mainstream scientific explorations were also ethically unacceptable from a modern perspective with their use of prisoners, autistic children, and psychiatric patients whose mental state made it impossible for them to understand properly the nature of the experiment.

Many neologisms were coined to describe these new drugs, including *phantastica, psycholytics, psychotogenics, psychodysleptics*, and some with even more syllables, as well as Humphrey Osmond's *psychedelics*. Osmond was an imaginative psychiatrist working in Canada at the forefront of clinical research with LSD. Visiting California, he corresponded with Aldous Huxley who agreed to act as an experimental subject in an investigation and analysis of the subjective effects of mescaline. The resulting experiences were published in the book *Doors of Perception* (1954), the title taken from the quotation by William Blake: '*If the doors of perception were cleansed, everything will appear to man as it is, infinite*'. Huxley thought that mescaline '. . . *lowers the efficiency of the brain as an instrument for focusing mind on the problems of life on the surface of our planet*'.

This interference with the brain's efficiency '. . . *seems to permit entry into consciousness of certain classes of mental events which are normally excluded because they possess no survival value*'. Huxley believed that the relentlessly materialistic focus of modern Western society had robbed its citizens of the spiritual dimension which is essential for true contentment. He came to believe that psychedelics could bring this within the reach of every citizen, and that permanent and beneficial changes in attitudes and values would result from allowing ordinary people access to them.

The use of psychedelics soon spread beyond the little world of clinicians and lofty aesthetes into the grasp of earthier souls. Writers such as Ken Kesey and Allen Ginsburg became high-profile users and protagonists, and William Burroughs boasted his experiences with yagé. Jazz musicians such as Thelonius Monk, Dizzy Gillespie, and John Coltrane were early consumers, and classical musicians also experimented with the effects of psychedelics on musical creativity and interpretation. Timothy Leary, a previously rather conventional Harvard psychologist, took psilocybin mushrooms in 1960 and was '*swept over the edge of a sensory Niagara into a maelstrom of transcendental visions and hallucinations*'. Feeling that his life had been changed fundamentally and irrevocably, he began a series of psychedelic experiments with friends, colleagues, and students. His catchphrase 'turn on, tune in, drop out' became a mantra for the hip generation and an excoriant for parents, teachers, and the rest of that great army of what he saw as robotic 'straights'. He also drew attention to the importance of 'set and setting' in determining the effects of drugs; the attitudes, personality, and expectations of the taker, and the nature of the environment in which the drug is taken. He launched a personal attack on convention and ritual. Accused of being a psychopath, he riposted that '*there is no such thing as personal responsibility*'. Introduced to LSD by Allen Ginsberg and Michael Hollingshead, he gained access through them to the musicians, writers, and millionaires who were spearheading the new cultural movement. The scandal generated by the Harvard connection was important in gaining the interest of the mass media and nurturing the growth of the hippy movement.

Sacked from Harvard in 1963, Leary founded with others the International Foundation for Internal Freedom (IFIF) to pursue the study and propagation of psychedelia. He foresaw a time when every student would be 'turned on' in order to spearhead a New World Order. Expelled from his base in Mexico, he returned to the US to set up the Millbrook Foundation in 1964 with the backing of a wealthy friend. Meanwhile, Michael Hollingshead had set up the World Psychedelic Centre in London, patronized by hip rock musicians and street poets of the emergent 'swinging London'. The dissolution of the amphetamine-driven Mod scene in favour of the hash and acid atmosphere of hippiedom had begun.

On the proceeds of his novel *One Flew Over The Cuckoo's Nest* (1960), Ken Kesey bought a large estate close to San Francisco which became a focus and magnet for like-minded writers, musicians, and acolytes. This was the setting for the notorious 'acid tests' in which gatherings of people drank Kool-Aid spiked with LSD and talked, played music, or made love. A folk–rock band called 'The Warlocks' was a frequent fixture at these happenings. Later the band changed its name to 'The Grateful Dead' and spearheaded the West Coast acid rock scene. Kesey's riotous and creative band of 'Merry Pranksters' voyaged in their ancient fluorescent bus in a stoned odyssey across America, shocking and outraging the straights and recording it all on 48 hours of uneditable film. They journeyed to Millbrook for a meeting of minds with the Leary group, but found them disappointingly staid and serious! Anyone wishing to pick up the flavour of these extraordinary times should read Tom Wolfe's account in *The Electric Kool-Aid Acid Test* (1969).

The hippie philosophy had at its heart an unstable mixture of straightforward hedonism, rejection of existing cultural values and conventional morality, snippets of Eastern religion, and repudiation of personal and institutionalized violence. Its epicentre in the early days was in the Haight-Ashbury area of San Francisco, but its cultural energy washed through Britain and mainland Europe. The psychedelic movement injected its unique style of music, art, and life-view into almost every level of Western culture. Scarcely a single segment of society could avoid reacting to it, even if this reaction took the form of disparagement or contempt. It generated its own journalistic voice; *Berkely Barb, International Times, Oracle, Oz.*

The Grateful Dead, Cream, Jefferson Airplane, Pink Floyd, Soft Machine, The Incredible String Band, Traffic, Donovan – the list of musicians reflecting the psychedelic influence is endless. The Beatles' musical style changed strikingly as they became caught up, as is clear from the album *Rubber Soul* onwards. The music industry was not slow to recognize the bonanza on the horizon; it was at this time that the long-playing record first came into sharp commercial focus. Some have even argued that the 'acid revolution' was largely funded and driven by the profit-seeking strategies of the record industry. Perhaps the peak, the heyday, of the hippie era was represented by the 1967 'Summer of Love' in Northern California, where flower power found its finest hour.

The consumption of LSD skyrocketed within this cultural revolution. In 1962 it was estimated that 25,000 Americans had tried it, and by 1965 this figure had leapt to four million. In the same year, the first federal law controlling its manufacture stopped short of outlawing individual possession, but more restrictive state laws soon followed and created the climate for the nation-wide ban introduced in 1968 making mere possession a felony offence. Britain had already proscribed it in 1966, and Sandoz simultaneously ceased produc-tion for the licit market. These developments stimulated the emergence of entrepreneurial underground chemists some of whom, such as Augustus Owsley Stanley III – 'the man who did for LSD what Henry Ford did for the motor car' – were ideologically involved and not driven primarily by the profit motive. These individuals were often skilled enough to make a high-quality crysalline, even piezo-luminescent product, one of Stanley's more memorable vintages being immortalized by Jimi Hendrix's chartbuster, *Purple Haze*.

After 1967, the tawdriness that was never far from the surface became more evident. The commercial exploitation of the hippie culture by both commerce and the criminal underworld grew rapidly in scale. Nowhere was this deterio-ration more evident than in Haight-Ashbury itself, with daily street violence over methamphetamine deals or poor-quality acid cut with phencyclidine (PCP) and busloads of gawping tourists patrolling the area as if it were some kind of wildlife theme park. Icons tumbled. In 1968, Timothy Leary was jailed on marijuana charges, and although his life remained no less colourful with escapes, recaptures, and eventual pardon, he never regained his former influence or prominence. Even the musical associations began to turn sour: at the post-Woodstock Altamont Rock Festival in 1969, Hell's Angels stabbed and beat a man to death in front of the stage where the Rolling Stones were performing. This and the subsequent free-for-all were blamed on the mixture of alcohol, amphetamine, and bathtub-quality LSD freely available at the concert.

Scare stories surrounding LSD gathered pace in the media. Sensationalized accounts of suicides, madness, blindness from staring into the sun, sexual orgies involving prominent people, and acid-head mothers giving birth to deformed babies began to change the public perception of psychedelics. Charles Manson shocked the world with his grotesque violence, his compul-sive hold over his 'family' apparently greatly enhanced by their shared use of LSD. Law enforcement became more determined, and a number of under-ground chemists were given long prison sentences in the early 1970s. From the middle of the decade until the early 1980s, LSD was in short supply and the trade in mushrooms and mescaline (usually PCP or similar artificial substitute in reality) took over. After this, the illicit industry recovered and reasonably pure LSD has been available in most UK and US cities to the present day. It is a Schedule I (US) Class A (UK) controlled drug. Interest in the pos-sible medical applications of psychedelics continued in a low-key manner: a temporary relaxation of the law in Switzerland in the late 1980s permitted some clinical research in the use of LSD in patients with emotional and personality disorders.

A number of synthetic molecules developed originally by the pharmaceutical industry have been diverted to recreational use in pursuit of their hallucinatory effects. Phencyclidine (PCP) was marketed in the 1950s as an anaesthetic free of respiratory or heart depression, but was soon restricted to veterinary use as its dissociative and hallucinatory side-effects became apparent. The most notable of these were delirium and confusion on emergence from anaesthetic. It was completely withdrawn in 1965 as awareness grew of escalating street use. Since 1978 it has been classified within Schedule II of the US Controlled Substances Act (CSA), and it is a Class A drug under the UK Misuse of Drugs Act (MDA). Gammahydroxybutyrate (GHB or GBH in UK) was developed in the US as a possible anaesthetic and premedicant for surgery, but its authorization for medical use was removed in 1990 because of unwanted effects. It was freely available as a health food product advertised for its sleep-enhancing and weight control activity until March 2000, when it was classified within Schedule I of the CSA. In the UK, it is restricted within Class C under the MDA. GHB is popular as a euphoriant on the club scene, and among body-builders as a muscle-bulking agent. Ketamine (Ketalar), a derivative of PCP, was synthesized in 1962. It is used in medicine as an intravenous anaesthetic, but its application is limited by a high incidence of hallucinations. It also increases muscle tone, speeds up the heart, and increases blood pressure. Its indication as a Schedule III controlled drug in the US for treatment of narcolepsy was approved in 2002, and in 2006, it became a Class C controlled substance under the MDA.

An indigenous agent of increasing notoriety and interest is *Salvia divinorum*, 'magic mint' or 'Sally D', whose leaves are chewed by the Mazatec tribe of the high Sierra in Oaxaca, Mexico as an aid to divination, and produce a dissociative hallucinogenic effect. Its use has spread to the US, Canada, and Europe, where it has developed an underground following. It is forbidden in Australia, controlled in Finland and Denmark, and has been rendered illegal in various American states and municipalities. *Salvia divinorum* is currently listed amongst 'Drugs and Chemicals of Concern' by the American Drug Enforcement Administration (DEA).

Preparation and distribution

Lysergic acid forms the nucleus of a group of chemicals called ergot alkaloids. Ergot is a fungus which colonizes rye grasses and has a fascinating history. When bread made from infected rye is eaten, two sets of symptoms may result.

Most commonly, there is excruciating pain in the hands and feet due to constriction of the arteries which can cause death of the tissue (gangrene). The popular name for this affliction in medieval times, St Anthony's Fire, derived from the observation that sufferers who travelled to pray at the shrine of the saint often recovered. Cynics may surmise that the saint's influence must have been boosted by a lack of fungus in the region of the shrine. The other effect was to produce fits, hallucinations, coma, and not infrequently death through heart failure or depression of breathing. Ergot was identified in the 17th century as the cause of these outbreaks which have continued into the modern era, the most recent being in France in 1951. Doctors found that some ingredients in ergot were useful in the treatment of migraine and for speeding up childbirth, but there are now much less toxic alternatives.

Hofmann synthesized LSD whilst searching among the derivatives of lysergic acid for a compound which might act as a breathing stimulant. It induces peculiar behaviour in many different animal species, but is not self-administered by animals in tests of dependence or reinforcement. It does not damage the brain or nerves and the lethal dose in animals is huge, death in such experiments being due to respiratory failure. Precursors are readily accessible, it is easy and cheap to manufacture, and the potency is extremely high so there is a strong economic incentive for black market production.

LSD belongs to the group of substances called indolealkylamines, which are similar in structure to the neurotransmitter 5-hydroxytryptamine (5HT, serotonin). The group also includes DMT, psilocin, psilocybin, the harmaloid alkaloids (such as William Burroughs' yagé), and ibogaine. The other major group of chemicals producing psychedelic effects are the phenylethylamines, which include mescaline, MDA, and MDMA. These last two have a distinct profile of activity and are discussed in Chapter 9.

LSD is a white, tasteless powder which dissolves easily in water to a colourless solution. It is immensely potent, being hallucinogenic in doses from 50 micrograms (0.05 mg) upwards. When used as an adjunct to psychotherapy, doses between 200 and 500 micrograms were usual. Current street doses range between 20 and 250 micrograms, more frequently at the bottom end of that range.

There are many species of hallucinogenic mushrooms to be found in Europe and the US, but the most easily recognized and widely used is *Psilocybe semilanceata*, popularly known as Liberty Cap. This can be found in abundance in autumn and early winter, and 20 or so will provide sufficient psilocybin for a hallucinatory experience. A more potent cousin, *Psilocybe azurescens*, has recently been discovered in the American Northwest, and is active following eight or more ingested caps. Another mushroom, *Amanita muscaria*

(Fly Agaric), also makes its appearance around September but its effects can be unpleasantly toxic.

Salvia divinorum plants seem to be sterile human cultigens that require cloned propagation by cuttings. Plants and dried leaves are available via the Internet and some 'head shops'.

PCP and GHB are manufactured in illicit laboratories, whilst ketamine is usually obtained from diversion of pharmaceutical supplies.

Scientific information

The psychedelic drugs produce changes in sensory perception, mood, intellectual and physical performance, and the pattern of thinking, all of this in the absence of an alteration in consciousness. Memory is relatively unimpaired. It is difficult to have much confidence in the results of psychological testing carried out on those under the influence. Either the subject lacks the concentration or inclination to participate, or fluctuations in one modality will interfere with another being tested; for example, a sudden shift in mood from elation to despair would greatly influence performance in a problem-solving task. For this reason, reliable non-subjective information on the effects of the psychedelics on intellectual functioning is not available.

Psychological effects begin to appear about 20 minutes after an oral dose of LSD, and the concentration in blood halves every five hours or so. The duration of action is variable but averages around 12 hours. Sensitivity to repeated doses rapidly decreases, but returns equally rapidly after a brief abstinence.

Only a tiny fraction of an oral dose actually reaches the brain, and even this has disappeared within 20 minutes. Since the duration of effect is many hours, the drug must cause some residual change in brain chemistry. As Huxley remarked, following the line proposed by the Cambridge philosopher C.D. Broad, the result seems to be an interference with the filtering and integrating function of the brain, so that the mind's eye is overwhelmed with a mass of unfamiliar material, often termed a 'flight of ideas'. It also has a 'dehabituating' effect: the familiar regains its power to generate a fresh sense of novelty. Sensory deprivation in a dark, soundproofed float tank greatly reduces the psychedelic potential of LSD, and totally blind people do not experience visual hallucinations or Leary's so-called 'magic theater'.

Psychedelics such as LSD, psilocybin, mescaline, and DMT probably act through stimulating three serotonin receptors in the brain, primarily $5HT_{2A}$ but also $5HT_{1A}$ and $5HT_{2C}$. It does this as a 'partial agonist', meaning that the activation effect is not so complete as following serotonin itself. These receptors are plentiful in the parts of the brain which deal with attending to and processing incoming information (thalamus), integrating this information (prefrontal cortex), and higher level decision making (frontal cortex). Dopamine receptors and certain adrenergic receptors are probably also affected within other structures (e.g ventral tegmental pathway, locus coeruleus). There is no physical dependence syndrome or withdrawal symptoms after ceasing regular use. Psychological dependence (see Chapter 13) is very rare. The 'fight and flight' mechanism of the sympathetic nervous system is mildly stimulated. This may result in dilation of the pupils, modest increases in blood pressure and heart rate, trembling, dizziness, loss of appetite, a small increase in body temperature, and sleeplessness. Death due to toxicity or overdose is almost unknown, and people have shown full recovery from documented doses as large as 100,000 micrograms.

PCP and ketamine are arylcycloalkylamines which freely cross the blood-brain barrier, and their pharmacology is markedly different from LSD. The primary action seems to be antagonism at the NMDA receptor, and since the resulting glutamate deficit produces symptoms similar to those found in schizophrenia these drugs have been used as a laboratory model of psychosis. However, cholinergic, adrenergic, and serotonergic neurotransmission is also profoundly affected. Along with a hallucinatory effect, these drugs produce an amphetamine-like stimulation, analgesia, and fearlessness, and this combination can result in sustained destructive behaviour. Tolerance and dependence can be demonstrated in laboratory animals, but the latter does not seem to be a feature in human use.

GHB is a naturally occuring substance which is present in the central nervous system of most animals (including humans) and various plants. It is also easy to synthesize. It acts within the brain as an inhibitory neurotransmitter at both the GABA receptor and also a newly-identified 'GHB receptor'. Activation of these receptors also produces effects within glutamate and dopaminergic systems.

Salvia divinorum acts primarily via salvinorin A, a non-nitrogenous diterpenoid and highly selective kappa (κ)-opioid agonist. The latter receptor shares certain pain-relieving properties with its better known sibling, the mu (μ)-opioid receptor, but in contrast seems to mediate anti-addictive properties in experimental models.

Medical uses

Ketamine is still in use as an analgesic and anaesthetic, particularly in children. A small US pilot study suggested that it could be useful in resistant depression, and in Russia a controlled trial showed improved rates of abstinence in heroin addicts. Its repetitive application has also been of occasional benefit in treatment of chronic pain states. GHB is licenced in the US for the treatment of cataplexy and narcolepsy.

Numerous anecdotal reports exist of therapeutic benefits in recreational psychedelic users. There is still considerable interest in scientific and medical circles in evaluating some of these leads in properly designed clinical trials using LSD or psilocybin. Particular areas of interest include obsessive-compulsive disorder, eating disorders, migraine and cluster headaches, post-traumatic stress disorder, intractable depression, and various addictions. The pharmacology of salvinorin A suggests possible utility for treatment of dependency on opiates, nicotine, cocaine, and alcohol. One case report claimed that Salvia produced long-term remission from an intractable severe chronic depression.

Modern ritualistic use

Use of hallucinogens for spiritual purposes and as a means of personal enlightenment persists in several countries. Ayahuasca is used within the defined rituals in the Church of Santo Daime which was founded in Brazil in the 1930s. The Brazilian government recognized this as a valid religion in 1992 and sanctioned its use of the drug. It also sponsored safety studies which revealed no apparent harmful long-term effects. Ahahuasca is also tolerated in the Netherlands. Use as a religious sacrament by adherents of the União do Vegetal (UDV) syncretic religion was sanctioned by the US Supreme Court in 2006, but is still being legally contested. It remains illegal in most other countries. Nevertheless, the Church has a few hundred followers in the UK.

The Native American Church continues to attract adherents in the US and peyote use remains legal for its members. It is widely considered a positive agent in these populations and modern research suggests that it has contributed to a lower recidivism rate of alcoholism.

While *Tabernanthe iboga*, the plant source of ibogaine, has continued usage as an ordeal poison by the Bwiti culture in West Africa (notably Gabon), it is gaining currency amongst some Western clinics as a last-ditch prolonged psychedelic mental purge in treating addictions.

Recreational use

The use of psychedelic drugs in the US has remained remarkably constant over the last four decades. In 1974, the proportion of college students who had ever used LSD (acid; blotter; paper; squares; lucy; dots; haze; rainbow) was reported to be 23%, and the figure for a similar group in 2006 was 20%. A slightly conflicting message is found when the annual number of new initiates to hallucinogens is examined: in the late 1990s numbers were quite stable at around 600,000 new users each year, but this has risen steadily in the last decade: 886,000 in 2003, 953,000 in 2005, and over one million in 2006. One million US citizens over the age of 12 are estimated to have used hallucinogens at least once during the previous year. This amounts to roughly 2% of students, since only a tiny proportion of these users are aged 26 or older. Similarly, in the UK use of hallucinogens seems to have been stable over the past decade, with approximately 9% of adults ever having used one, and 1% in the past year. As would be expected, highest rates of recent are to be found in the age groups 16 to 19 (3%) and 20 to 24 (3.6%). Rates decline rapidly thereafter. These levels of usage are mirrored across other European countries, although somewhat higher prevalences are noted in Hungary and Latvia. Among school pupils aged 11 to 15, 26% had been offered psychedelics at some time and 2% had used one at least once within the previous year. This principally reflects use by 14 (4%) and 15 year-olds (5%). Again, levels are similar across Europe with slightly higher levels in the Czech Republic. Notably an outlier in this respect, Canadian Addiction Surveys actually showed a doubling of lifetime prevalence of psychedelics in the decade 1994–2004 from 5.2 to 11.4%.

PCP (angel dust; hog; wack; ozone; dipper; elephant; goon) was widely abused in the US in the 1960s, but went into a decline as its toxic potential was appreciated on the street. It has re-emerged since the 1970s and is once again widely available. Although rarely described as a drug of first choice, it remains a popular stand-by when other, more desirable substances are in short supply, and finds its way covertly into other street drugs as a cheap, active adulterant. In 2006–2007, it was estimated that around 1.6 million Americans (2.7%) have taken PCP at least once in their lives, including 2.1% of high school seniors. Fortunately, the use of PCP has never really caught on in Europe. It sometimes crops up as a contaminant of MDMA (ecstasy) on sale in British nightclubs, and people who say they have only smoked cannabis have sometimes tested positive for PCP, suggesting that it may occasionally be added as a deliberate adulterant. Such chemical trickery is common in the US where only one in seven Americans testing positively for PCP in their urine were aware of having taken it.

In years gone by, illicit LSD was often available as a clear liquid in small bottles wrapped in foil to protect it from light, or absorbed into sugar cubes in huge doses by today's standards of 250 micrograms or more. These days it is generally supplied on squares of impregnated paper (blotters) or tiny tablets (microdots), costing between £2–5 for a single dose of between 20 and 80 micrograms.

Possession or consumption of magic mushrooms (shrooms; magics; mushies; liberties; caps) is illegal in the US and became illegal in the UK in 2005.

Approximately 20 Liberty Caps (or half that amount for *Psilocybe azurescens*) will produce a mildish trip, and a bagful can be bought for a few pounds or dollars. They are occasionally sold ground up as a brown powder or pressed into tablets. Of course, the buyer can never be at all sure what the powder or tablets contain. Occasionally, 'mescaline' is also available as a dark-brown powder, but this is likely to be heavily adulterated if indeed it contains any genuine material at all. In the US, it may well contain LSD or much more toxic substances such as PCP. Those who sample Morning Glory seeds obtained from garden centres in the UK risk toxic side-effects since they are routinely doused in fungicide. Ketamine (K; Special K; Vitamin K; cat valium; green; jet) is supplied as tablets or a powder to be snorted or smoked, and costs around £25 per gram or $65–100 per gram ($20–40 per dose unit) in the US. GHB (liquid ecstasy; soap; GBH; georgia home boy) usually takes the form of a colourless, odourless, tasteless liquid containing around 20% active material and costing between £5 and £10 for a small bottle ($5–25 in the US), but is also encountered as a powder or capsule. Statistics related to ketamine and GHB use are lacking but the impression is that they are gaining popularity, especially amongst the clubbing generation.

The DMT-containing plants are most commonly used as snuffs or brewed teas. When pure DMT is smoked, an intense and colourful phantasmagoria of morphing geometric patterns is typical. It is of short duration and has been termed the 'businessman's trip', being a cosmic journey that can be experienced within the lunch hour.

Salvinorin A is inactive orally, and requires leaf chewing to allow absorption via the oral mucous membranes. Its use, however, demands a steep learning curve and large measure of devotion, as it may prove difficult to achieve a threshold dose, and its effects are often subtle and evanescent. Devotees recommend usage in complete darkness, and will most often employ concentrated extracts for chewing. Smoking is also quite popular, but inhalation of large volumes of acrid smoke are necessary. If successfully attained, the salvia trip is a brief and often awesome experience which seems to defy accurate description and is infrequently considered enjoyable or even attractive for a repeat performance.

The expectations and mood of the user and the setting in which LSD or a related drug is taken have a profound influence on the experience that results, as Timothy Leary pointed out. There are hundreds of subjective accounts in the literature; a good selection can be found in Grinspoon and Bakalar's *Psychedelic Drugs Reconsidered* (1979). Typically, the subjective experience gets underway about 20 minutes or so after an oral dose. After an initial sharpening of perception, visual distortion, and a sense of detachment, apprehension, elation, or fear are the first signs of take-off. Thoughts begin to follow strange pathways, sparking off rapid shifts in mood. After this the shape of the experience becomes almost infinitely variable. Time seems to stand still.

Regular attitudes or viewpoints dissolve, and the familiar and hackneyed become novel, fascinating, or terrifying. Not only do hallucinations, illusions, and distortions of sight or sound tantalize or terrify, but one sense may seem to blot out all the others, or they may blend together so that a voice is felt or music experienced as a visual sensation. When the eyes are closed, swirling colours or images fill the mind (the 'magic theater'). Memories long suppressed spring into consciousness. Body image may be grossly distorted, or boundaries between the self and the external world seem to evaporate. Objects sometimes seem to loom immense or shrink away, with loss of perspective.

This psychedelic phase, with its twists and turns, its dread and delight, its mixture of pain and wonder, ebbs and flows in intensity. After a few hours there is a gradual drift into a more relaxed, sensual phase. Every random thing or event has a meaning, a subtle significance. Gradually this magical aura recedes and small windows of ordinary reality intrude and expand until all that is left is the memory of the journey. The average duration of the trip is around 12 hours, but it may persist for a day or more.

PCP is usually smoked, although some people stir it into a drink, others snort it, and the lunatic fringe injects it. Many Americans take it inadvertently when it is sold as mescaline, psilocybin, or ecstacy (MDMA), cut into other drugs as a filler, or sprayed on to indifferent cannabis to give it a bit more bite. In a recent screen of attenders at a US drug clinic, only 14 out of 100 people whose urine tested positive for PCP were aware that they had taken it.

Whichever way it is absorbed, PCP gives quite a jolt to the system. For the infrequent user 10 mg is an active dose, but regulars find they need bigger and bigger amounts to get the same effects. Within 15 minutes or so a warm, relaxed feeling gives way to dreamy euphoria, with or without hallucinations, lasting for several hours. Tingling in the limbs precedes a numb feeling and insensitivity to pain, whilst coordination and self-concern are greatly impaired. These effects gradually pass off to be replaced by a lingering sense of irritable depression.

A small dose of ketamine snorted into the nose generally results in a brief and usually mild hallucinogenic experience lasting a couple of hours, but there is a risk that larger doses may produce an effect similar to that of PCP. GHB has growing popularity among clubbers who enjoy its ability to produce euphoria and alcohol-like intoxication which can be quite long-lasting. It is also used by body-builders because the increased slow-wave sleep it produces is associated with the secretion of growth hormone. Both ketamine and GHB (along with Rohypnol) are frequently implicated as 'date-rape drugs'.

Salvia divinorum when chewed may produce effects within 10 minutes and last one hour, but quite often less. When smoked, effects commence in 30 seconds and last for 15 to 30 minutes. Marked variability is reported.

Most users of psychedelics allow weeks or months to elapse between trips, but some have runs of a few days at a time. People who have been in the habit of using psychedelics regularly for long periods may seem to have only a rather tentative grasp on reality. However, such investigations as were done in the 1960s and 1970s suggest that their intellect and brain functioning remained pretty much unimpaired. The sort of compulsive use that may be associated with stimulants or opiates is almost unknown. These are not 'addictive' drugs—it just isn't that sort of experience.

Unwanted effects

Death due directly to overdose of LSD, psylocybin, or mescaline is incredibly rare, if indeed it has ever occurred. People are on record as surviving vast unintended overdoses, and fatal cases usually seem to involve other drugs as well as LSD. Physical collapse following toxic doses also seems very uncommon. Convulsions have been reported following big doses. Death resulting from accidents sustained under the influence of LSD are well documented, especially when the drug has been given to someone who is unaware. These may be related to lack of self-concern, impaired performance of tasks requiring concentration and coordination such as driving, the acting out of fantasies such as a feeling that one can fly, or simply a sense of omnipotence and invulnerability. Reports of people going blind as a result of staring into the sun seem largely apocryphal. There is no good evidence that LSD damages chromosomes or the unborn baby but taking it during pregnancy would not be wise. A recent review of drug harms by a panel of experts actually rated LSD dangers below those associated with cannabis, cocaine, amphetamines, opiates, tobacco and alcohol.

The biggest risk is the occurrence of a 'bad trip', and individual differences in sensitivity means that a comfortable dose for one person may be far too much for another. Any encounter with LSD is likely to have some frightening or unpleasant moments, but most people find most trips rewarding overall. Sometimes, however, terror or distress dominate the whole experience. A bad trip is much more likely if the setting is unsuitable, if there are no sympathetic and trusted straight friends at hand, or if the pre-existing mood was a negative one.

A strong conviction that the mind is breaking up or that one is losing control may lead to intense agitation and panic. Thoughts may turn toward suspiciousness and a sense of persecution, which then shapes subsequent hallucinations. Destruction of mental defence mechanisms can unleash profound feelings of hopelessness, emptiness, or futility. Occasionally, such feelings may find expression in self-harm or suicide, or even more rarely outwardly directed violence. Religious or other delusions may lead to ritualistic or symbolic self-mutilation, for example by emasculation or eye-gouging, but again this is very rare. Most people recover from bad trips in a day or so, but occasionally it persists for longer. It has been estimated that around 1% of regular LSD users will seek professional help at some time as a result of a bad trip.

Much more serious are the prolonged psychological disturbances which can follow the use of psychedelics. These consist either of prolonged psychosis with delusions and hallucinations, or persistent anxiety or depression. Some idea of the level of risk can be obtained from the reports of large-scale studies carried out when use of LSD in psychiatry was legal. Prolonged psychosis seems to have occurred in between 0.1–1% of all patients exposed, and from 0.05–0.1% of healthy experimental subjects. Bearing in mind the large numbers of people who regularly take LSD, this is by no means a negligible risk. Suicide was reported in 0.03–0.07 % of patients. Major complications with LSD occurred in just over 2% of psychiatric patients who received the drug.

When prolonged psychosis does occur, it usually resembles schizophrenia in its pattern of symptoms, though wide swings of mood are sometimes more prominent than would be usual. Most people recover gradually over the course of a few days or a week with symptomatic treatment only, but some remain ill for weeks or months. It remains an open question as to whether these drugs are capable of inducing a long-term psychosis in a person who was previously completely normal. The current consensus is that this happens very rarely, if at all. In most reported cases of illness persisting more than a week or so after the last exposure to the drug there are usually vulnerability factors such as pre-existing psychological problems or a family history of psychosis. The outlook for such cases is similar to schizophrenia, with a fairly high likelihood of further attacks. Persistent anxiety and depression usually respond in time to standard treatments, and again the drug's relation to causation is uncertain.

'Flashbacks' are sudden recurrences of psychedelic experiences occurring when no drug has been taken, sometimes after many months of abstinence. About a quarter of LSD users experience them at one time or another, and some find them quite pleasant ('free trips'!). Most people are frightened and disturbed by the experience and may think it is a sign of impending madness. They last for seconds or hours and usually come on in association with tiredness, stress, the *déjà-vu* phenomenon, or the use of another drug such as cannabis. They may be sparked off by the sight, sound, or smell of something or somebody associated in the individual's mind with LSD use in the past. A number of neurological explanations have been proposed, but none are entirely convincing. In most people, the experience seems to bear a close similarity to a panic attack. There is no connection at all with mental illness and flashbacks usually become less and less frequent, disappearing completely within a few weeks or months of abstinence. Occasionally, they coalesce into an almost continuous experience lasting weeks, months, or even longer and the label 'post hallucinogenic perceptual disorder' has been attached to this phenomenon.

PCP is a much more toxic substance in overdose, and there are many reports of delirium, coma, brain damage, and death. Muscle stiffness, difficulty in walking and speaking, and constant drooling from the mouth may result from brain damage caused by impurities arising during illicit manufacture. Memory may be permanently impaired. The combination of a strong sense of invulnerability and omnipotence, insensitivity to pain, impaired judgement, and reduced tolerance of frustration is fraught with danger for users and those who interact with them. Unpredictable sudden violence or self-harm may occur, as may psychotic reactions with prominent delusions and hallucinations which are usually brief in duration but occasionally become longstanding. Persistent mood disorders following abstinence have also been reported. Unlike the psychedelics repeated use can sometimes lead to features of addiction such as craving and compulsive use. Physical effects include depression of blood pressure and respiration, nausea and vomiting, sweating, numbness, confusion, and loss of coordination.

Ketamine in large doses may produce a similar pattern of effects although usually much less severe. Nevertheless, ketamine-related fatalities have been reported. Users may feel depersonalized or cut off and remote from their surroundings. Nausea and vomiting, clumsiness, limb numbness, visual impairment, and slurring of speech are all quite likely to occur, so accidents are always possible. There is no information on the possible consequences of long-term use.

Too much GHB can result in sleep disturbances, mood disorders, dizziness, nausea and vomiting, muscle weakness, visual problems, agitation, hallucinations, convulsions, and coma. The ratio between a euphoriant and a toxic dose is very small. A withdrawal syndrome consisting of cramps, anxiety, and insomnia has been reported following heavy regular use. It may interact with MDMA to produce psychosis, amphetamine to cause convulsions, and alcohol to bring about dangerous respiratory depression. It seems to antagonize the effects of cannabis. Case reports of fatal overdoses exist in the scientific literature.

Salvia divinorum and salvinorin A have no identified direct tissue toxicity. A fair proportion of those who try it may become scared by the experience, and frequent repetitive use is rare. Because affected individuals may totally lose their objective appreciation of their surroundings, a sober guide is an absolute necessity to prevent accidents. A few episodes of prolonged depression and rare suicides after usage have been reported in the lay press.

Selected references

Abraham, H. D., Aldridge, A. M. (1993). Adverse consequences of lysergic acid diethylamide. *Addiction*, **88**, 1327–34.

Abraham, H. D., Aldridge, A. M., Gogia, P. (1996). The psychopharmacology of hallucinogens. *Neuropsychopharmacology*, **14**, 285–98.

Abramson, H. A., Jarvik, M. E., Kaufman, M. R. et al. (1955). Lysergic acid diethylamide (LSD–25): 1. Physiological and perceptual responses. *Journal of Physiology*, **39**, 3–62.

Boire, R. G., Russo, E., Fish, A. R., Bowman, J. (2002). *Salvia divinorum.* Information concerning the plant and its active principle. H.R. 5607. Davis, CA: Center for Cognitive Liberty & Ethics http://www.cognitiveliberty.org/pdf/salvia_dea.pdf

Bowers, M. B. (1977). Psychoses precipitated by psychotomimetic drugs: a follow-up study. *Archives of General Psychiatry*, **34**, 832–5.

Budd, R. D., Lindstrom, D. M. (1982). Characteristics of victims of PCP-related deaths in Los Angeles County, *Journal of Toxicology and Clinical Toxicology*, **19**, 997–1004.

Crowley N., Edwards G., Read T., Sandison R., Sessa B. (2005). A role for psychedelics in psychiatry? (correspondence). *British Journal of Psychiatry* **187**, 483–90.

Drug Enforcement Administration Intelligence Division Drug Intelligence Brief (2003). *PCP: the threat remains.* DEA: Springfield, VA.

Eisner, B. G., Cohen, S. (1958). Psychotherapy with lysergic acid diethylamide. *Journal of Nervous and Mental Diseases*, **127**, 528–39.

Grinspoon, L. (1979). The major psychedelic drugs: sources and effects *and* psychedelic drugs in the twentieth century. *Psychedelic drugs reconsidered.* Basic Books, Inc. New York.

Hofmann, A. (1980). *LSD: my problem child.* McGraw-Hill, New York.

Javitt, D. C., Zukin, S. R. (1991). Recent advances in the phencyclidine model of schizophrenia. *American Journal of Psychiatry*, **148**, 1301–8.

Isbell, H., Belleville, R. E., Fraser, H. F., Wikler, A., Logan, C. R. (1956). Studies on lysergic acid diethylamide (LSD–25). *Archives of Neurology and Psychiatry*, **76**, 468–78.

Matefy, R. E. (1978). Psychedelic drug flashbacks. *Addictive Behaviour*, **3**, 165–78.

Milhorn, H. T. (1991). Diagnosis and management of phencyclidine intoxication. *American Family Physician*, **43**, 1293–302.

Nichols D. E. (2001). LSD and its lysergamide cousins. *Heffter Review of Psychedelic Research* **2**, 80–7.

Nichols D. (2005). *The scientific and therapeutic potential of psychedelics.* Beckley Foundation Global Drug Policy Seminar, House of Lords, November 2005.

Pierce, P. A., Peroutka, S. J. (1990). Antagonist properties of d-LSD at 5-hydroxytryptamine$_2$ receptors *Neuropsychopharmacology*, **3**, 503–8.

Rudgley, R. (1995). The archaic use of hallucinogens in Europe: an archaeology of altered states. *Addiction*, **90**, 163–4.

Sanders-Bush, E., Burris, K. D., Knoth, K. (1988). Lysergic acid diethylamide and 2,5-dimethoxy-4-methylamphetamine are partial agonists at serotonin receptors linked to phosphoinositide hydrolysis. *Journal of Pharmacology and Experimental Therapeutics*, **246**, 924–8.

Sessa B (2005). Can psychedelics have a role in psychiatry once again? *British Journal of Psychiatry* **186**, 457–8.

Yesavage, J. A., Freeman, A. M. (1978). Acute phencyclidine (PCP) intoxication: psychopathology and prognosis. *Journal of Clinical Psychiatry*, **44**, 664–5.

Weil, A. T. (1977). Observations on consciousness alteration: some notes on Datura. *Journal of Psychedelic Drugs*, **9**, 165–9.

Chapter 8

The inhalants

Historical background

It is evident from cave drawings in Australia and Mexico, and from the writings of Greek and Persian scholars, that the inhalation of naturally occuring mind-altering gases or vapours is a practice which extends back into prehistory. Mystics, including the Delphic Oracle, used such emissions along with other mind-altering miasmas such as fumes from perfumes and burning spices to induce visions and enhance contact with the spirit world.

Modern recreational enjoyment of inhalants has its roots in the 19th century. At that time pain relief in surgery relied upon alcohol, opium, cannabis, or even, for some unfortunate patients, concussion or partial suffocation. Sir Humphry Davy, writing at the very beginning of the century to deplore this state of affairs, was the first to propose the use of nitrous oxide gas as an anaesthetic and painkiller. He also extolled the experience of inhaling the gas for pleasure, describing how one could summon up exciting visions without untoward effects upon sleep or appetite. He introduced this pastime to a number of his affluent friends, and their enthusiasm extended to the idea of establishing a 'nitrous oxide tavern'.

A landmark event in the history of anaesthesia took place in 1844 with the painless removal of a molar tooth from the mouth of one Dr Wells, who had prepared himself for the ordeal by breathing nitrous oxide in the manner recommended by Sir Humphry. Ether was first tried in 1846 and chloroform the following year. These early efforts were rather hit and miss, not least because of the potential toxicity of these last two compounds, and there was some opposition on religious grounds. Despite this, the practice of anaesthesia gained ground rapidly. The royal seal of approval was given by Queen Victoria, who was delivered of her eighth child in 1853 with the aid of chloroform.

News of the recreational possibilities of these substances spread rapidly, and nitrous oxide or chloroform parties became quite fashionable during the remainder of the century. Physicians and dentists gained new popularity because of their ready access to the necessary pharmaceuticals. From that time to the present day, a professional proximity to such powerful mind-altering substances has caused some individuals to give way to the temptation to sample their own wares. In modern times abuse of anaesthetics such as trichloroethylene and halothane comes to light sporadically, sometimes through the tragic consequences of their very high potency. Nitrous oxide still makes an appearance at medical student parties from time to time, and has sometimes been made more widely available at such events as rock concerts, conveniently packaged in balloons.

Petrol sniffing was first discussed in the newspapers in 1942, but it wasn't until the 1950s that solvent inhalation began to cause serious concern, with reports appearing of the increasing popularity of the practice among teenagers throughout the US. Similar reports emanated from the UK, Australia, and India. This publicity fuelled the popularity of the habit dramatically. Sniffers were typically economically deprived and therefore less able to afford alcohol or other more conventional intoxicants.

At the same time, another form of inhalant was becoming popular in show-business circles, and soon afterwards within the gay community on North America's West Coast. This was the pungent amyl nitrite, a volatile liquid which had been introduced into medical practice in 1867 for the relief of cardiac pain (angina) through its ability to dilate the coronary arteries. It underwent a resurgence for this indication in the 1960s when it became available over the counter in pharmacies. Small gauze-covered glass ampoules or 'vitrellas' (poppers) were designed to be crushed between finger and thumb to release the vapour. Apart from the usual inhalant 'high', poppers soon got the reputation of enhancing the joy of sex.

Amyl nitrite was made a prescription-only medicine in 1969, and its place in the pleasure market was largely taken over by butyl-, octyl-, and isobutyl nitrite. Virtually the only remaining legal source of amyl nitrite these days is in emergency kits for the treatment of industrial cyanide poisoning. Isobutyl nitrite was and still is widely available in small bottles as a 'room odorizer', though trade names such as *Rush, Ram, Locker Room, Bullet, Thrust*, and *Lightning Bolt* indicate that the manufacturers had more than an inkling of the true appeal of their products. Between 1973 and 1978, more than 12 million such bottles were sold in US discotheques, pornography shops, and hardware stores.

By the 1980s it was clear that volatile substance abuse (VSA) was a worldwide problem and in some neighbourhoods as many as one in two children admitted to trying it at least once. As indicated by the historical perspective above, inhalant abuse has always been endemic on a variable scale throughout the world whenever the opportunity has arisen. In the UK, the habit spread most rapidly among teenagers in the larger towns, especially those in Scotland, Northern Ireland, and Northern England. By 1980, surveys indicated that as many as 15% of 14 to 17 year-olds in Britain and the US had used inhalants at some time. Apart from childhood experimentation, some adult occupations apart from medicine have carried a special risk because of the ready availability and daily contact with volatile substances. These include shoe making, carpentry, printing, carpet laying, dry cleaning, painting and decorating, and hair styling.

As the spotlight was turned on VSA the risk involved became all too apparent. More than 300 solvent-related deaths had been reported in the US by 1972, and in 1978 alone 1,800 American adolescents required emergency medical treatment as a result of VSA. Nearly 300 deaths were recorded in Britain between 1971 and 1983, and by 1990 this figure had passed the 1,000 mark. More than 80% of these deaths occurred in teenagers, 60% of them under seventeen and the youngest only ten. Fatalities were much more common in boys and peaked at 15 to 16. In the early 1980s, three teenagers were dying weekly in the UK as a direct result of VSA, but over the following decade the mortality steadily declined to a yearly average of around 50 where it remains to the present day. The reason for this may or may not be related to a high-profile and continuing public health campaign which began in 1985, and passage in the same year of the Intoxicating Substances Supply Act which made it an offence to supply an underage person with a substance the supplier knows, or has reason to believe, will be used to 'achieve intoxication'. Successful prosecutions have been few and far between. In the UK, as in most other countries, possession of poppers and inhalable solvents is not illegal, though attempts have been made to limit availability of butane products to children since this has been consistently the most lethal abusable product.

VSA today remains a serious concern throughout the world, particularly among the 100 million or so street children among whom the prevalence exceeds 80% in some African, South American, and Eastern European cities.

Preparations available

Some examples of everyday products containing volatile solvents are glues and adhesives (toluene, benzene, xylene, acetone, heptanes); cleaning fluids (trichloroethylene, tetrachloroethylene, carbon tetrachloride); aerosols (fluorocarbons, hydrocarbons); petrol (hydrocarbons); rubber solution (benzene, n-hexane, chloroform); typewriter correcting fluid (trichloroethylene); paint (toluene); varnish and lacquer (trichloroethylene, toluene); nail polish and its remover (acetone, amylacetate); dyes (acetone, methylene chloride); fire extinguishers (fluorocarbons); and 'room fresheners' (butyl and isobutyl nitrites). The solvents themselves are usually relatively simple hydrocarbon compounds.

Butane cigarette lighter refills have been responsible for more than half of VSA deaths, and the gas is also contained in camping stoves and as a propellant for food dispensers.

The average home contains at least 30 different products capable of producing intoxication when inhaled.

Scientific information

A typical solvent such as toluene is absorbed rapidly when the vapour is inhaled, and peak blood levels occur within a few minutes. It enters the brain very quickly and has a high affinity for fat stores throughout the body. For this reason, solvents disappear from the blood within six hours of the last inhalation but may reappear days later as they are released gradually from these stores. Some of the absorbed solvent evaporates away through the lungs, but much of it is metabolized in the liver then excreted in the urine, in the case of toluene as hippuric acid. The highest acceptable concentration of toluene in the air for industrial workers is 100 parts per million; 'sniffers' can exceed this level many hundredfold. Once the concentration in blood reaches the modest level of 0.5 micrograms per gram, it can easily be smelt on the breath.

Solvents probably achieve their intoxicating effect through a similar action to alcohol and inhalational anaesthetics. The permeability of nerve membranes to electrically charged chemicals (ions) passing in and out of the cell is altered by an effect on the gating mechanism operated at receptor sites for neurotransmitters such as GABA and glutamate. The balance of these ions across the membrane determines whether or not the nerve is receptive to transmitting an impulse. Tolerance to the intoxicating effect occurs on repeated exposure.

Recreational use

In the US and UK, sniffing ('huffing') inhalants is the commonest form of illicit drug use in children under 14. Prevalence rates among 12 year-olds in 2007 were 4% and 6% respectively, ahead of cannabis (1% and 3%), and these levels have remained fairly constant over the past decade. Among European school children the average lifetime prevalence rate is 10%, ranging between 1% (Romania) and 22% (Greenland). US surveys suggest that three quarters of huffers initiate the practice before the age of 18, and there were an estimated 780,000 new initiates aged 12 or older during 2006.

Although individuals from deprived backgrounds, ethnic minorities, and inner cities are over-represented in most samples, solvent inhalation (with the exception of petrol) occurs among people from all social backgrounds. There is some indication that it is more widespread in the summer months.

Epidemics in closed societies such as boarding schools and prisons are reported from time to time. The most obvious motive for huffing is the immediate and intense intoxication, but other reasons include peer pressure, to boost confidence, to relieve boredom, or to blot out other worries. As with most illicit drug use, almost everyone's first exposure is initiated and supplied by a friend. In developed countries, the practice is now marginally more prevalent in girls in the 11 to 15 age bracket yet a fatal outcome is twice as common in boys. Almost three-quarters of those who try sniffing only do so once or twice, a further 20% huff for a few weeks or months, and only about 10% persist long term. Heavy users are likely to be abusing a range of other substances as well as solvents, and are much more likely to be suffering from psychological problems or a seriously disrupted home life.

A young adolescent who inhales solvents at any time is 10 times more likely to try other illegal drugs in the future than non-huffing peers, and three times more likely to inject a drug at some time. There is also a strong link with delinquent behaviour of one sort or another.

The extent of use of the volatile nitrites is difficult to quantify, but it is clearly considerable. Millions of bottles of butyl nitrite are sold each year in Britain and the US.

Inhalants have a limited place as 'party drugs'. When taken on the dance floor they may provide a brief blast of energy, but unpleasant dizziness or nausea is always possible. There are dangers in combining physical exertion with huffing solvents, as will be described below. Volatile nitrites may be used specifically for sexual enhancement by both hetero and homosexuals.

Since the average home contains such a range of inhalable products, the would-be sniffer has plenty of choice. Typically, a globule of suitable material such as glue or rubber solution is dropped into an empty crisp packet or small plastic bag which is then held over the mouth and nose so that the fumes can be deeply inhaled ('huffed') 10 or more times. This is often a group activity, and the bag is passed round from hand to hand. 'Sniffing' is not a term which accurately conveys the vigour of the technique.

Alternatively, a volatile liquid can be inhaled directly from the container, or poured on to a rag or coat-sleeve for easier or more surreptitious access. Sometimes the user may seek to enhance the effect by enclosing the head completely, for example under the bedclothes or within a larger plastic bag. Suffocation or overdose are all too possible in such circumstances.

Small brown bottles of butyl nitrite or similar are available from some sex shops and gay clubs in Britain and the US, costing a few pounds or dollars. If kept in the fridge with the cap firmly applied between episodes, a single bottle will provide several highs before completely evaporating.

Gas lighter fuel (butane) can be sprayed into a balloon or bag before inhalation, but all too often the plunger is pressed against the teeth and the contents projected straight down the throat. Aerosols, for example spray paints, are usually inhaled indirectly, but it is impossible to avoid absorbing droplets of paint (or whatever dissolved material the product contains) along with the solvent vapour.

Euphoric effects come on extremely rapidly with a distinct 'rush'. The user feels exhilarated and excited, 'high', disinhibited, and powerful. This is often accompanied by blurred vision, slurred speech, a buzzing in the ears, and marked clumsiness. Time seems to pass slowly. Interesting visual illusions or hallucinations sometimes occur, and can often be 'steered' or harnessed in an enjoyable way. Inhibitions disappear and during sex orgasm is, or at least seems, prolonged and intensified. As with all psychoactive drugs, the user's expectations and the nature of the environment shape the experience very considerably.

These peak effects usually last only for a few minutes or so, and are followed by a more relaxed sense of well-being for half an hour or more. Some seasoned users have remarked that the intensity of the pleasurable effects increases with subsequent exposure, contrary to experience with most euphoria-producing drugs for which the opposite is normally the case. Tolerance (increasing resistance to the euphoric effects leading to consumption of ever-larger doses) is likely to occur in regular sniffers.

Unwanted effects

During the high, most users feel dizzy and lightheaded, may be aware of their heart pounding rather quickly, and look a bit flushed and flustered. Clumsiness not infrequently leads to accidents. About a third report an unpleasant headache, there may be buzzing in the ears or episodes of double vision, nausea is not uncommon, and vomiting may occur. Some experience chest or abdominal pain. An observer may note quivering eyeballs (nystagmus) and enlarged pupils. Irritant fumes may cause coughing bouts, sneezing, and streaming eyes. If the concentration of vapour is intense, there may be disorientation, drowsiness, and even unconsciousness at very high doses.

After the high has passed, there often follows a hangover period characterized by lethargy, depression, irritability, restlessness and agitation, poor appetite, and altered sleeping pattern. The user may experience chills, aches, and pains. The mood swings unpredictably and memory and concentration can be impaired. Parents of regular sniffers sometimes notice that their child seems more secretive or suspicious, that hobbies and established interests are being abandoned, that patterns of friendship are altering, and that school performance is deteriorating. Regular users at times develop spots or ulcers round their mouths or noses ('glue sniffer's rash'), cracked lips, and seem to suffer from a perpetual cold, sore throat, or bronchitis. They may exude a characteristic odour, spill marks are sometimes evident on clothes (especially cuffs) or around their room, and smelly bottles, bags, or rags may be left lying about. Regular, heavy huffers, or first-timers who have completely misjudged the dose, occasionally require hospital admission if they become very confused, have fits, or lapse into complete unconsciousness. Recovery is usually rapid (within a few hours) and complete.

One study indicated that school children who sniff solvents perform less well on tests of vocabulary, IQ, and impulsivity. However, when measures of background social disadvantage were taken into account, the difference disappeared. Also, the performance deficit did not correlate with the amount or frequency of sniffing. The authors concluded that there was no evidence of neuropsychological impairment in this particular sample of glue-sniffing adolescents. However long-term sniffers probably run the risk of some memory loss and attention deficits.

In the very large majority of sniffers for whom the activity is a one-off or transient phase, no long-term harm ensues. People who do suffer harm are much more likely to be those using large amounts over prolonged periods, with other drug use and risky or deviant behaviour contributing to the picture. There is a risk of damage to the liver or kidneys in heavy, chronic sniffers. Toluene and benzene can depress the blood cell production in the bone marrow leading to anaemia, sometimes irreversible. Benzene is thought to be associated with increased risks of cancer and leukaemia. The brain is also vulnerable to structural damage which can cause people to tremble, slur their speech, become clumsy and lose their balance, or develop memory problems. There may be injury to the nerves in the limbs, giving rise to 'glove and stocking' anaesthesia. A part of the brain concerned with balance and coordination (cerebellum) is particularly at risk from toluene. Occasionally, the optic nerve (which relays messages from the retina to the brain) can be affected, leading to progressive blindness. Additives such as lead in petrol may contribute greatly to the toxic potential.

Inhalation of solvents by pregnant women is dangerous because these chemicals freely cross the placenta into the fetal circulation. There have been reports of such babies being born with abnormalities comparable to those of the fetal alcohol syndrome. The absence of more conclusive evidence of damage to the unborn baby may simply reflect a lack of appropriate research.

Heavy use of solvents is more common in people with psychiatric problems, and was found to be the major factor in 3.5% of referrals of under-16-year-olds to one London psychiatric hospital. It seems likely that these problems usually predate the solvent use rather than result from it and there is no evidence that solvent misuse directly causes mental illness. The sort of person who is seeking to blot out unpleasant emotions or thoughts is likely to be a solitary, daily user of larger and larger quantities, who is a regular attender at general practices or hospital emergency units with repeated social or medical crises.

Although rare in relation to the level of use, more children die as a result of VSA than from all the other illicit drugs combined. Between a quarter and a half of the deaths in recent years have occured in first-time huffers, and male fatalities outnumber female by three to one. The use of butane gas is particularly risky: its use accounted for 34 out of the 49 VSA-related fatalities which occured in the UK in 2006. Lighter fuel sprayed directly into the mouth may cause the throat to swell sufficiently to cause suffocation. Aerosols are the second most dangerous, since they tend to deliver toxic chemicals as droplets along with the vapour and have a particular propensity to cause the heart irregularities.

Most butane-related deaths are caused by direct toxicity, but as many as half of the deaths associated with glue sniffing are caused indirectly. The combination of disorientation, clumsiness, a sense of invulnerability, and lack of self-concern is potentially lethal and any alcohol taken at the same time greatly increases the risk. Injury from accidents, suffocation by the plastic bag or as a result of throat damage, sudden fire or explosion when people mix sniffing with smoking cigarettes, or choking on vomit whilst semi-conscious or comatose all contribute to the tragic catalogue.

Most of the other acute deaths result from irregular beating and decreased efficiency of the heart. Many inhalants exert a direct effect on the heart's muscle and nervous control, and the heart is made much more sensitive to the effects of adrenaline released in response to exercise or emotion. A sudden scare or abrupt physical exertion can provoke a potentially fatal dysrhythmia. For this reason, it is essential not to threaten or over-react to intoxicated sniffers. The vulnerability of the heart is further enhanced by reduced oxygen levels in the blood when air is rebreathed in a plastic bag.

Intermittent and even quite regular sniffers will not be troubled by a withdrawal syndrome on stopping, apart from the hangover described above. Very heavy regular users may experience a cluster of symptoms and signs similar to those suffered by people dependent on alcohol: trembling, sweating, and agitation, sometimes progressing in those who do not receive treatment to disorientation, hallucinations, delusions, and fits.

Selected references

Anderson, H. R. (1990). Increase in deaths from deliberate inhalation of fuel gases and pressurised aerosols [letter]. *British Medical Journal*. **301**, 41.

Chadwick, O., Anderson, R., Bland, M., Ramsey, J. (1989). Neuropsychological consequences of volatile substance abuse: a population-based study of secondary school pupils. *British Medical Journal*, **298**, 1679–84.

Cooke, B. R. B., Evans, D. A., Farrow, S. C. (1988). Solvent misuse in secondary school children: a prevalence study. *Community Medicine*, **10**, 8–13.

Davies, B., Thorley, A., O'Connor, D. (1985). Progression of addiction careers in young adult solvent misusers. *British Medical Journal*, **290**, 109–10.

Department of Health (2007). *Volatile Substance Abuse* http://www.dh.gov.uk/en/ Publichealth/Healthimprovement/Drugmisuse/Substancemisusegeneralinformation/ DH_4136708

Dinwiddie, S. H. (1994). Abuse of inhalants: a review. *Addiction*, **89**, 925–39.

Editorial (1990) Solvent abuse: little progress after 20 years. *British Medical Journal*, **300**, 135–6.

Field-Smith ME, Butland BK, Ramsey JD, Anderson HR (2008). *Trends in death associated with abuse of volatile substances 1971–2006.* Report 21: St George's, University of London.

Ives, R. (1990). Helping the sniffers. *Druglink*, **5**(5), 10–12.

Ives, R. (1990). The fad that refuses to fade. *Druglink*, **5**(5), 12–13.

King, M. D., Day, R. E., Oliver, J. S., Lush, M., Watson, J. M. (1981). Solvent encephalopathy. *British Medical Journal*, **283**, 663–5.

MORI (2005). *Volatile substance abuse today: a qualitative study.* Department of Health, London.

Nicholi, A. M. (1983). The inhalants: an overview. *Psychosomatics*, **24**, 914–21.

Lynn, E. J., Walter, R. G., Harris, L. A., Dendy, R., James, M. (1972). Nitrous oxide: it's a gas. *Journal of Psychedelic Drugs*, **5**, 1–7.

Ramsey, J., Bloor, K., Anderson, R. (1990). 'Dangerous games: UK solvent deaths 1983–1988. *Druglink*, **5**(5), 8–9.

Re-Solv (2009) *Factsheets.* http://www.re-solv.org/factsheets.asp.

Richardson, H. (1989). Volatile substance abuse: evaluation and treatment. *Human Toxicology*, **8**, 319–22.

Ron, M. A. (1986). Volatile substance abuse: a review of possible long-term neurological, intellectual, and psychiatric sequelae. *British Journal of Psychiatry*, **148**, 235–46.

Schwartz, R. H., Peary, P. (1986). Abuse of isobutyl nitrite inhalation (Rush) by adolescents. *Clinical Pediatrics*, **25**, 308–10.

Westermeyer, J. (1987). The psychiatrist and solvent inhalant abuse: recognition, assessment, and treatment. *American Journal of Psychiatry*, **144**, 903–7.

Chapter 9

Ecstasy and other 'party drugs'

The club scene

Multiple drug use has always been much more prevalent within the world-wide dance club subculture which emerged from the 'rave' scene of the 1980s in comparison with other young people. For example, a recent British survey revealed that whereas 50% of 16 to 29 year-olds had used an illicit drug at least once in the past, the figure for 'clubbers' was 79%. For many of these, drug taking might only be an occasional event, but 44% agreed that 'taking drugs is an integral part of my social life'. The breadth of drug use is also staggering. A group of Scottish dance club attenders interviewed in the 1990s had each consumed an average of 11 different drugs. Drug use within the past year was as follows: alcohol 96%; cannabis 96%; Ecstasy 87%; tobacco 86%; LSD 79%; amphetamine 77%; cocaine 59%; nitrite 'poppers' 51%; psilocybin 47%; temazepam 39%; diazepam 26%; codeine 19%; heroin 11%; ketamine 7%; solvents 6%; and buprenorphine 6%.

In trying to understand the effects, both wanted and unwanted, of Ecstasy and other party drugs, it is essential to keep in mind the fact that they are generally being taken as one among many other drugs, declared or covert.

Ecstasy

Historical background

Methylenedioxyamphetamine (MDA) was synthesized in 1910, then lay dormant until 1939 when it underwent testing in animals. It was launched in 1941 as a treatment for Parkinson's disease, without any great success. Gordon Alles, discoverer of amphetamine, wrote about his experiences with MDA in the 1950s, and perhaps it was this work which suggested some military potential to the organizers of the US chemical warfare research programme. MDA (the 'love drug') became available on the streets from the mid-1960s, and was subsequently brought under the control of the US Drug Abuse Prevention and Control Act (1970) and the British Misuse of Drugs Act (1971).

Methylenedioxymethamphetamine (MDMA, Ecstasy) is a phenylisopropylamine derived from aromatic oils from various plants, including nutmeg.

It was patented by the pharmaceutical company E. Merck in 1914. It too underwent toxicology studies courtesy of the US military in the 1950s and began to be used for its psychoactive effects from around 1970. This non-medical use grew steadily, particularly in Texas and California. In the UK an amendment to the Misuse of Drugs Act was introduced in 1976 to outlaw all amphetamine-like compounds, but in the US it remained legal and its use expanded steadily. One Californian laboratory alone produced 10,000 doses monthly in 1976, 30,000 monthly in 1984, and 500,000 in 1985. This enormous escalation may have been related to the easing of the cocaine epidemic and some eulogizing publicity for MDMA in journals such as *Time* and *Newsweek*.

In 1976, reports were appearing of the successful use of MDMA as an adjunct to individual, marital, and group psychotherapy. Leo Zeff, a psychologist who had used LSD in therapy sessions 10 years earlier, found that it helped people to communicate their feelings more effectively and tolerate criticism. It was also said to be helpful in the treatment of drug and alcohol abuse. Many favourable scientific publications appeared over the next few years, and more than 4,000 people received the drug as an adjunct to psychotherapy.

At the same time, concern about MDMA's abuse potential was growing, and the US Drug Enforcement Administration (DEA) sought to bring it under legal control in the early 1980s. Strong counterarguments were put forward by psychiatrists and others, but in 1985 the DEA terminated the discussion abruptly by invoking the Comprehensive Crime Control Act to bring MDMA under Schedule 1 control. Appeals brought a temporary reprieve, but DEA lawyers attacked the quality of the scientific evidence for efficacy and safety. MDMA was restored to Schedule 1 control in 1988, where it still resides. Publicity surrounding these protracted legal disputes was probably responsible for a spectacular increase in the non-medical consumption of the drug. The ban in 1985 also led to a flurry of 'designer drugs', chemical variants on the theme which did not fall within the scope of the law, one of which was methylenedioxyethamphetamine (MDEA, 'Eve'). This loophole was plugged in 1986 by the Controlled Substance Analogue Enforcement Act, which proscribes drugs similar in structure or psychological effect to those already banned.

Ecstasy took off in Britain in the mid-1980s through its association with the 'acid house' music phenomenon from which the rave culture and modern club scene have evolved. There are no reliable prevalence surveys, but it seems likely that it has been a familiar commodity to many hundreds of thousands of young people over the last decade. As a Class A controlled drug, the penalties for using or selling the drug are similar to those for heroin and cocaine. The UK Advisory

Council on the Misuse of Drugs reviewed the evidence of MDMA's harmfulness and recommended in 2008 that it should be reclassified to Class B. The Home Secretary rejected this advice in February, 2009.

Preparation and distribution

Ecstasy production peaked in the 1990s but began to decline early in the 21st century. The UN estimated that global production was around 103 tons in 2006. Western Europe continues to be the main source, but production has now spread to North America and South-East Asia. The Netherlands remains the principal European source, followed by Belgium, Poland, and the UK. Pure MDMA is a white powder, but its form on the streets is very varied. Most commonly it is sold as tablets or capsules of many different colours, often imprinted with an image such as a dove, heart, face, or other logo.

Around 80% of Ecstasy tablets manufactured in Europe contain MDMA (or a close variant such as MDA or MDEA) as the sole psychoactive ingredient, but the potency varies very widely between batches of tablets: the MDMA content of recently seized tablets has ranged from 2 mg to 130 mg. In batches which contain other psychoactive substances, methylamphetamine is the most frequent component but caffeine, ephedrine, ketamine, LSD, and PCP sometimes crop up.

Scientific information

The 'entactogens' or 'empathogens' produce a pleasurable combination of amphetamine-like stimulation and mild sensory distortion, but their particular characteristic is to induce a general feeling of empathy and goodwill. Although they interact with several monamine neurotransmitter systems, the unique profile of these drugs is related to their ability to cause the release of large amounts (far greater than the amphetamines) of serotonin (5-HT) from nerve endings in the brain. Serotonin plays an important role in regulating mood, sleep, aggression, hunger, and sexual activity. The primary, sought-after effects of MDMA seem to be related to the initial flood of serotonin through the brain, and the residual hangover to a subsequent depletion. It may also be relevant that MDMA can activate (albeit with low potency) a particular serotonin receptor subtype, 5-HT_{2A}, through which some hallucinogens (e.g. LSD, psilocybin) appear to work. Effects on the hormones oxytocin, vasopressin, and cortisol may contribute to this unique profile. Animals given MDMA show increased mobility, body temperature, heart rate, and salivation. These patterns of behaviour are different from those seen characteristically with stimulants or hallucinogens. MDA is reported to be longer acting and a 'rougher ride' than MDMA. It is supposedly less euphoriant and more amphetamine-like, and had a reputation on the street of being less well toler-ated by women than men.

MDMA is well absorbed when taken by mouth and metabolized by the liver, with a plasma half-life of around eight hours. Its pharmacokinetics are non-linear in that larger doses produce much greater increases in blood (and brain) levels than would be predicted. Reduced sensitivity to the pleasurable effects comes with repeated use, alongside more prominent amphetamine-type stimulation possibly due to a relatively greater degree of dopamine release. The amphetamine-like effects cause stimulation of the sympathetic nervous system 'fight or flight' mechanism. Heart rate and blood pressure go up, blood is diverted to the muscles away from the guts, the body's chemical processes speed up, and more oxygen is absorbed through the lungs.

Animal experiments have shown consistently that MDMA and MDA deplete the brain of serotonin and are directly toxic to serotinergic nerves, some of which actually die off. After several months some evidence of regeneration is usually evident, but at least a part of the damage appears permanent. The dam-age is proportional to the size and frequency of the doses and animal species vary considerably in their susceptibility. Monkeys, for example, are much more vulnerable than mice. They sustain damage at doses as low as 2 mg per kg of body weight twice daily, a level that is worryingly close to doses typically taken recreationally by party-goers. However, most animal studies have been conducted at very much greater doses than ever achievable by humans, or by routes of administration (e.g. intravenous, intraperitoneal) which produce much higher brain levels than the oral route.

There have been a number of studies in humans exploring serotonin func-tion by means of brain imaging, sampling its metabolites in cerebrospinal fluid, or pharmacological challenges of one sort or another. Stress response and cognitive function have been compared between MDMA users and nor-mal controls. The interpretation of this literature is unclear, and experts remain divided on whether or not there is convincing evidence of long-term human neurotoxicity following recreational use of MDMA.

MDMA gives positive results in animal models of dependency, but compulsive use or 'addiction' in humans seems unusual.

Medical uses

Although its current controlled drug status precludes any medicinal use, the therapeutic potential of MDMA has recently come under active review. Positive results have been reported in laboratory models of Parkinson's disease, and at the time of writing pilot studies of its use in the treatment of post traumatic stress disorder are underway in the US, Spain, Israel, and Switzerland. A further

US study of its utility in treating anxiety arising from a cancer diagnosis has begun, and it has been proposed as a possible alternative to electroconvulsive therapy in severe depression. Ketamine is being piloted as an adjunct to psychotherapy in the treatment of alcohol and heroin addiction.

Recreational use

The average lifetime prevalence of MDMA (Ecstasy; E; adam; bump; hug; doves; XTC) use amongst adults in developed countries is between 3–4%, with regional variations which fluctuate from time to time. Rates in Europe currently range between 1% (Finland, Malta, Romania, Ukraine) and 8% (Czech Republic). Figures for the US and UK are 5% and 7% respectively. Unsurprisingly, much of this consumption is concentrated in young adults, with lifetime use for those aged 18 to 24 19% in the Czech Republic, 10% in the UK, and 9% in the US. However, there is some evidence that the numbers of new initiates has declined in recent years in several countries, for example down from 1.2 million in the US in 2002 to 860,000 in 2006. Three quarters of new initiates are over the age of 18 with an average age of 21. Ecstasy use is ten times commoner in clubbers than non-clubbers, and twice as prevalent in males. Average prices have declined in Europe to around €4/tablet, but remain much higher in the US ($20–30/tablet).

The drug is almost always swallowed, but may occasionally be snorted into the nose. There are two distinct classes of user. By far the most numerous are young dance-clubbers who take it for the pleasure of the high and the enhanced sense of togetherness. Many of these will also be regular users of a range of other drugs, including alcohol, amphetamine, LSD, and cannabis, which will certainly modify the profile of effects. The other, much smaller group is made up of more spiritually inclined people in their thirties or beyond, perhaps exploring a 'New Age' philosophy of life, or seeking personal insights alone or within a relationship.

As with all drugs, the effects of MDMA depend to a large extent upon the characteristics of the taker, and the setting in which it is taken. It is hardly surprising that the experiences of a middle-aged psychiatrist who takes MDMA in the company of professional colleagues might contrast sharply with those of a young 'raver' grooving the night away with a thousand others to the beat from a sound system producing more decibels than a jumbo jet.

There are some common strands, however. Half an hour after taking a tablet, both the psychiatrist and the raver might have noticed increased alertness, possibly accompanied by a dry mouth, skin tingling, and an awareness of the heart beating faster. A sense of closeness and empathy with other people appears gradually and peaks after a couple of hours or so. A change in the quality of light perception (luminescence) usually occurs, and some people may experience actual visual hallucinations. The jaw often feels tight, sometimes with involuntary grinding of the teeth (bruxism).

Reports differ on the effects upon sexual behaviour. Concern has been expressed that MDMA and variants might release inhibitions and lead to an upsurge in promiscuous, 'unsafe' sex, alarming to those concerned about the spread of sexually transmitted diseases. The drug certainly seems to enhance the sensual enjoyment of sex, but whether or not it increases sex drive is unclear. The amphetamine-like component of the drug's activity may cause erectile failure in men, and inhibit orgasm in both sexes.

Some American psychiatrists have reported their personal experiences with Ecstasy. They described enhanced powers of communication, feelings of intimacy, improved 'interpersonal skills', and euphoria. Most also experienced perceptual enhancement (for example, increased musical appreciation), reduced fear and feelings of alienation, increased awareness of emotions, and suppression of aggressive impulses. Some said that the experience had caused them to rethink their priorities in life, whilst others felt that their social functioning had been improved significantly.

The most rewarding effects of MDMA seem to come from the first exposure, with diminishing returns for most people thereafter. Increasing the dose ('stacking') may recapture the pleasure and also enhance the likelihood of hallucinations, but more often it just increases the ratio of unwanted to wanted effects.

Unwanted effects

Certain pre-existing diseases, of which a person may be unaware, increase the likelihood of unpleasant or dangerous reactions to MDMA. These include diabetes mellitus, liver disease, high blood pressure or heart disease, epilepsy, glaucoma, hyperthyroidism, or a history of psychiatric illness. Pregnant women would be wise to avoid it; the lack of direct evidence of toxicity to the foetus may simply reflect the lack of appropriate research, and there is always the risk of toxic adulterants in black-market drugs.

MDMA produces a lot of transient unwanted effects, including clumsiness, incoordination, and poor concentration which may lead to accidents; drowsiness or restless agitation; fear or anxiety sometimes escalating into panic attacks or a sense of loss of control; depression; a racing heart and increased blood pressure, dizziness, or fainting; dry mouth and thirst; nausea and vomiting; headaches; tingling extremities; and persecutory feelings or unpleasant hallucinations.

Many people experience hangover effects which last for a day or two. These usually consist of tiredness, lethargy, insomnia, irritability, or low mood. The muscles may ache and feel stiff. One study showed that weekend use was associated with memory impairment and a dip in mood mid-week approaching the sort of severity seen in clinical depression. Flashbacks have been reported.

There are well-documented reports of serious physical and psychological reactions to MDMA. Whilst a proportion have occurred in people at risk because of pre-existing conditions or taking large doses of other drugs as well as MDMA, it is clear that idiosyncratic reactions to modest doses do occur, though rarely, and that these may prove fatal. The amphetamine-like effect may overstretch the heart and circulatory system, especially if there is unrecognized narrowing of the arteries or other cardiovascular disease. Convulsions have been reported, and blood pressure changes may be enough to cause a stroke. Interactions with other illicit or prescribed drugs that either inhibit a particular liver enzyme key to MDMA metabolism (CYP 450 2D6: e.g. ritonavir, methadone, bupropion) or also target serotonin (e.g. stimulants, SSRI antidepressants, MAO-inhibitors) may cause a dangerous reaction (serotonin syndrome). An association with liver damage has been suggested.

A rare but particularly serious physical reaction is a sharp rise in body temperature (hyperthermia) associated with damage to muscle fibres and blood clotting inside arteries and veins. This can lead to liver or kidney failure, coma and convulsions, and death. A hot environment, vigorous exercise, and dehydration may combine with the direct effects of the drug to increase the risk of this reaction. Provision at clubs of adequate ventilation with access to water and soft drinks, rest areas, and cool retreats where people can 'chill out' is essential. On the other hand, overdoing the water may cause a loss of salts from the body and Ecstasy may itself heighten this effect leading to overhydration or 'water intoxication', and at least one death has been attributed to this. The best advice is to sip water regularly rather than gulp it in huge amounts, and try to include some isotonic drinks and salty snacks.

Although these risks are genuine, it is important to keep them in perspective. Deaths and serious reactions are very rare in relation to the large amounts of the drug which have been consumed over the years. Some of the deaths attributed to MDMA, and other serious but non-fatal reactions, may be due at least in part to pre-existing physical disease, other drugs, or adulterants in the black-market supplies. One study has estimated that somewhere between three and nine emergency hospital visits may occur from every 10,000 uses of Ecstasy. In the UK, approximately 20 deaths per year are attributed to the drug in the context of an estimated 100 million tablets consumed. This contrasts with

7,000 deaths associated with alcohol consumption each year, and 106,000 caused directly by tobacco smoking.

Serious psychological reactions to MDMA can also occur. These usually take the form of prolonged anxiety or depression, but a few cases of persistent psychotic illness with hallucinations, delusions, and loss of contact with reality have been reported. In almost all of these cases, an important contribution from pre-existing mental disorder, or the regular use of other street drugs clearly associated with the risk of psychosis such as amphetamine, cannot be ruled out. Again, these reactions seem few and far between when viewed in context of the millions of doses consumed world-wide. One study showed that subjects who developed psychiatric problems associated with Ecstasy were more likely to have had mental state abnormalities which preceded their drug use. Treatment is symptomatic with antipsychotic medication and psychological support. MDMA does not cause physical dependence and its propensity to psychological dependence seems to be much less than the amphetamines but a bit more than the hallucinogens.

Gammahydroxybutyrate (GHB)

GHB (liquid Ecstasy; soap; GBH; Georgia home boy) is a naturally occurring fatty acid widely distributed in the brain. As a synthetic preparation it was developed in the US as a possible anaesthetic and premedicant for surgery, and was also used in the treatment of alcohol and opioid addiction and sleep disorders. It stimulates release of growth hormone and protein synthesis and therefore became popular amongst bodybuilders. Its over-the-counter availability was terminated in the US in 1990 because of concerns over abuse potential, and it was made a controlled drug in the US and UK in 2000 and 2003 respectively. It remains prescribable (as Xyrem) for the treatment of narcolepsy, but since it is easily synthesized from precursors widely available as industrial solvents almost all street supplies are manufactured illicitly.

GHB probably acts as an inhibitory neurotransmitter in the brain, and it has structural similarities to naturally occuring neurotransmitters such as GABA and glutamic acid. It is absorbed rapidly by mouth, reaches peak levels in blood within an hour, and is broken down quite rapidly to carbon dioxide and water.

Black market GHB is available in the form of powder, capsules, or more usually in small bottles of colourless, odourless liquid containing up to 20 grams of drug costing around £15 or $40, and enough for three or four doses. It is increasingly popular among clubbers for the euphoria and alcohol-like disinhibition and intoxication which come on within 30 minutes and last a few hours.

Unwanted effects, which can also be persistent, include dizziness, nausea and vomiting, muscle weakness, blurred vision, agitation, blackouts and memory lapses, hallucinations, fits, respiratory depression, and coma. The drug has been incriminated in several deaths in the EU. The ratio between a euphoriant and a toxic dose is very small. Variation in potency of black market preparations aggravates the risk. Regular users will find they need increasing doses to achieve the same effect and risk physical and psychological addiction. A very unpleasant withdrawal syndrome consisting of cramps, anxiety, and insomnia has been reported following heavy regular use and may escalate to hallucinations and delirium. GHB can interact with alcohol to bring about dangerous respiratory depression.

Gamma-butyrolactone (GBL) and 1,4-butanediol (1,4-BD)

GBL and 1,4-BD are widely used as solvents and components in the manufacture of paints, plastics and industrial cleaning agents. When taken orally, they are very rapidly converted in the body to GBH and appear to be growing in popularity as party drugs in many countries throughout the world. At the time of writing they are not generally subject to the same legal controls as GHB although this is under active review in the UK and US.

Because of its widespread industrial use, GBL is easily obtainable and a recreational dose (1ml of industrial strength material) costs only a few pence or cents. However, concentrations of different preparations vary widely, so accidental overdoses are a constant risk. Onset of action is reputed to be faster than GBH, but subsequently the profile of wanted and unwanted effects is identical. Since only GBH is detectable in body fluids following dosing with GBL or 1,4-BD it is difficult to estimate the morbidity and mortality associated with these drugs, but several deaths directly attributed to GBL are on record in the UK.

Ketamine

Ketamine (Ketalar; K; Special K; Vitamin K; cat valium; green; jet) is used in medicine as an intravenous anaesthetic which does not depress respiration and has a relatively benign safety profile. It is particularly useful as a battlefield drug and is also widely used in veterinary practice. However, it does have a propensity to cause hallucinations, and this has led to its recreational use. This was at a low level until the 1990s, when it became popular in the dance club scene and is now used by as many as 20% of clubbers. A separate and much smaller group of people use it as a tool for greater self enlightenment.

Black market supplies emanate from diverted pharmaceutical material, and the major sources are Mexico, the US, and Europe. It is available on the street in the form of powder, tablets, capsules, or liquid costing around £30 or $70 for a gram, and can be taken orally, snorted, or injected. It produces hallucinogenic and painkilling effects which are similar to those of PCP, but is shorter lasting and considerably less toxic. Small doses ('bumps') of around 100 mg produce a pleasant dreamy effect with mild perceptual changes. Users can feel depersonalized or cut off and remote from their surroundings, but the duration of action is usually only an hour or so. Ketamine increases heart rate, cardiac output and blood pressure, and impairs cognition and coordination. Nausea and vomiting, clumsiness, limb numbness, visual impairment, and slurring of speech are all quite likely to occur, and accidents are always possible. Because of its action in the brain as a glutamate antagonist, concern has been expressed that it may precipitate schizophrenia and other psychotic disorders. As yet, there is no reliable information on the possible consequences of long-term use.

mCPP

1-(meta-chlorophenyl)piperazine (mCPP) is a powerful releaser of brain serotonin, and thus has a pharmacological similarity to MDMA. It is the active metabolite of a widely used antidepressant, trazodone. It is not currently illegal and some tablets marketed as Ecstasy actually contain mCPP.

Selected references

Advisory Council on the Misuse of Drugs Technical Committee (2004). *Report on ketamine*. Home Office, London.

Advisory Council on Misuse of Drugs (2006). *GBL & 1,4-BD: Assessment of risk to the individual and communities in the UK*. Home Office, London. http://drugs.homeoffice.gov.uk/publication-search/acmd/report-on-gbl1

Barnes, D. M. (1988). New data intensify the agony over Ecstasy. *Science*, **239**, 864–6.

Chadwick, I. S., Linsey, A., Freemont, A. J., Doran, B., Curry, P. D. (1991). Ecstasy, a fatality associated with coagulopathy and hyperthermia. *Journal of the Royal Society of Medicine*, **84**, 371.

Creighton, F. J., Black, D. L., Hyde, C. E. (1991). Ecstasy psychosis and flashbacks. *British Journal of Psychiatry*, **159**, 713–15.

Curran, H. V., Travill, R. A. (1997). Mood and cognitive effects of MDMA: weekend 'high' followed by mid-week low. *Addiction*, **92**, 821–31.

Deehan A., Saville E. (2003). *Calculating the risk: recreational drug use among clubbers in the South East of England*. Home Office Online Report 43/03; Home Office, London.

De Win, M. M. L., Jager, G., Booij, J. et al. (2008). Neurotoxic effects of ecstasy on the thalamus. *BJPsych*, **193**, 289–96.

Dorn, N., Murji, K., South, N. (1991). Abby, the Ecstasy dealer. *Druglink*, **6**(6), 14–15.

Forsyth, A. J. M. (1996). Places and patterns of drug use in the Scottish dance scene. *Addiction*, **91**, 511–21.

Galloway, G. P., Frederick, S. L., Staggers, F. E. et al. (1997). Gamma-hydroxybutyrate: an emerging drug of abuse that causes physical dependence. *Addiction*, **92**, 89–96.

Gonzalez, A. and Nutt, D. J. (2005) Gamma hydroxy butyrate abuse and dependency. *J.Psychopharmacol.*, **19**, 195–204.

Greer, B., Tolbert, R. (1986). Subjective reports of the effects of MDMA in a clinical setting. *Journal of Psychoactive Drugs*, **18**, 319–27.

Hayner, G. N., Mckinney, H. (1986). MDMA: the darker side of Ecstasy. *Journal of Psychoactive Drugs*, **18**, 341–7.

Henry, J. A. (1992). Toxicity and deaths from Ecstasy. *Lancet*, **340**, 384–7.

Lenton, S. Boys, A., Norcross, K. (1997). Raves, drugs, and experience: drug use by a sample of people who attend raves in Western Australia. *Addiction*, **92**, 1327–37.

Mcguire, P., Fahy, T. (1991). Chronic paranoid psychosis after misuse of MDMA (Ecstasy). *British Medical Journal*, **302**, 697.

Molliver, M. E., Berger, U. V., Mamounas, L. A., Molliver, D. C., O'Hearn, E., Wilson, M. A. (1990). Neurotoxicity of MDMA and related compounds: anatomic studies. *Annals of the New York Academy of Sciences*, **600**, 640–64.

Muetzelfeldt L., Kamboj S. K., Rees H. et al. (2008). Journey through the K-hole: phenomenological aspects of ketamine use. *Drug & Alcohol Dependence* **95**, 219–29.

Oesterheld J. R., Armstrong S. C., Cozza K. L. (2004). Ecstasy: pharmacodynamic and pharmacokinetic interactions. *Psychosomatics* **45**, 84–7.

Pearson, G., Ditton, J., Newcombe, R., Gilman, M. (1991). An introduction to Ecstasy use by young people in Britain. *Druglink*, **6**(6), 10–11.

Price, L. H., Ricaurte, G. A., Krystal, J. H., Heninger, G. R. (1989). Neurendocrine and mood responses to intravenous L-tryptophan in MDMA users. *Archives of General Psychiatry*, **46**, 20–2.

Sessa B., Nutt D. J. (2007). MDMA, politics and medical research: have we thrown the baby out with the bathwater? *Journal of Psychopharmacology* **21**, 787–91.

Shapiro, H. (1989). The speed trip: MDMA in perspective. *Druglink*, **4**(2), 14–15.

Solowij, N., Hall, W., Lee, N. (1992). Recreational MDMA use in Sydney: a profile of Ecstasy users and their experiences with the drug. *British Journal of Addiction*, **87**, 1161–72.

Steele, T. D., McCann, U.D., Ricaurte, G. A. (1994). 3, 4-Methylenedioxymethamphetamine (MDMA, 'Ecstasy'): pharmacology and toxicology in animals and humans. *Addiction*, **89**, 539–50.

Whitaker-Azmitia, P. M., Aronson, T. A. (1989). Ecstasy-induced panic [letter]. *American Journal of Psychiatry*, **146**, 119.

Chapter 10

Anabolic steroids

Historical background

The effects of testosterone on muscle growth and development were first reported in 1938 and and the relevance of this discovery for improving sports performance was appreciated within a year. Derivatives were used by the German military in World War II to enhance aggression among new recruits. Body-builders began to give public endorsement to various brands of anabolic steroid in the 1940s and 1950s and they were openly used by Olympic weight-lifting teams at that time. Since then, millions of pounds have been spent by official sporting bodies in an attempt to eliminate their use, but with only limited success.

Anabolic steroids have been used in a wide range of medical conditions including osteoporosis, metastatic breast cancer, testicular deficiency, and as an aid to recovery from burns, surgery, or trauma, but alternatives with better side-effect profiles are now generally preferred. A small list of current indications remains (see below). They are Schedule III (US) and Class C (UK) controlled drugs. In most countries steroids are available on prescription and possession for personal use remains legal, but illicit importation or supply may attract a prison sentence.

Preparation and distribution

Anabolic steroids which can be prescribed legally in the US and UK include nandrolone, oxandrolone, oxymetholone, and stanozolol. However, over a hundred variants are available illicitly, some of which are manufactured in 'underground' laboratories and may therefore be of dubious purity. The most common black market products currently available are the pharmaceuticals listed above diverted from legitimate use, methandrostenolone, and injectable preparations of nandrolone, Depo-testosterone, and boldenone. Some of the illegal supplies entering the US emanate from Mexico where no prescription is required for their purchase, but the bulk of illicit production seems to be centred in Eastern Europe.

Scientific information

The term 'anabolism' is derived from the Greek *anabole* which means 'a raising up'. In physiology it refers to the building up in the body of complex chemical compounds by the bringing together of clusters of simpler ones, and particularly the creation of proteins from collections of amino acids. An androgen is a substance which stimulates the male genital organs, and all anabolic steroids have some androgenic effect.

The most important natural androgen is testosterone, and when secreted at puberty this hormone produces a growth spurt and stimulates development of the masculine sexual equipment and general appearance. In females and prepubescent boys the testosterone levels in plasma are generally less than 60 mg per 100 ml, while those in adult men are usually more than 10 times greater than this. In animal studies there is a clear link between testosterone levels and aggression, but the correlation is not so clear-cut in humans.

Anabolic steroids increase the proportion of protein laid down as tissue, especially in the muscles. They also stimulate the growth of bone but at the same time hasten the process which terminates the extension of the long bones in the arms and legs (epiphyseal closure). This can result in a stunting of growth if they are taken by children or adolescents.

Volunteers given test doses describe euphoric effects, increased energy, and sexual arousal, but also irritability, mood swings, and raised feelings of hostility. In the brain they bind to androgen and oestrogen receptors and influence gene expression. They are not directly euphoric, but long-term use seems to influence dopamine, serotonin, and endorphin pathways. They are active in some animal models of reinforcement, suggesting some addictive potential.

Anabolic steroids are taken by male and female athletes because they increase lean muscle mass and strength if taken alongside intensive exercise and a high-protein, high-calorie diet. They also stimulate production of red blood corpuscles, thereby increasing the oxygen-carrying capacity of the blood and enhancing the capacity for intensive training. The androgenic component boosts competitiveness and determination.

Medical uses

Medical indications are now limited to treatment of life-threatening aplastic anaemia, chronic muscle wasting associated with AIDS or other major disease, severe itching due to certain types of jaundice, the rare condition of hereditary angio-oedema, and endometriosis or fibrocystic breast disease unresponsive to other drugs.

Recreational use

Prevalence rates for anabolic steroids (roids; gym candy; juice; arnolds; pumpers; stackers) in the general adult population of developed countries are quite modest, generally 0.6% lifetime experience and 0.1% current use. Rates are higher among young people, with almost 5% of high school students in the US admitting having used them at least once. In Europe the average within the same age group is 2%, with a range between 1% (several countries including UK) and 5% (Poland, Turkey). These figures probably represent a small decline in use over the last twenty years. Reasons for using them are to increase strength and muscle bulk, to improve appearance, and peer pressure. However, the real concern is the level of use aimed at improving athletic performance. Recent surveys among gym attenders and bodybuilders have indicated prevalence rates up to 30% and 50% respectively. Among such users, there is resistance to giving them up despite a clear awareness of the risks to health. Athletes are on record as saying that serious illness in the future or even a premature death would be an acceptable price to pay for sporting excellence now.

Steroids are usually taken by mouth, though injection is by no means uncommon, and are easily obtained at gyms and weight-training clubs. Prices vary between products, but average around £10 ($20, €13) for 20 tablets and £2 per ampoule. Athletes typically consume them in cycles of three months on alternating with three months off, and doses way beyond recommended maximums are the norm. The practice of combining several different steroids to enhance the effect is known as stacking. There are many other performance-enhancing drugs which are likely to be taken in addition, including clenbuterol (promotes muscle growth and fat metabolism), growth hormone (not detectable on urine testing), human chorionic gonadotrophin (stimulates secretion of testosterone), diuretics such as spironolactone or frusemide (for muscle shaping), and thyroxine (promotes fat metabolism). For sprinting and other 'explosive' sports stimulants such as caffeine or amphetamine may be used, and erythropoietin boosts stamina by enhancing the oxygen-carrying capacity of the blood. When extra steadiness is required, beta-blockers such as propanolol may be effective. Corticosteroids, anti-inflammatories, and even opioids are used to suppress the pain that comes from excessive exercise, and female gymnasts have been known to take endocrine agents to delay the inconvenience of puberty. Diuretics are used by boxers and jockeys to lose weight—artificially, since this is only due to a temporary voiding of fluids—just before a fight or a race.

Although most steroid use is in the context of enhancing sporting performance, some young people take them simply for the euphoric and confidence-boosting effect. Injecting in this context is not unusual, and the majority of needle-exchange clinics have steroid injectors amongst their clientele.

Unwanted effects

Anabolic steroids produce many unpleasant or dangerous effects but there have been no long-term studies to quantify this risk accurately in young, healthy people. In one survey less than a fifth of users escaped with no unwanted effects at all, while two-thirds had experienced two or more at some time. The commonest effects described by this sample were shrinking testicles, menstrual problems, raised blood pressure, and nosebleeds.

The most obvious cosmetic problems in men include a puffy face and spotty skin, breast enlargement, and a bulkier penis offset by shrinking testicles and a propensity to impotence. Women risk masculinization and hair loss. Headaches, nausea, and vomiting are common. Gum swelling can be a problem for both sexes.

In regular users blood pressure is increased alongside fluid and electrolyte retention, giving a risk of strokes. Raised plasma LDL and lowered HDL cholesterol levels could contribute to heart attacks and atherosclerosis. Liver damage may result in jaundice (particularly with stanozolol) as may a particular form of inflammation (peliosis hepatitis), and there is a raised incidence of liver cancer. Sex drive is often boosted but fertility declines in both men and women as a result of suppression of sperm production and motility and disruption of the menstrual cycle. The immune system may be impaired, and it is possible that injectors who share equipment are more than usually vulnerable to infection with HIV or hepatitis. In adolescents, growth and pubertal changes are inhibited through direct effects on bone growth in the arms and legs and suppression of hormones such as gonadotrophin. Large doses can produce diabetes and the hormonal disorder acromegaly.

Anabolic steroids can induce a wide range of unpleasant psychological symptoms. Depression, confusion, chronic fatigue, psychosis, emotional instability, grandiose delusions, and impulsive aggression have all been described. The phenomenon of 'roid rage' is particularly associated with the more androgenic agents or with large doses ('stacking'), and the 'steroid defence' has been used in a number of rape, assault, and homicide cases in the US. Sleep patterns are often interrupted and memory and concentration may suffer. Some cases of addiction have been reported.

Selected references

Korkia, P. (1994) Anabolic steroid use in Britain. *Drug Policy*, **5**, 6–10.

Korkia, P. (1997). Anabolic–androgenic steroids and their uses in sport and recreation. *Journal of Substance Misuse*, **2**, 131–5.

National Institute on Drug Abuse (2006). *Anabolic steroid abuse.* NIDA Research Report Series; NIH Publication Number 06-3721

National Institute on Drug Abuse (2009). *NIDA Infofacts: steroids (anabolic-androgenic)* http://www.drugabuse.gov/Infofacts/Steroids.html.

Wiefferink C.H., Detmar S.B., Coumans B. et al. (2008). Social psychological determinants of the use of performance-enhancing drugs by gym users. *Health Education Research* **23**, 70–80.

Williamson, D. (1994). The psychological effects of anabolic steorids. *Drug Policy*, **5**, 18–22.

Chapter 11

Tranquillizers and sleeping pills

Barbiturates

Historical background

Insomnia, or at least the subjective impression that one is not getting enough sleep, is a perennial human blight. Modern surveys suggest that between 30–40% of the adult population of Europe, the US, and Japan are experiencing poor sleep at any one time, and half of these have measurable daytime deficits in performance as a result. Herbal potions, opium, and alcohol have all served as sleeping-draughts in their time. In the middle of the 19th century, the sleep-inducing property of bromide was discovered, and its derivatives became very popular. It was not until the 1930s that recognition of their neurotoxic effects led to their disappearance.

Advances in organic chemistry in the 19th century resulted in the introduction of paraldehyde and chloral but the most significant discovery was that of barbituric acid in 1864 (named by its originator, von Baeyer, after 'a charming lady named Barbara'). Barbitone was marketed in 1903, phenobarbitone quickly followed and quite soon there were more than 50 'barbiturates' commercially available. These were soon prescribed widely for insomnia and anxiety and later, in combination with amphetamine, for depression. Cases of dependence were reported in Europe as early as 1912, but it was not until 1950 that physical dependence on barbiturates was fully recognized.

Until the late 1950s, the morbidity and mortality associated with barbiturates was mainly confined to people receiving legitimate prescriptions and those members of their households with access to the bathroom medicine cupboard. This changed when young people discovered that barbiturates were effective in slowing the pace of life back down to a controllable tempo after partying with amphetamine. Heavier users of stimulants came to realize that taking barbiturates simultaneously mellowed out the sharp edges of the high and eased the crash which eventually has to be faced at the end of a binge. For heroin users their easy availability and low price made them an invaluable stand-by when supplies ran short, and dealers cut them into street opiates as a cheap alternative to the real thing. Oblivion seekers found in them the ultimate prize.

This rapid growth in non-medical use of barbiturates was facilitated by the huge amounts being manufactured for the legal market. In 1960, one billion tablets were dispensed from pharmacies in Britain, 2,000 tons were manufactured in the US and several hundred thousand US citizens were physically dependent. Combinations with amphetamine, such as Purple Hearts (Drinamyl), became very popular for recreational use. Mandrax (methaqualone—not a barbiturate but very similar in profile—plus diphenhydramine) appeared in Britain and the US in 1965, and by 1968 was the most widely prescribed sleeping tablet. Although withdrawn as a medicine in the 1980s methaqualone still has its devotees, particularly in South Africa where it is widely smoked in combination with marijuana.

By the late 1960s, there were more than 2,000 barbiturate-related deaths each year in Britain, including high profile musicians such as Brian Jones, Jimi Hendrix, and even Elvis Presley. Injection of barbiturates was common among heroin addicts and responsible for many fatal accidental overdoses. Barbiturates were second only to coal gas as the instrument for suicide, accounting for 8,000 deaths yearly in Britain.

These sombre statistics did little to stem the enthusiasm of doctors or their insomniac and anxious patients. British doctors wrote 16 million prescriptions for barbiturates in 1964. Five hundred thousand people were reckoned to be taking them legitimately, with almost a quarter of these dependent on them. It was only the introduction of a safer alternative, the benzodiazepines, that stemmed the tide. This sent the barbiturates into a rapid decline during the 1970s, and their use in medicine became highly restricted. There was a small upsurge in illicit use in the early 1980s, and they retain a limited though toxic presence within today's street drug scene.

Preparation and distribution

Almost all black market barbiturates are diverted from legitimate medical practice. Drugs currently available include phenobarbital, amylobarbital (Amytal), pentobarbital (Nembutal), butobarbital (Soneryl), quinalbarbital (Seconal), and a mixture of amylobarbital and quinalbarbital (Tuinal). It is possible to buy drugs such as mephobarbital and secobarbital via the internet.

Scientific information

The barbiturates are categorized according to their duration of action. Use of short-acters such as thiopentone is confined to the operating theatre or intensive care unit. Long-acting drugs, which include phenobarbitone and allobarbitone, remain in the bloodstream for days and so rapidly accumulate in the body if taken regularly. Blood levels of the medium-acting group (pentobarbitone, quinalbarbitone, butobarbitone, and amylobarbitone among others) halve every 30 to 40 hours. All are absorbed well by mouth and are gradually broken down by the liver. Barbiturates stimulate drug-metabolizing enzymes in the liver, and this can result in reduced effectiveness of other drugs such as the contraceptive pill, blood thinning agents, and corticosteroids.

Resistance develops to the hypnotic and tranquillizing effects but less so to the depressant effect on respiration, which can lead to accidental overdose with fatal consequences. This tolerance generalizes to other brain depressants such as alcohol.

Barbiturates work by enhancing the activity of the inhibitory neurotransmitter, γ-aminobutyric acid (GABA). They interact with the GABA receptor complex on the cell membrane to increase the flow of chloride ions through its channel (ionophore), increasing the polarization and thereby inhibiting cellular excitation. The duration of opening of the ionophore is also increased, causing prolonged depression of the cell. Larger doses directly activate GABA receptors and block CNS glutamate (excitatory) receptors. A small dose of barbiturate produces calmness and relaxation that is comparable to three or four units of alcohol, but since the ratio between therapeutic and toxic doses is very low it may also cause clumsiness, slurred speech, and unsteady gait. People taking barbiturates are notoriously accident prone. Subclinical depression of breathing at therapeutic doses increases vulnerability to bronchitis and pneumonia.

Medical uses

Apart from the use of short-acting compounds in anaesthesia, the only current medical indications are for epilepsy and severe intractable insomnia in patients already taking barbiturates.

Recreational use

Statistics are lacking on current non-medical use of barbiturates (barbs; yellow jackets; red birds; goof balls). In comparison to benzodiazepines they are not easily accessible on the black market but are still prized by serious oblivion seekers. Such people may grind up tablets or dissolve the contents of capsules and inject the resulting sludge into a vein. Pill injecting is always risky but with barbiturates it is particularly dangerous. Heroin addicts sometimes inject barbiturates unknowingly when they are used as adulterants to boost inferior material. The combination of barbiturate and amphetamine has a timeless appeal which transcends the current lack of a ready-formulated product.

It seems that the stimulant's effect on energy, confidence, and strength, and the depressant's suppression of fear and anxiety combine to produce a particularly desirable high. The shortage of barbiturates makes it much more likely that the infinitely safer benzodiazepines will fulfill this role, and opiates are another alternative.

Unwanted effects

Mild toxicity at low doses is characterized by clumsiness, quivering pupils (nystagmus), slurred speech, and emotional instability. Alcohol and other brain depressants will potentiate these toxic effects. Minor side-effects include skin rashes, growth of hair in the wrong places, and swelling of the gums. Larger doses may cause respiratory or cardiovascular depression, pneumonia, or kidney failure, any of which can prove fatal. Confusion may progress to delirium or coma, sometimes after a delay of several days.

Long-term users often exist in a state of chronic impairment with symptoms of mild toxicity ebbing and flowing. They will exhibit unpredictable emotional states, switching between euphoria, depression, or irritability with little warning or provocation. Behaviour may be disinhibited and impulsive, and if influenced by a feeling of persecution dangerous aggression can result. Social deterioration is often apparent.

When tablets or the contents of capsules are ground up, mixed in water, and injected into a vein, the resulting suspension is highly irritant. Local tissue damage may be intense, and injury to the vein, or even worse to the nearby artery or nerve, can threaten the viability of the limb. Because of the rapid destruction of superficial veins, intravenous users may be forced to go for the large veins in the groin or neck, with disastrous consequences.

Sudden withdrawal of barbiturates will produce anxiety, agitation, trembling, stomach cramps, and sleeplessness. The sufferer may vomit, develop circulatory disturbances, or a fever. Without treatment, disorientation may be accompanied by delusions and hallucinations. There is a serious risk of convulsions which are often difficult to bring under control. Because of the potential seriousness of the barbiturate withdrawal syndrome, the procedure should be conducted in hospital or under close medical supervision.

There are several drugs which are not actually barbiturates but have very similar effects. Ethchlorvynol (Placidyl) is a tranquillizer with a characteristic mint-like aftertaste, whose effects begin around 30 minutes after oral dosing, peak at 90 minutes, and last between four and six hours. A hangover the next day is the usual sequel when it is used as a sleeping pill, and facial numbness is not uncommon.

Glutethimide (Doriden) enters the brain with particular rapidity, but is broken down in the body rather slowly. Apart from the usual barbiturate-like effects, it blocks the neurotransmitter acetylcholine which, in the graphic phraseology of a 1940s article, makes you '... hot as a hare, blind as a bat, dry as a bone, and mad as a hen'. It can also cause loss of calcium from the bones or anaemia.

Meprobamate (Miltown) is an effective muscle relaxant and tranquillizer, and in 1957 became the most widely used sleeping pill in the US because of effective marketing as a safer alternative to the barbiturates. It soon became a great favourite with opiate addicts for intravenous use. Its popularity waned as its true toxic potential emerged: fatalities were reported after as few as 15 tablets.

Although methaqualone (Qaalude—ludes; sopor) was withdrawn from legal supply many years ago, it is still prized on the black market and manufactured illegally in South America, China, India, and South Africa. In the latter it remains a major problem, although this is now said to be diminishing. It is famed for its ability to produce a dreamy 'dissociative high' without sedation, an effect similar to that described following heroin. There have been a number of deaths resulting from lack of attention, clumsiness, or disinhibition. There is also the possibility of rare but serious toxic effects, including nerve damage, life-threatening anaemias, and fits.

Benzodiazepines

Historical background

Extensive research in the 1950s fuelled by the need for a less toxic and addictive alternative to the barbiturates led to the serendipitous synthesis of chlordiazepoxide. This was shown to have a 'taming' effect in animals and increased exploratory behaviour, eating, and drinking which had been suppressed by new or frightening experimental conditions. It was marketed as Librium in 1960, and was soon followed by diazepam (Valium) in 1963. Both products were marketed aggressively by their manufacturer, Hoffman La Roche, and prescription sales accelerated rapidly as more analogues appeared and the barbiturates were swept aside.

Repeat prescriptions became commonplace, a process aggravated by the fact that most benzodiazepines were prescribed by hard-pressed family doctors confronted daily by large numbers of patients demanding treatment for sleeplessness and worry. Medicinal use peaked in the mid-1970s: in 1978 30 million benzodiazepine prescriptions were written in Britain and 2.5 billion Valium tablets consumed in the US. Since this zenith a slow decline has been noted, more recently reinforced by growing awareness among doctors of their limitations and addictive potential when used for longer periods, and publicity campaigns in the media. This process has been given momentum by lawsuits brought against doctors and pharmaceutical companies by individuals who feel they have been turned into addicts. Most doctors now try to limit their prescribing to carefully selected patients for no more than a few weeks, although others argue that the reaction against them has been excessive. Anxiety and insomnia remain as common as ever, and in comparison to other anxiolytic drugs their safety profile is impressive. Psychological treatments such as cognitive therapy are at least as effective but are unavailable in many parts of the world. There is some evidence that when benzodiazepine availability is reduced, self-medication with more toxic depressants such as alcohol increases.

Non-medical consumption of benzodiazepines mirrored prescription use and peaked around the same time. In the 1980s they were used regularly by around 4% of the US and UK populations, with much higher levels among adolescents and young adults. Usually they were taken by mouth, but tablets and the contents of capsules were sometimes ground up and snorted into the nose, or less commonly injected into a vein. Temazepam (temazzies; eggs; jellies) was and is a particularly popular black market choice in some countries (particularly the UK), but less so in the US. The intravenous injection of benzodiazepines intended for oral use, especially temazepam, became a significant problem with as many as 70% of injecting drug users in some parts of the UK admitting having done this at some time. The manufacturers of temazepam did not welcome the publicity, and in 1989 reformulated their liquid capsules as a hard gel in an attempt to make them uninjectable. Determined addicts found they could overcome this hurdle by warming the gel and using larger needles. This practice carried terrible health risks since the gel tends to harden up again in the bloodstream and can easily block vessels.

Preparation and distribution

Black market benzodiazepines emanate mainly from forged prescriptions or diverted pharmaceutical products. Availability thus reflects the contemporary commercial sucesses within the licit market. At present, the most popular products are lorazepam(Ativan), alprazolam (Xanax), clonazepam (Klonapin, Rivotril), diazepam (Valium), and temazepam (Restoril). Flunitrazepam (Rohypnol) is sought after but no longer commercially available, and is therefore manufactured illegally. There is a thriving internet business in benzodiazepines, with several hundred sites offering a variety of products.

Scientific information

As with the barbiturates, benzodiazepines work by enhancing the effects in the brain of the inhibitory neurotransmitter γ-aminobutyric acid (GABA). By acting at a specific site on the $GABA_A$ receptor complex on membranes of nerve cells they facilitate the binding of GABA to its own receptor, which increases the flow of chloride ions into the cell through its ionophore and thereby inhibits cellular excitation. Recently it has become apparent that there are several subtypes of $GABA_A$ receptor with different functions. Differences in activity at the various subtypes might account for subtle differences in pharmacological profile between benzodiazepines The abundance of GABA receptor complexes throughout the brain and spinal cord accounts for the diverse effects of the benzodiazepines. Stimulation of GABA receptors produces sedation, reduction of anxiety and agitation, muscle relaxation, a raised convulsion threshold, decreased cardiac contractility, and dilation of blood vessels.

From a safety viewpoint, benzodiazepines are not toxic to nerves and there are virtually no adverse effects outside the nervous system. However, respiration can be depressed by larger doses and there are currently 5.9 fatalities per million prescriptions (= toxicity index (TI)). The danger is greater in drugs which are very long-acting (flurazepam: TI = 150 or rapidly absorbed (temazepam: TI = 12), and a higher affinity for the receptor complex may also increase risk. In many cases with a fatal outcome there may have been coadministration with other brain depressants such as alcohol. Benzodiazepines cross the placenta and do seem to be associated with a small increase in risk of birth defects. When taken late in pregnancy they may produce the 'floppy infant syndrome', and since they enter breast milk they may sedate the baby.

Benzodiazepines are not very potent in laboratory models of dependency, but greatly reduce the suppressive effects of punishment on animal behaviour. Their hypnotic effect depends on an alteration in the pattern of 'rapid eye movement' and 'slow wave' phases of sleep. When they are discontinued this alteration is reversed with a degree of overshoot, giving rise to 'rebound insomnia'.

All benzodiazepines are well absorbed by mouth and most are broken down in the liver to active and inactive metabolites, some of which may be very long-acting. Depending upon rate of metabolism and profile of metabolites they can be conveniently categorised as short-acting (temazepam, oxazepam, loprazolam), medium-acting (lorazepam, alprazolam), and long-acting (nitrazepam, flunitrazepam, chlordiazepoxide, diazepam, clobazam, flurazepam, ketazolam). There is a complicated chemical interrelation between the drugs. For example, one of the metabolites of diazepam is temazepam, which in turn has oxazepam as one of its breakdown products.

Medical uses

Benzodiazepines are still widely prescribed for sleeplessness and anxiety. Other common indications include supplementation of anaesthesia and sedation for diagnostic or dental procedures; muscle relaxation in patients with spasticity or involuntary movements; various forms of epilepsy; detoxification from alcohol, stimulants and other drugs; and agitation caused by psychiatric disorders or drugs.

Recreational use

Most black market benzodiazepines (moggies; benzos; blues; downers; tranx; sleepers) are taken for their intoxicant effect but other important reasons include the need for sleep or rest, to limit the unwanted effects of stimulants or hallucinogens, to gain confidence to carry out criminal activities or other stressful tasks, and to boost the effects of opiates. They are cheap, costing around 50 pence or $1 a tablet and much less in bulk. Average prevalence of lifetime use among school students in Europe is 6%, with a range of 2% (Denmark, Germany, Ireland, UK) to 17% (Poland). High levels were also reported in Lithuania (14%), France (13%), Czech Republic (11%), and Hungary (10%). In most countries the prevalence in girls exceeds that in boys, although in the UK the opposite is the case. A very similar average pertains in the countries of South America. Amongst adults in the UK and US lifetime prevalence is around 3%, a level unchanged over the past 10 years. Prevalence is higher among young adults in both countries, with 1% and 2% respectively having taken them within the previous year.

At low doses the intoxication is similar to that of alcohol, but increasing tolerance to the desired effects causes some people to escalate their intake to 20 or 30 times the manufacturer's recommended limits. Such an intake is possible to maintain because the drugs are relatively cheap and easy to come by. Apart from criminal suppliers tablets can be obtained from enterprising pensioners whose repeat prescriptions for insomnia generate a useful income supplement, from alcoholics who prefer alcohol to the Librium or Chloral they are prescribed for withdrawal symptoms, or amongst the leftovers in family medicine cupboards.

Most people dependent upon opioids or stimulants use benzodiazepines from time to time, often in huge doses. A survey in Oxford revealed that 81% of the heroin addicts in contact with the drug dependency unit had used them in the previous year, and 27% were using them daily. Benzodiazepines augment the euphoric effect of heroin and methadone, and relieve agitation and dysphoria caused by amphetamine or cocaine. Intravenous administration using ground up tablets or gel extracted from capsules is by no means unusual in this context. Heroin addicts who also use benzodiazepines show higher levels of psychological and social impairment and are harder to treat. They are more likely to share injecting equipment, use multiple drugs, and inject more frequently; to be infected with hepatitis C; to be of low educational status and unemployed; to be more criminally active; and to have fewer friends.

Flunitrazepam (Rohypnol; roofies: rope) has developed a sinister reputation as a 'date rape drug'. It is a potent and rather long-acting agent which dissolves rapidly in fluids and is then tasteless and colourless. Combination with alcohol further enhances its ability to produce disinhibition or semi-consciousness, and someone who has received a covert dose may have little or no memory of what happens subsequently. In 1998 the legal manufacturer of Rohypnol altered the formulation to reduce its solubility and included a blue dye which is released when the tablets dissolve, but the drug in its original form is still available in generic formulations. Flunitrazepam is an illegal drug in the US, but still available on prescription in most other countries.

Unwanted effects

Apart from the possibility of accidents as a consequence of cognitive impairment, the only significant physical risk is respiratory depression and coma following overdose (or combination with other brain depressants) with the possibility of pneumonia or death resulting from inhaled vomit. This accounts for 5.9 fatalities per million prescriptions, although this figure underestimates the risk among illicit users who are often coadministering other psychoactive drugs. Very rarely, reversible abnormalities in liver function may occur.

Cognitive impairment with increased reaction time, clumsiness, and memory problems commonly occurs during short-term use. Almost half the users in one survey thought tranquillizers made them more violent and disinhibited. Chronic use is usually associated with diminishing benefits and numerous unwanted effects. These include increasing problems with concentration and memory; depression, tiredness, and apathy; clumsiness and accident proneness; fluctuating and unpredictable disinhibition; and instability of mood. The ability to cope with everyday problems is impaired and the elderly are particularly prone to all these effects. From time to time, withdrawal symptoms may emerge due to altered sensitivity to the regular dose. With toxic doses, confusion and memory deficits worsen and control over bodily activity deteriorates.

Anyone taking benzodiazepines regularly for longer than three weeks or so risks developing both psychological and physical dependence, particularly in the context of chronic stress, a history of dependence on other drugs or alcohol, poor coping skills, or a propensity to unpredictable mood swings.

Well over 50% of people coming off long-term benzodiazepine use will experience a withdrawal syndrome, although this is often difficult to distinguish from re-emergence of the pre-existing anxiety state. Abrupt termination results in more symptoms than tapering the dose off gradually. Shorter-acting drugs cause more intense withdrawal symptoms, and are associated with greater rates of relapse. Relapse occurs in up to half of those trying to give up, but successful quitters report lower levels of anxiety than when they were still taking the drugs. Symptoms come on after a day or two of abstinence in the case of short-acting compounds such as temazepam or lorazepam, but can be delayed for a week or more following more slowly metabolized drugs such as diazepam. Patients complain of anxiety, restlessness and irritability, heightened sensitivity to noise and other environmental stimuli, twitches and shakiness, weakness and lack of motivation or energy, stomach cramps, headaches, poor concentration or confusion, sleeplessness, and a craving for tranquillizers. These symptoms vary greatly in severity, and usually last for about two weeks. Convulsions may result from abrupt withdrawal from substantial doses.

Injecting benzodiazepines is associated with all the usual risks of this practice: septicaemia, hepatitis, HIV, and other infections; blockage of veins, damage to nearby arteries or nerves which can lead to loss of the limb; and abscesses or ulcers at the injection site. Injecting tranquillizers has a particular association with a self-destructive, chaotic, deviant lifestyle. People whose lives have taken this course are more likely to share injecting equipment, have unprotected sex, and take more accidental and deliberate overdoses.

There are a number of drugs which are not benzodiazepines but have a very similar effect. Chloral hydrate (or chloral betane, 'Welldorm') is a hypnotic first synthesized in the early 19th century, and was the original 'Mickey Finn' for slipping into someone's drink to knock them out. It is rapidly absorbed by mouth and the sedative effect lasts for a few hours. It has a characteristic bitter taste and is irritating to the stomach, and so should be avoided by those prone to indigestion or gastric ulcers. People with heart, liver, or kidney disease and breast-feeding mothers should avoid it. Chloral is still prescribable, though little used, and is sometimes available on the black market.

Chlormethiazole (Heminevrin) is another sleeping pill, and is structurally related to vitamin B_1 (thiamine). It is broken down rapidly in the body and is therefore quite short-acting. It has similar contraindications to chloral, and should be avoided during pregnancy and by breast-feeding mothers. It seems to cause sneezing and itchy, red eyes. It is used to treat severe insomnia and agitation in the elderly, and is often prescribed to alcoholics to relieve their withdrawal symptoms. Unfortunately it potentiates the toxic effects of alcohol in those who continue to drink, and is fairly easy to obtain on the black market.

Selected references

Buckley N. A., Dawson A. H., Whyte I. M., O'Connell D. L. (1995). Relative toxicity of benzodiazepines in overdose. *British Medical Journal* 310, 219–21.

Busto, U. E., Sellers, E. M., (1991). Anxiolytics and sedative/hypnotics dependence. *British Journal of Addiction*, 86, 1647–52.

Darke, S. (1994). Benzodiazepine use among injecting drug users: problems and implications. *Addiction*, 89, 379–82.

Darke, S., Ross, J., Cohen, J. (1994). The use of benzodiazepines among regular amphetamine users. *Addiction*, 89, 1683–90.

Higgit, A. C., Lader, M. H., Fonagy, P. (1985). Clinical management of benzodiazepine dependence. *British Medical Journal*, 291, 688–90.

Klee, H., Faugier, J., Hayes, C., Boulton, T., Morris, J. (1990). AIDS-related risk behaviour, polydrug use, and temazepam. *British Journal of Addiction*, 85, 1125–32.

Lader, M., File, S. (1987). The biological basis of benzodiazepine dependence. *Psychological Medicine*, 17, 539–47.

Lader, M., Morton, S. (1991). Benzodiazepine problems. *British Journal of Addiction*, 86, 823–8.

Leonard, B. E. (1989). Are all benzodiazepines the same? An assessment of the similarities and differences in pharmacological properties. *Psychiatry in Practice*, (Special Issue), April, 9–12.

Livingston, M. G. (1991). Benzodiazepine dependence: avoidance, detection, and management. *Prescribers Journal*, 31, 149–56.

Longo LP, Johnson B (2000). Addiction: Part 1. Benzodiazepines - side effects, abuse risks and alternatives. *American Family Physician* 61, 2121–8.

Lynch, S., Priest, R. (1992). Insomnia: who suffers, when, and why? *Prescriber*, 5th March, 37–44.

Nutt, D. (1991). Actions of classic and alternative anxiolytics. *Prescriber*, 19th May, 31–4.

Perera, K. M. H., Tulley, M., Jenner, F. A. (1987). The use of benzodiazepines among drug addicts. *British Journal of Addiction*, 82, 511–15.

Petersson, H., Lader, M. (1984). Dependence on tranquillizers. *Maudsley Monograph No. 28*. Oxford University Press, Oxford.

Rickels, K., Schweizer, E., Case, W. G., Greenblatt, D. J. (1990). Long-term therapeutic use of benzodiazepines: effects of abrupt discontinuation. *Archives of General Psychiatry*, 47, 899–907.

Schweizer, E., Rickels, K., Case, G., Greenblatt, D. J. (1990). Long-term therapeutic use of benzodiazepines: effect of gradual taper. *Archives of General Psychiatry*, 47, 908–15.

Seivewright, N., Donmall, M., Daly, C. (1993). Benzodiazepines in the illicit drugs scene: the UK picture and some treatment dilemmas. *International Journal of Drug Policy*, 4, 42–8.

Warneke, L. B. (1991). Benzodiazepines: abuse and new use. *Canadian Journal of Psychiatry*, 36, 194–204.

Chapter 12

Heroin and the opioids

Historical background

The opium poppy has provided humankind with one of the most important of all medicines. For thousands of years its products have been harnessed to soothe and sedate, and folklore evolved into descriptions in the great pharmacopoeias of the Egyptians, Sumerians, Greeks, Persians, and Romans.

Each age has spun its myths around opium. Theophrastus defined its medical applications in 320 BC but the Ancient Greeks also knew that when the goddess Demeter discovered the poppy's secret she forgot all her sorrows. What else could Helen of Troy's nepenthe have been but opium?

Today, the need and desire for the fruits of the poppy remain as great as ever. Strict international legal control of supply has created the basis for a worldwide, multi-billion dollar crime network built upon the exploitation and misery of millions of heroin addicts. Opioids remain central to pain control in Western medicine, but underdosing because of the fear of inducing dependency results in thousands of patients suffering needlessly.

From its roots in the ancient world, knowledge of opium was borne along the arteries of commerce. Arab traders introduced it into India in the seventh century AD, and to the shores of China a couple of hundred years later. Another messenger was the common soldier. Opium found its way to Europe in the pouches of returning Crusaders at the start of the new millennium.

Paracelsus (1490–1541), the first European to recommend the targeting of specific symptoms with specific remedies (for which he has been called the 'father of modern pharmacology'), invented a mixture of opium, alcohol, and spices which he called laudanum ('worthy of praise'). With minor modifications to the formula, laudanum was to soothe and torment millions of Europeans over the next 400 years.

The possibility of addiction to opium was recognized from the earliest times, but the first occasion this escalated into a national concern occurred in 18th-century China. When Britain conquered Bengal in 1773 it acquired a monopoly of Indian opium, which the East India Company began exporting to China in vast quantities. Opium smoking became widespread, and the failure over several decades to limit the habit led in 1839 to the seizure and destruction of large amounts of the drug at the instruction of Emperor Daoguang. Lord Palmerston promptly despatched 16 warships to besiege Nanjing, and so began what later became known as the First Opium War. It ended in 1842 with massive concessions to the British, including the ceding of Hong Kong island as a colony 'in perpetuity'. Further fighting took place between 1856 and 1860, but this simply led to more humiliation for the Chinese. By this time, there were between 15 and 20 million opium addicts in the country.

Opium was eulogized in European medical textbooks of the 18th and early 19th centuries. It was even recommended for use by those in the pink of health because of its ability to 'optimize the internal equilibrium of the human body'. In England, it became a popular home remedy comparable to aspirin today with consumption peaking in the middle of the 19th century.

Use of opium for pleasure or the relief of anxiety or insomnia was widespread throughout society, not least among such literary figures as Thomas de Quincy, S.T. Coleridge, Wilkie Collins, Charles Dickens, and Elizabeth Barrett Browning among many others. Less well publicized were those politicians and members of the professions who were also dependent upon laudanum. Nor was its use restricted to the rich and famous, since its modest cost brought opium within the financial reach of all but the destitute. And even the latter could always fall back on a bowl of poppy-head tea. The risk of dependency was recognized, but carried little social stigma for the most part. This tolerance was generally restricted to opium 'eaters' ('drinkers' would be a more appropriate term, since laudanum or patent medicines were by far the commonest form in which the drug was available). Opium smoking seems always to have been regarded as a rather vile alien indulgence.

Opium-containing medicines were widely used as child-calmers, and the mortality associated with this became a major concern in the middle of the 19th century. Most at risk were the small children of those women whose labours fuelled the industrial revolution. Inflexible working hours meant leaving children unattended for long periods and recorded fatalities (likely to be a considerable underestimate) were running at around 80 each year. In the population at large, fatal poisoning with narcotics made up about a third of all poisoning deaths.

Growing concern led to the introduction of the Pharmacy Act in 1868, which restricted sale of opium and its derivatives to registered chemists but had little or no impact on the volume of sales. This only began to decline significantly towards the end of the century as public perception of the drug became less favourable. This period saw a rapid decline in popularity of patent medicines and some expensive lawsuits against their manufacturers. The Act was made more restrictive in 1908.

Opium was brought to North America by the early European settlers, and quickly became familiar to most households as in Britain. With characteristic energy and enthusiasm, entrepreneurs were quick to see the commercial possibilities and America's first opium-containing patent medicine appeared in 1796. The dangers of excess were recognized just as quickly and were described in the Dispensatory of 1818 but, as in Europe, the drug soon became central to mainstream medicine. A prominent American physician wrote in 1846 that *'opium is undoubtedly the most important and valuable remedy of the whole materia medica'.* Laudanum could be bought for a few cents an ounce, and Americans took to patent medicines even more enthusiastically than Europeans. The foundations of some collosal modern fortunes were laid in those unregulated times, and by the end of the century more than 50,000 products were on the market. Poppies were cultivated throughout the land, and business was booming. Opiate addiction at that time was said to be much more common in women, possibly because social restrictions limited their access to alcohol.

Two 19th-century advances laid the foundation for the scale of problems we face today. First, the active ingredients of opium were identified, paving the way to the creation of immensely potent synthetic opioids. Second, the technique of intravenous injection was perfected.

In 1805, a German pharmacist's apprentice called Sertuerner isolated a chemical from raw opium which he initially called *principum somniferum.* Later, he hit upon the snappier name of morphine, after Morpheus, Greek god of dreams. This chemical was found to make up 10% of the weight of opium, and to be 10 times more potent. Isolation of codeine followed in 1832, thebaine in 1833, and papaverine in 1868. In 1874, di-acetyl morphine was synthesized in London but was not marketed by Bayer until 1898. It was initially considered an effective remedy for morphine addiction and its trade name was derived from the German word *heroisch,* meaning powerful.

The architect Christopher Wren was one of the first to experiment with injecting substances into the bodies of both animals and humans. In the early days, a blob of material would be placed on the skin, and repeatedly jabbed with a quill or something similar. Then came the idea of inserting a hollow tube into a vein and later in the 17th century there were even attempts at blood transfusions. The outcome of these early experiments was disappointing, particularly for the recipients. Interest was revived in the 19th century, and in 1858 a Scottish surgeon adapted an instrument which had been designed to drain blood from birthmarks to deliver a dose of morphine as closely as possible to the point of pain. This device became known as the hypodermic syringe. Administering drugs by injection very rapidly transformed medical practice, and the face of addiction too. Casualties in the American Civil War generated a big increase in opioid usage, and morphine addiction became known as 'the soldier's disease'.

Despite the widespread use of opium and its derivatives in 19th-century America, opium smoking remained socially unacceptable as in Britain. It was associated in the public mind with the Chinese immigrants who had been brought over in large numbers to work on the railroads in the 1850s. When a deep recession arrived soon after this with large-scale unemployment, these hard-working foreigners were deeply resented. Their habit of opium smoking became symbolic of a perceived degeneracy, and in an era of almost totally unrestrained drug and alcohol use opium smoking was made illegal in San Francisco in 1875.

Attempts to regulate the booming patent medicine business were slow in coming to the US. Not until 1906 did the Federal Pure Food and Drug Act require the ingredients to be specified on the label. Public concern mounted in the early years of the 20th century, and action to stem misuse of opioids suddenly became a political vote-winner. In 1909, importation of smoking opium became illegal, and the US was instrumental in bringing about a series of international conferences on narcotic abuse, first in Shanghai then at The Hague. In 1912, it was agreed that the participating countries (by then numbering more than 30) should enact domestic legislation to restrict the use of opioids to medical indications on prescription from a doctor. In the same year, the importation of opium into the US was banned.

The Harrison Act entered the statute books in 1914. A lengthy debate began as to whether the maintenance prescription of opioids to confirmed addicts constituted acceptable medical practice. In 1919, the Supreme Court ruled that it did not, thereby setting in motion a punitive response to drug addiction which remained unchanged until the AIDS epidemic forced a partial reconsideration of policy in the 1980s.

The public alarm which drove these legal moves is understandable given the size of the problem at the time; it was conservatively estimated that there were at least 275,000 opioid addicts in the US in 1920. In Britain, the situation seemed rather different. Despite the extensive use of opium and morphine throughout the previous century, opioid addiction was not a pressing problem in the early 20th century. The British were in no hurry to ratify the Hague agreement, a position which may possibly have been influenced by Britain's position as the world's foremost producer of morphine.

This *laissez-faire* approach was quickly abandoned during the First World War when it became clear that British soldiers on leave in London were keen to get hold of drugs which might make life in the trenches more tolerable. There was a roaring London black market in cocaine, but the fashionable shops were getting in on the act too. Harrods, for example, sold morphine and cocaine kits complete with syringe and spare needles labelled 'A Useful Present for Friends at the Front'. An order from army HQ forbidding the supply of drugs to soldiers on active service merely fuelled the black market. The order was then given teeth by the introduction of Defence of the Realm Act Regulation 40B in June 1916. This primarily targeted cocaine, but also restricted opium.

After the war, there were lurid newspaper stories of drug-fuelled debaucheries in London's West End. The death of a well-known actress and subsequent high-profile prosecution of her supplier gave the Home Office the opportunity to press for immediate civil legislation. This was unsuccessfully resisted by the Ministry of Health, and in 1920 the DORA 40B was enacted with many extra restrictions as the first Dangerous Drugs Act.

At first it looked as though the British response to drug problems would follow the penal route chosen by the US, but in 1926 a committee chaired by the President of the Royal College of Physicians was asked to examine the logic and practicalities of this course. The Rolleston Committee recommended that addiction should be regarded as an illness requiring treatment, rather than a crime deserving punishment. Long-term maintenance on an opioid prescription was recommended for addicts who were unable to give up but who could lead a 'useful life' when so maintained. The 'British System' for the treatment of opioid addiction thus came in to being.

Whether this humane approach would have found support if addiction had been other than a thoroughly middle-class affair has often been questioned. There were very few working-class opioid addicts known to doctors in the Britain of that era. Most came from the professional classes, and for some reason morphine injecting was particularly prevalent among respectable housewives. This stable, almost complacent state of affairs remained in place right through to the 1960s when it was suddenly and rudely disturbed.

In the US after the Great War the situation was very different. The visible plight of large numbers of opioid addicts led many doctors to hope that the Harrison Act would not be vigorously enforced. Addiction clinics were set up and large numbers of patients maintained. The Narcotics Division within the Bureau of Prohibition had other plans. In 1922, agents began a clamp-down on the clinics, and initiated prosecutions against addicts, doctors, and pharmacists. At first many physicians were prepared to contest these prosecutions in the courts, but after a number of careers had been ruined most were deterred and by 1925 the medical profession had withdrawn from the addiction field. By this time heroin had also been banned from use in medicine, and its legal manufacture in the US ceased entirely.

Half a million opioid addicts were thus abruptly cut off from their drug supply. Racketeers who had already grown fat on the proceeds of bootleg whisky couldn't believe their luck. Opium was cheap and easy to come by, morphine and heroin were simple to manufacture in backstreet laboratories, and the black market in narcotics was soon a nationwide business. When alcohol prohibition was repealed in 1933 the mobsters were unconcerned, because by this time undreamed-of profits were being achieved in the most lucrative criminal enterprise of all time. Since the 1920s, no world event has ever seriously interfered with the flow of heroin into North America.

American addiction rates probably fell during the Second World War and for a time thereafter, but rose steadily in the 1950s as the Mafia reopened trade routes from Turkey and South East Asia. Urban Black and Puerto Rican communities became key targets for the Mob. The penal response became more savage in an attempt to reverse the trend. The 1951 Bogges Act had already defined mandatory jail terms for possession with no possibility of parole in some cases. In 1956, the Narcotic Control Act doubled maximum sentences and made it possible to award dealers the death penalty.

By this time, it was becoming noticeable that the average age of American addicts was falling steadily: in the 1930s, fewer than 20% of male addicts were less than thirty, but by 1962 more than half were in their twenties.

Observing this trend with concern, the British government decided to review the situation in the UK. The Brain Committee's first report in 1961 was reassuring. Nothing had changed since the 1920s, just a small number of well-behaved professional types plodding along quietly on their scripts, and a handful of bohemian addicts in Soho and West Kensington.

Barely was the ink dry on the parchment when it became obvious to anyone visiting a jazz club or a coffee bar in West London that things were changing fast. The Brain Committee was hurriedly reconvened, and its second report pointed to a growing problem requiring drastic measures. These included restrictions on heroin and cocaine prescriptions, compulsory notification of opioid and cocaine addicts by doctors to the Home Office, and the establishment of special drug dependency units. The Misuse of Drugs Act was passed in 1970.

Why had the drug culture suddenly exploded? Economic stability meant money in people's pockets, better international communications were leading to the emergence of a powerful and independent youth culture, and a number of established addicts escaping the repressive policies of their own countries arrived in England to take advantage of the British System.

In an attempt to keep their patients out of the clutches of criminal suppliers, or more occasionally for simple monetary reward, a handful of London physicians were prepared to prescribe awesome quantities of heroin, cocaine, or injectable amphetamine to their young clients. One infamous doctor prescribed at least 600,000 heroin pills (for injection) to addicts in 1962. It was apparently not unusual for her to give an addict as many as 900 pills on a single occasion, and be prepared to replace them a few days later if they were reported 'lost'. She went on a lecture tour of Canada to describe her philosophy, resulting in a sudden wave of addicted immigrants to Britain. Some 'drug doctors' held their surgeries in pubs or station buffets. When the restrictions on heroin prescribing were introduced, some were undeterred or simply switched their addicts to other drugs. One who was later barred from practice prescribed more than 25,000 ampoules of methamphetamine in one month alone. By 1967, there were 2,000 registered heroin addicts in the UK.

The irony is that there was virtually no criminally organized black market in Britain at that time. Almost all drug seizures up to the end of the 1960s were of pharmaceutical heroin, cocaine, or amphetamine—overspill from this orgy of prescribing.

In both the UK and US there was a further upsurge of heroin use as the hippie movement degenerated, in the wake of an outbreak of methamphetamine injecting which swept the big cities. Heroin was one way of coming down from this harsh drug. Two peaks of prevalence occurred from 1968–72 and 1974–76: at these times, the drug was unusually plentiful, of relatively high quality, and cheap. Heroin use became endemic in provincial cities during the 1970s and 1980s. Street dealing was associated with increasing violence and some inner-city areas became virtual no-go areas to law-abiding citizens at certain times. The Iranian revolution in 1979 brought a large influx of refugees into Britain, many of whom transported their wealth in the form of heroin. The practice of smoking the drug off foil ('chasing') gained popularity as a result.

In periods of relatively short supply, 'designer drugs' tend to be marketed as an alternative, especially in the US. These have often been based on fentanyl, a synthetic compound 200 times more potent than morphine. Alpha-methyl fentanyl appeared on the streets in 1979 as 'China White', so-called because of its similarity in appearance to Chinese heroin of a particular type. Within 10 years, backstreet chemists had come up with at least ten variations of this basic drug, and perhaps a quarter of California's heroin addicts used a fentanyl variant at some time. One potential advantage for the user of these drugs is that they do not show up in standard laboratory tests for heroin. Unfortunately, fentanyl's high potency poses a potentially lethal risk and it has been directly responsible for well over a thousand deaths in the US. Analogues of pethidine (meperidine) also appear from time to time. Between 1982 and 1985, methyl-phenyl-propionoxypiperidine (MPPP) was marketed as 'synthetic heroin', and a toxic by-product of manufacture resulted in more than 500 cases of brain-damage.

In recent years diversion of prescription opioids has become a major problem in several countries, particularly the US. Around seven million US citizens used them illicitly in 2007, an increase in 80% from the numbers in 2000. Those most frequently diverted include codeine, dextropropoxyphene, oxycodone, hydrocodone, methadone, fentanyl, pethidine, and morphine. In one study, a third of all patients in receipt of an opioid prescription violated controlled drug policy in some way. One third of all new prescription drug abusers are teenagers, and diverted pharmaceuticals are now the most frequently abused drugs for 12 to 13 year-olds. In some countries, particularly France, Ireland, Scotland, New Zealand, and Mauritius, buprenorphine (an opioid receptor partial agonist) has become a frequent substitute for heroin. It is often used intravenously, and combination with a benzodiazepine seems particularly popular.

Preparation and distribution

Raw opium is obtained from the seed capsule of the poppy, *Papaver somniferum*. When this is slit after the petals have fallen, a white juice oozes out which soon thickens and darkens to a tar-like substance with a bitter taste and pungent smell. This is scraped off and boiled in water for several hours, then strained and evaporated to a thick paste called prepared opium which can be rolled into balls or squashed into bricks. Active ingredients, including morphine, codeine, papaverine, and thebaine, make up about a quarter of this material by weight. When smoked, up to half of the material is left behind in the pipe as a charred powder. This 'opium dross', rich in carcinogens, can be recycled by boiling it up with the next batch of raw opium.

In 2007 global production of illegal opium was estimated at 8,870 tons, up from 4,691 in 2000. Around 90% of this now originates from Afghanistan with a total export value around $4 billion, a quarter of which goes to the opium farmers. Myanmar (Burma), which used to be joint lead producer, accounted for around 5% and other producer countries include Columbia and Mexico which together produced most of the heroin imported into the US. Morphine is extracted in local laboratories by a simple process involving solubilizing with lime then precipitation by ammonium chloride. The resulting crude morphine base is further purified by adding hydrochloric acid to produce morphine hydrochloride, which in turn can be converted to heroin in a simple 12-hour process involving acetic anhydride. Two thirds of illegal raw opium is processed in this way, and the remainder is prepared for smoking by cooking in boiling water and straining to remove soil and plant material. The resulting solution is evaporated to a thick paste and dried in the sun, then compressed into tablets or sticks.

Heroin from Afghanistan reaches Europe mainly via Turkey, but also through Central Asia into the Russian Federation or less commonly by air or sea from Pakistan. New markets are being opened up in China, and West Africa has become a conduit to compete for US custom. Mexican heroin reaching the US is known as 'black tar' because of its texture and colour, the result of crude processing methods. South American 'white heroin' is regarded as a superior product. Heroin base (diamorphine not attached to a hydrochloride salt) vaporizes at a much lower temperature and is therefore preferred for smoking or 'chasing' (see below), and is often mixed with barbitone or caffeine which both increase the diamorphine content of the vapour. Purified diamorphine hydrochloride is sometimes known as No. 4 heroin, whereas brown heroin cut with caffeine is No. 3. Street heroin is cut with bulking agents such as starch, sugar, powdered milk, mannitol or glucose and sometimes active adulterants such as fentanyl, barbiturates, or even strychnine. It passes down the user chain in a sort of pyramid-selling operation, becoming more adulterated at each stage. Potentially lethal substances may be used as bulking or colouring agents including talcum powder, flour, brick dust, or detergent. Street purity used to be much higher on average in Europe than the US, but although the range remains very wide (1–70% in seized samples) 30–40 % is now usual in most big cities in the Western World.

Methadone is used with increasing frequency as a substitute opioid in the maintenance treatment of heroin addicts. The US, Spain, Germany, UK, Italy, Iran, and Canada together account for over 80% of the world's methadone consumption, and the drug is easily accessible on the black market of these countries. Buprenorphine is an alternative to methadone as a maintenance treatment. Its use was pioneered in France and it is now used in many countries including the US (since 2002). A small number of heroin addicts in the UK and the Netherlands receive pharmaceutical diamorphine on prescription as a white powder in 'dry amps', since diamorphine decays quite quickly in solution. These appear on the black market from time to time. Pharmaceutical morphine is not very popular with addicts unless formulated with the antivomiting drug cyclizine, but Palfium and Diconal tablets are sought after. Milder opioids as found in proprietary cough medicines all have some black-market value.

Europe and the US account for the vast majority of the world's consumption of legal prescription opioids, and 180 million prescriptions are dispensed by US pharmacies each year. There are many internet sites offering to provide drugs such as hydrocodone, oxycodone, codeine, propoxyphene, hydromorphone, and meperidine (pethidine) without a prescription. Most fentanyl available on the black market is manufactured illicitly rather than diverted.

Scientific information

Terminology for the derivatives of opium can be confusing. 'Narcotic' (derived from the Greek word meaning stupor) is a misleading term because it does not reflect the principal activity of the drug. 'Opiate' is sometimes used to describe drugs directly obtained from opium, as distinct from 'opioid' for synthetic morphine-like compounds. For simplicity, the author uses the latter term to represent all drugs, natural or synthetic, with a morphine-like action.

It was first suggested in the 1960s that opioids might act through binding with specific receptors in the nervous system, and several were identified soon after. The functional significance of these receptors was clarified by the discovery of the 'brain's own opiates' in 1975. These peptides are synthesized in response to pain and act as short-acting neurotransmitters in the brain and elsewhere, modifying and shaping the effects of serotonin, dopamine, and noradrenaline. These endogenous opioid-like peptides fall into three groups: alpha-, beta- and gamma-endorphins; leu- and met-enkephalins; and dynorphins. Since there are several different types of opioid receptor (designated δ-, μ-, or κ-) the response profile is complex. Exogenous opioids interact with these receptors to produce their effects and the picture is further confused by the fact that opioids vary in the way they affect a receptor. Some predominantly stimulate it and produce a positive effect (agonists), others sit on the receptor and block it without turning the system on (antagonists) and a third group bring about a mixture of these two actions (partial agonists). It is sometimes difficult to predict which effect will predominate in this third group. For example, if buprenorphine (partial agonist) is given to a heroin (agonist) addict, it may induce either intoxication or a withdrawal reaction. Regular long-term use of opioids causes a decrease in the number of μ-opioid receptors, and this may be a factor in the production of some of the unpleasant symptoms of acute withdrawal.

Opioids exert a mainly inhibitory effect within the brain and nervous system. Perception of, and concern about, pain is reduced; the pupils are constricted; drowsiness or sleep is induced with larger doses; anxiety, panic, and fear are inhibited, as is the 'fight and flight' mechanism; the cough reflex is suppressed; breathing is depressed; and body temperature is reduced.

Sex hormones are inhibited, whilst prolactin and growth hormone are increased. Peripheral blood vessels relax and blood pressure falls, intestinal peristalsis slows down, skeletal muscles loosen, and the sphincters tighten. Most opioids are not very effective when taken by mouth because the liver neutralizes most of the dose before it can reach the brain. An exception to this is methadone (synthesized in 1941 by German chemists) which also lasts much longer in the body. It takes 24 hours or more for the level in the blood to fall by half, compared with four hours for most other opioids. These properties have led to methadone being the most widely prescribed substitute opioid for addicts in treatment.

There is no evidence that opioids directly damage the foetus but they do cross the placenta, so neonates may be slow to breathe, or show withdrawal symptoms if the mother was taking them regularly. They also enter breast milk and may sedate the infant.

Medical uses

The more commonly used opioids (with equivalent dose to 10 mg morphine, a low analgesic dose) are as follows: codeine (120 mg); hydromorphone (Dilaudid, 1.5 mg); hydrocodone (10 mg); oxycodone (OxyContin, 5 mg); pethidine/meperidine (Demerol, 100 mg); dextromoramide (Palfium, 7.5 mg); dipipanone (Diconal, 10 mg); methadone (10 mg); buprenorphine (Temgesic, 0.4 mg); diamorphine (heroin, 4 mg). Opioids are widely used for the relief of moderate to severe pain, premedication for surgery, suppression of cough and diarrhoea, and for the alleviation of pulmonary oedema resulting from left ventricular failure. Methadone and buprenorphine (and diamorphine in the UK and Netherlands) are used as substitute opioids in the maintenance of heroin addicts.

After an adequate dose by intravenous or intramuscular injection (at least 10 mg for an average-size adult), morphine is effective against pain within minutes and lasts for three or four hours. Many patients suffer needlessly in hospital because of a fear amongst doctors of inducing addiction. In reality this is quite rare in patients treated for pain, approximately one in 100,000 treatments in one published series.

Opioids are very safe drugs in ordinary medical practice except in overdose when depression of breathing may be life-threatening. If recognized, this can easily be reversed by injections of the opioid antagonist naloxone. Since this has a very short duration of action, it may have to be given repeatedly until the opioid has worn off. The danger of fatal respiratory depression is greatly increased if other brain depressants such as alcohol, tranquillizers, or antidepressants have been taken as well. People with lung complaints or liver disease are particularly vulnerable to this dangerous effect.

Repeated doses may be associated with increasing resistance to many effects of the drug (tolerance), necessitating larger doses to achieve the same result. Some effects, such as constipation and pupillary constriction, do not exhibit tolerance.

Diamorphine is still used in medical practice in Britain (accounting for 95% of this use), Canada, and Hong Kong. The most common indications are pain in myocardial infarction, palliative care, pulmonary oedema, and postoperative pain. Reasons for preferring it to morphine by the parenteral route in these indications is greater potency, quicker onset of action, more sedation, less vomiting, and greater solubility (useful when very large doses are needed). It is pointless to give it orally since the liver will deacylate it instantly into morphine.

Recreational use

There are currently over 16 million non-medical users of opioids globally (0.4% adult population), three quarters of whom are heroin users. Over half of this use occurs in Asia, with Europe (22%), the Americas (13%), and Africa (8%) acounting for most of the rest. Most statistics are based upon problem users made visible by arrest or the need for treatment, but the real prevalence is much higher. For example, in the US in 2007 there were 335,000 heroin addicts in treatment, but the number of occasional users was estimated at 3.5 million. This invisibility of 90% heroin users makes it difficult to monitor prevalence of heroin use over time but it seems to have been quite stable in recent years in most countries. Exceptions include some countries of Eastern Europe where current use has escalated to over 1% of the adult population. Street price of heroin (gear, smack, skag, H, junk, brown, horse, blacktar) in the US and Europe is roughly half what it was ten years ago in real terms (average price per gram £50 UK, $170 US, €60 mainland Europe).

Lifetime non-medical use of opioids is reported by 0.9% and 1.5% of the adult populations of the UK and US respectively, with use within the previous year running at around 0.1% in both countries. Last year 106,000 North Americans tried heroin for the first time. In Europe around 1% of school students have tried heroin, ranging from 0% in several countries to 4% in Italy. Other countries reporting above average levels were France, Poland, Portugal, and Turkey.

In recent years, non-medical use of prescription opioids has become a serious problem in some countries, particularly the US. Last year over half a million US citizens used oxycodone non-medically for the first time with an average age of first use of 24. Around 10% of final year school students in the

US abused an opioid-containing prescription drug, and in children aged 12 to 13 these are the most prevalent recreational drugs.

Opioid use is common in the prison population of most countries, and one study revealed that 28% of Scottish prisoners were intravenous (IV) drug users prior to their current incarceration. A third of these continued to inject drugs in prison, and of these three-quarters had shared injecting equipment. Heroin is not difficult to come by in many prisons, but injecting equipment can be in short supply. Ex-prisoners say that dozens of inmates will sometimes share a single needle and syringe, a terrifying prospect in the era of HIV and hepatitis C.

Heroin is by far the most sought-after opioid throughout most of the world, though opium remains dominant in Asia. Brown heroin is generally cheaper and less pure than white, and much easier to come by. The popularity of injecting as the preferred route has declined steadily in many countries with many users preferring to vapourize the drug off silver foil ('chasing the dragon'), for which purpose brown Afghan heroin is ideal. This involves heating the powder on creased foil and inhaling the fumes through a tube of rolled foil or the outer case of a match box. It requires dexterity as the amount of heat applied has to be just sufficient to cause the heroin to liquefy and run along creases without charring. At the same time the tip of the tube has to follow and inhale the wisp of vapour that resembles a dragon's tail. Deposits within the foil tube can be vaporized in their turn to minimize waste. The rush or flash achieved by this method is almost as powerful as that by injection, but less economical since some smoke is lost into the atmosphere. Brown heroin can also be snorted nasally or rolled in a cigarette with tobacco. White (salt) heroin is water-soluble and therefore preferable for injecting, but is rarely available to most users. To inject brown or base heroin, it must first be placed in a spoon and acidified by addition of lemon juice or Vitamin C then heated to liquefy it. The fluid is then drawn into the syringe through a small piece of cotton wool or a cigarette filter to get rid of the larger chunks of undissolved matter. This is a particularly important operation when ground-up tablets are being used since these contain large amounts of chalky material. When supplies are short addicts may boil up their 'cottons' to extract every last bit of intoxication from their investment. The next step is to apply a tourniquet ('tie off'), tap up a vein, and 'shoot up'. Blood is sometimes drawn back and forth once or twice ('booting') to ensure that all the drug has been absorbed.

Mexican black tar heroin is a particularly toxic product. It tastes horrible if smoked, yet in order to liquefy it for injection quite intense heat is needed. It rapidly gums up syringes and causes much more damage to blood vessels than brown heroin. Ironically, areas where its use is prevalent seem to have lower levels of injection-related HIV infection, presumably because syringes are ruined and needles blocked before they can be shared.

There are thousands of first-hand descriptions of the opioid experience in print. Here is one from a 19th-century physician who was a frequent indulger: *'A sensation of fullness is felt in the head, soon followed by a universal feeling of delicious ease and comfort, with an elevation and expansion of the whole moral and intellectual nature which is, I think, the most characteristic of its effects ... the intellectual faculties are raised to the highest point compatible with individual capacity. It seems to make the individual, for the time, a better and greater man. The hallucinations, the delirious imaginings of alcoholic intoxication are, in general, quite wanting. Along with this emotional and intellectual elevation, there is also increased muscular energy; and the capacity to act, and to bear fatigue, is greatly augmented'.*

An injection of heroin will produce a powerful rush of extreme pleasure as the drug washes over the brain. This subsides into a relaxed, dreamy, cocooned feeling as anxieties and fears melt away. The user's head may droop and his eyes close as he goes 'on the nod' or 'gouches out'. The body feels heavy and warm. If problems come into the mind at all, they are suffused with optimism and confidence that all will turn out well. Unless overdosed into unconsciousness the mind remains active, though it may appear otherwise to an observer. Nausea and vomiting may occur, especially in the inexperienced. Diconal has a particular 'wiring' stimulant effect. The best high of all is said by some to be produced by a mixture of heroin and cocaine in the same syringe—the infamous and potentially lethal 'speedball'.

It is difficult to estimate what proportion of regular opioid users successfully avoid addiction or other problems. Little is known about such people since those coping successfully with their lives do not need the help of doctors or social workers or merit the attention of the police, and so remain invisible to researchers. It would be a mistake to build a picture of a typical opioid user based on those who become visible as a result of a visit to a police cell, hospital emergency department, or drug dependency unit. This would be like trying to understand social drinking on the basis of conversations with skid-row alcoholics.

So what do we know about these non-addicted opioid users ('chippers')? First, we have no real idea how many there might be. It has been suggested that there are more chippers than addicts, and certainly most dependent users say they know people who can use heroin intermittently. Population surveys suggest that ten times more people experiment with heroin than ever become a treatment statistic. It must be the case, therefore, that many people are able to experiment a few times and avoid going on to regular use. What is less certain is whether it is possible to use intermittently for long periods without becoming hooked. Are longer-term intermittent users simply in a transitional state on a path to either giving up or becoming addicted? Most chippers retain jobs, homes, and families. They are unlikely to be involved in criminal activities, except a minority who take part in some drug dealing, usually on a small scale. Most restrict their heroin to once or twice a month, with 20% using less frequently and 20% using weekly. Around one in five give a history of addiction at some time in the past.

Knowledge gained from observations of heroin use by US servicemen in Vietnam is relevant to this discussion. Heroin was accessible and cheap, and large numbers of GIs snorted, smoked, and even injected it during their active service. Moreover, with a purity of over 90% (compared with 5–10% on the streets of New York at that time), this was highly potent material. Despite this easy availability of high-quality heroin, most of these individuals never became hooked and did not use it on leave in the US, or when their tour of duty finished. Of those that did become addicted in Vietnam, only 20% ever used in the US. Even among those who did go on to use back home, only about 12% were addicted there and only 1% were still using a year after their return.

Many users who do become addicted say that the euphoric effects become much less rewarding, and claim they continue to take the drug just to 'stay straight'. Emotions are suppressed in the dependent user who is detached and insulated from routine cares and worries. Instead of the usual array of problems that life presents to the rest of us, the addict must face only one—where's the next hit coming from?

Unwanted effects

When used medically, opioids are remarkably safe drugs whose beneficial effects for patients with serious pain vastly outweigh the nuisance of the commoner side-effects. These include nausea and vomiting, reduced appetite, constipation, drowsiness, and apathy. Much more rarely patients may experience dry mouth and sweating, allergic reactions, difficulty in urinating, or spasm of the bile ducts or ureters. Non-medical users may also experience these effects.

In overdose the opioids are anything but safe. Depression of breathing can easily lead to a fatal outcome if not recognized and treated, drowsiness may progress to unconsciousness, and the blood pressure may fall so low that vital organs are starved of oxygen. Some opioids have particular risks in overdose; for example, pethidine can induce convulsions.

The uncertain strength and purity of street drugs make accidental overdose or poisoning by toxic adulterants an ever-present hazard. On average three out of four long-term, regular injectors have experienced this at least once, and four out of five have been present when someone else has seriously overdone it. This is particularly likely if other depressants such as alcohol or sedatives have also been taken. Unfortunately, there is a reluctance to summon help in such circumstances and well over half the deaths among heroin addicts are due to overdose, accidental or otherwise. Onlookers often attempt a home-remedy approach with cold showers or injections of amphetamine or cocaine, and 80% of those with a fatal outcome are already dead when the ambulance arrives. A typical victim would be a man in his late twenties with many years experience of heroin use, but about one in five fatalities occur in non-addicted users. Opioid overdose is still a leading cause of death among young people in Europe, particularly males. Most studies suggest an annual mortality among injecting opioid users of between 1% and 3%, which represents a six- to 20-fold excess in mortality rate for that age-group. In the US there were 2,011 heroin related deaths in 2005, an annual rate which has remained remarkably consistent since the 1980s. In contrast, deaths associated with prescription opioids (excluding methadone) have risen frighteningly from 2,757 in 1999 to 5,789 in 2005, an increase of 110%. Methadone associated deaths are even more astonishing: up 468% over the same period to 4,462 in 2005. In one state (West Virginia), over 90% of all unintentional overdose deaths were due to non medical use of prescription opioids. Oxycodone, hydrocodone and methadone are also responsible for rapidly increasing numbers of fatalities in Europe, Australia, and Canada.

Opioids carry a high risk of severe psychological and physical dependency. The number of people in treatment for opioid addiction has increased steadily in Europe and the US over the past two decades. For example, in the UK the number last year was over 140,000 compared to 61,689 in 1989 and 13,905 in 1985. In the US in 2007 there were 335,000 heroin addicts in treatment, but even this figure was dwarfed by the 558,000 seeking help for prescription drug problems, up 321% over the past 10 years.

The typical characteristics of the dependency syndrome include intrusive craving, preoccupation with maintaining a supply, compulsive use, impaired control, tolerance to the effects necessitating escalating doses, continued use despite physical and psychological problems, and withdrawal symptoms if supplies are interrupted. Once addiction is established, people will go to extraordinary lengths to maintain their habit.

You have to work at building up a physical dependence on heroin as it is not something which develops after a few fixes. People vary in their vulnerability, but a couple of weeks at least of daily use are likely to be needed. The usual pattern is gradually increasing intermittent use over many months, with increasing doses in response to subtle tolerance. Early signs of dependence may be explained away as sinusitis or a stubborn head cold.

Even when addiction has taken hold, historical analysis and some modern case histories demonstrate that as long as a regular supply of pharmaceutically pure drug is available, and the personality of the addict is adaptive, a productive lifestyle remains possible. A number of doctors are known to have sustained distinguished medical careers whilst addicted to huge doses of IV morphine or heroin. Indeed, one famous example asserted that his illustrious achievements would have been impossible *without* morphine, which he believed increased his stamina and capacity for hard work.

When an addict is denied heroin a predictable withdrawal syndrome develops. A few hours after the last dose the person becomes aware of increasing anxiousness, restlessness, and irritability. There is intense desire for another hit or chase. The victim yawns, stretches, sweats, and the eyes and nose begin to stream, with frequent sneezing. Cramping pains in the abdomen gather momentum, nausea comes on in waves, and the sufferer may be embarrassed by uncontrollable diarrhoea. Trembling, deep aching in the bones and muscles, terror, and insomnia complete the wretched picture. The skin is pale, clammy, and covered in goosebumps ('cold turkey') and the legs twitch and thrash in the bed ('kicking the habit'). Very rarely, there may be convulsions or a confusional state with delusions and hallucinations.

These unpleasant but not life-threatening symptoms are at their zenith for two or three days then gradually pass off over the next couple of weeks, although sleep disturbance and a feeling of malaise sometimes persist for many weeks. Onset and recovery can be delayed if the addict has been taking regular methadone because of its long duration of action. Although the syndrome is certainly unpleasant, most addicts have a disproportionate fear of 'clucking' and their whole life is organized around ensuring at all costs that it doesn't occur. Unfortunately, the exigencies of street life mean it will have to be faced on numerous occasions in an average addiction career.

The lifestyle of an addict often involves poor nutrition and living conditions, and a general lack of self-concern. Women may exchange sex for drugs, or take up prostitution to support a habit or keep a family together. It can be very hard for addict parents to give their children the physical and emotional nurturing they need, but many somehow manage to achieve this. Some could benefit from seeking assistance and support from their local drug service but hesitate to do so for fear that their children will be taken into care, though this is unusual.

It is not surprising with all these hardships that addicted IV users have a high incidence of physical and mental health problems. Quite apart from the risks of overdose and poisoning, they are susceptible to accidents and serious infection. If a group of addicts is followed up for 10 years or so, around 15% can be expected to have died. A study in Rome showed that the death rate among male addicts was 10 times higher than among men of the same age in the general population; for women, the ratio was 20 times.

Even intermittent injectors of street heroin expose themselves to considerable immediate risk. Variations in diamorphine content may result in accidental overdose and people who have either not developed tolerance or have lost it by cutting back on their intake may actually be more vulnerable to this. This risk was confirmed by a study which compared morphine content of the hair of individuals who had died of heroin overdose with that of active heroin addicts and a sample of ex-addicts (hair analysis gives a measure of average drug intake over several months). Morphine content from the hair of the fatalities was similar to that of the ex-addicts and very much lower than that of the addicts who were still using. Poisoning by adulterants and impurities is always possible, and life-threatening infections can fulminate in the bloodstream (septicaemia) or take hold within the heart, liver, lungs, bones, or brain. Local skin infection leading to abscesses is commonplace. Sharing needles or syringes is one of the most important ways in which infectious hepatitis and HIV are passed on.

Heroin suppresses ovulation and makes pregnancy less likely, but if conception does occur the addict lifestyle is not conducive to a relaxed pregnancy or good antenatal preparation. Poor nutrition can cause anaemia and increased susceptibility to infection. The strain of coping alone can lead to depression with a risk of self-harm.

There is no evidence that opiates cause direct damage to the foetus, although impurities in street heroin pose a threat. The main danger is premature delivery of a low birth-weight baby, and there is some increase in the risk of perinatal mortality. It is essential that an addicted mother receives coordinated care and support throughout the pregnancy, and that steps are taken to get her off street drugs whilst avoiding withdrawal symptoms (which may cause miscarriage). This is usually achieved by switching her to methadone, and then either withdrawing this very cautiously or maintaining her at the lowest dose possible. If the birth takes place while the mother is still receiving methadone or taking street opioids, paediatric input is advisable because the baby may exhibit withdrawal symptoms such as irritability, twitching, diarrhoea and vomiting, or repeated sneezing during the first few days of life. The onset may sometimes be delayed for days or weeks if the mother was taking methadone. Usually the syndrome responds to simple measures such as gentle handling, demand feeding, and possibly swaddling, but tiny doses of morphine or chlorpromazine are sometimes required. If the mother has been taking large doses of opioids up to delivery, the baby may not breathe adequately or develop convulsions. With appropriate medical management the immediate prospects are excellent, but the lifestyle of an addicted mother may prove hazardous to the physical and mental welfare of the developing child.

Psychiatric symptoms are common among opioid addicts presenting to drug units, but true psychiatric illness is unusual. The symptoms usually disappear spontaneously when immediate addiction-related problems are alleviated. True mental illness when it does occur usually antedates the addiction.

Many people who seek help for heroin addiction have experienced a disrupted and deprived childhood, possibly with physical or sexual abuse, and give a history of emotional or behavioural problems which predate the drug problem. Unless these inherent problems are addressed following detoxification, repeated relapses will be almost inevitable.

Selected references

Ball, J. C., Lange, W. R., Myers, C. P., Friedman, S. R. (1988). Reducing the risk of AIDS through methadone maintenance treatment. *Journal of Health and Social Behaviour,* **29**, 214–26.

Bennett, T., Wright, R. (1986). The impact of prescribing on the crimes of opioid users. *British Journal of Addiction,* **81**, 265–73.

Blackwell, J. S. (1983). Drifting, controlling, and overcoming: opiate users who avoid becoming chronically dependent. *Journal of Drug Issues,* **13**, 219–35.

Caviston, P. (1987). Pregnancy and opiate addiction. *British Medical Journal,* **295**, 285.

Chugh, S. S., Socoteanu, C., Reinier, K. et al. (2008). A community-based evaluation of sudden death associated with therapeutic levels of methadone. *Am J Medicine,* **121**, 66–71.

Darke, S., Zador, D. (1996). Fatal heroin overdose: a review. *Addiction,* **91**, 1765–72.

Farrell, M., Neeleman, J., Griffiths, P., et al. (1996). Suicide and overdose among opiate addicts. *Addiction,* **91**, 321–3.

Hall, A. J., Logan, J. E., Toblin, R. L. et al. (2008). Patterns of abuse among unintentional pharmaceutical overdose fatalities. *JAMA,* **300**, 2672–3.

Jansson, L. M, Choo, R., Velez, M. L. et al. (2008). Methadone maintenance and breast-feeding in the neonatal period. *Pediatrics,* **121**, 106–14.

Kalant, H. (1997). Opium revisited: a brief review of its nature, composition, non-medical use, and relative risks. *Addiction,* **92**, 267–77.

Kramer, J. C. (1980). The opiates: two centuries of scientific study. *Journal of Psychedelic Drugs.,* **12**, 89–103.

Levinthal, C. F. (1985). Milk of paradise, milk of hell: the history of ideas about opium. *Perspectives in Biology and Medicine,* **28**, 561–77.

Martindale Pharmacopoeia (29th edn). Chlorpromazine – use in neonates withdrawing from opiates. p. 724.

Musto, D. F. (1991). Opium, cocaine, and marijuana in American history. *Scientific American*, **July**, 40–7.

Porter, J., Jick, H. (1980). Addiction rare in patients treated with narcotics [letter]. *New England Journal of Medicine*, **302**, 123.

Rounsaville, B. J., Weissman, M. M., Crits-Christoph, K., Wilber, C., Kleber, H. (1982). Diagnosis and symptoms of depression in opiate addicts. *Archives of General Psychiatry*, **39**, 151–6.

Shields LBE, Hunsaker JC, Corey TS et al. (2007). Methadone toxicity fatalities: a review or Medical Examiner cases in a large metropolitan area. *Journal of Forensic Science*, **52**, 1389–95.

Skidmore, C. A., Robertson, J. R., Roberts, J. J. K. (1989). Changes in HIV risk-taking behaviour in intravenous drug users: a second follow-up.*British Journal of Addiction*, **84**, 695–6.

Sternbach, G. I., Varon, J. (1992). Designer drugs. *Postgraduate Medicine*, **91**, 169–76.

Strang, J., Griffiths, P., Gossop, M. (1997). Heroin smoking by 'chasing the dragon': origins and history. *Addiction*, **92**, 673–83.

Swift, W., Williams, G., Neill, O., Grenyer, B. (1990). The prevalence of minor psychopathology in opioid users seeking treatment. *British Journal of Addiction*, **85**, 629–34.

Tagliaro, F., De Battisti, Z., Smith, F. P., Marigo, M. (1998). Death from heroin overdose: findings from hair analysis. *Lancet*, **351**, 1923–5.

Thomson, J. W. (1984). Opioid peptides. *British Medical Journal*, **288**, 259–60.

Wood, P. L. (1982). Multiple opiate receptors: support for unique mu, delta, and kappa sites. *Neuropharmacology*, **21**, 487–97.

Zinberg, N. E. (1979). Non-addictive opiate use. In: *Handbook on drug abuse* (ed. R. L. Dupont, A. Goldstein, and J. O'Donnell), pp. 303–14. N.I.D.A., Washington.

Zinberg, N. E., Jacobson, R. C. (1976). The natural history of 'chipping' (controlled use of opiates). *American Journal of Psychiatry*, **133**, 37–40.

Chapter 13

The Nature of addiction

Introduction

Addictus—a citizen of ancient Rome who had built up debts that could not be repaid and was therefore delivered by the courts into slavery under his creditor. There is some confusion about the terms 'addiction' and 'dependence'. They are often used interchangeably, but addiction is more properly taken to refer to psychological dependence and drug-seeking behaviour as distinct from physical dependence (see below). Whatever term is preferred, the addictive potential of heroin and cocaine is taken for granted but are alcohol and tobacco to be feared in the same way? And what about tea, or sugar, or gambling, or computer games?

The International Classification of Diseases (Revision 10) defines substance dependence by the presence of at least three of the following during the previous year:

- a strong desire or sense of compulsion to take the substance;
- difficulty in controlling intake in terms of onset, termination, or levels of use;
- a physiological withdrawal state when substance use has ceased or been reduced;
- evidence of tolerance (the need for bigger doses to achieve the same effect);
- progressive neglect of alternative pleasures or interests;
- persisting with use despite clear evidence of overtly harmful consequences.

Being 'addicted' is to be caught up in the following sequence: an increasingly pressing desire to carry out some activity; growing anxiety and ever-increasing mental preoccupation to the exclusion of other important priorities if this is resisted or prevented; a sudden and highly rewarding elimination of tension and desire as the act is carried out; as the glow of satisfaction wears off, a resumption of the cycle all over again. It is apparent that the basic biological drives of eating, drinking, sleeping, and having sex all conform to this sequence. Leaving aside natural functions essential for life, there are quite a lot of human activities which fulfill the addictive sequence but do not involve the ingestion of any substance. People can get overinvolved in activities as diverse as body-building or on-line poker and there are some whose work ethic is as devastating to family life as any heroin habit. Elements of obsessional compulsive behaviour shows some similarities to the addictive sequence.

Two independent components of chemical dependency (or addiction) are recognized. Physical dependence can be diagnosed if a consistent pattern of bodily symptoms and signs, the 'withdrawal syndrome', develops when the drug is withheld or the dose reduced after a period of regular use. It is characteristic of drugs whose primary effect is to inhibit or depress brain function, and these include alcohol, tranquillizers and sleeping pills, and opioids. It is often associated with tolerance, when escalating doses are required to achieve the same effect in either a medicinal or recreational context. Psychological dependency is manifested by a powerful preoccupation and intense longing for the drug (craving) touched off or modified by elements of the environment (cues) which have become associated in the person's mind with drug-related experiences. Physical dependence can occur in people who exhibit no drug seeking behaviour or other elements of the psychological syndrome, for example patients on long-term opioid prescriptions for pain relief. Use of the term addiction in such cases is inappropriate.

Labelling addiction or dependency is a good deal easier than explaining it. This remains a controversial area. Some authorities (e.g. US National Institute of Drug Abuse) regard it as a chronic, relapsing disease in which drug-related changes in both the structure and function of the brain rob the sufferer at least in part of the ability to exert self control. This putative helplessness has influenced the legal response to drug-related criminal behaviour in some cases. Guidelines issued to British courts in late 2008 recommended that addiction should be treated as a mitigating factor in cases of burglary or theft, such that the normal custodial sentence be replaced by a more lenient community order or fine. A contrasting perspective (e.g. as persuasively formulated by the psychologist Stanton Peele among others) is that this perceived helplessness in the face of biological drives is a myth, and what is really required is for problem drug users to accept moral responsibility for their actions.

In attempting to understand the forces which cause in some people a progression from controlled, non-problematic consumption into the phenomenon of addiction, four categories of causation require consideration.

Neurobiological mechanisms

This approach centres on the many ways in which drugs and their metabolites can interfere with the transmission of chemical or electrical messages in the central nervous system (CNS), alter the connections between groups of neurones, or even cause structural brain changes over time.

The discovery of the endorphins (the brain's own opiates) in the 1970s raised the possibility that drugs may compensate for an inborn or acquired neurochemical deficiency. Endorphins are polypeptides which are released in response to painful, frightening, or satisfying experiences and act as neurotransmitters interacting with opioid receptors. They turn off aversive (unpleasant) messages and mediate reward. If you are constitutionally deficient in endorphins and happen to be exposed to opioids, (or short of dopamine and exposed to amphetamine or cocaine), it is plausible that you may be particularly sensitive to the rewarding or aversion-reducing effect. There are precedents for this scenario: for example, deficiency of serotonin may increase susceptibility to suicide. This deficiency could be genetically programmed, and its possibility has prompted the suggestion that some addicts may be no more to blame for their state than diabetics. Just as a diabetic needs insulin to maintain normal functioning, perhaps the endorphin-deficient junkie needs heroin and the dopamine-starved cocaine snorter must have his stimulant. Very recent research has shown that specific gene clusters influence the level of response to alcohol, which in turn determines susceptibility to alcohol abuse.

Biological systems are programmed to restore themselves to their original state when perturbed (homoeostasis). When the balance is upset by an external agent such as a drug, compensatory mechanisms cut in to restore the status quo. These might include activation of feedback mechanisms, alterations in receptor numbers or sensitivity, and release of compensatory neurochemicals.

Messages in the brain cross the gaps (synapses) between nerves by means of chemical messengers (neurotransmitters), which are manufactured and stored in the end of the nerve and released by changes in the electrical charge across the nerve membrane. They pass into the synapse, latch on to receptors on the other side, and cause changes in the permeability of the post-synaptic membrane. As a result of this, electrically charged elements (ions) such as sodium, potassium, and calcium are allowed to move in or out of the cell, which reconverts the impulse to an electrical wave. There are also receptors on the proximal side of the gap (pre-synaptic receptors) and when the neurotransmitter combines with these, further discharge from the nerve is inhibited. So the greater the flow of chemicals into the gap, the greater the activity of these pre-synaptic receptors in inhibiting further release. This sort of mechanism is called a 'negative feedback loop'. Drugs such as cannabis, heroin, and cocaine can induce shortages or malfunction in the neurotransmitter systems they are hijacking and produce a secondary deficit state which drives drug-seeking behaviour.

The number of the various receptors, and their sensitivity, are not fixed. They can be influenced by drugs themselves, or by the effect these have on naturally occurring brain chemicals. If a drug produces a push in one direction, the brain may increase its output of a chemical which is directly oppositional. This chemical merry-go-round finds tangible manifestation in a wide variety of symptoms, behaviours, or emotions. It is also what causes tolerance, a progressively reduced response to the drug necessitating ever bigger doses to achieve the same effect.

Withdrawal syndromes may be due to the chemical imbalance left behind as a drug wears off. For example, one of the effects of opioids is to suppress the activity of noradrenaline (norepinephrine) in the brain. If an opioid such as heroin is taken regularly over a long period, the noradrenergic system becomes hypoactive. As the drug wears off and the restraint is removed, it springs back into life with an initial overcompensation leading the system to become hyperactive for a while before settling back to its pre-drug level. This period of hyperactivity accounts for many of the unpleasant symptoms making up the withdrawal syndrome.

The neurotransmitter which is boosted or suppressed by a drug may express itself through psychological rather than physical manifestations. Drugs such as cocaine and amphetamine are not so obviously associated with physical dependency but can induce very powerful mental effects on withdrawal. These are just as closely related to chemical changes in the brain as the 'cold turkey' of opiate addiction.

But what if these homeostatic mechanisms fail, either due to the slow recovery rate of suppressed systems or some sort of permanent damage within nerves as has been noted in laboratory studies with amphetamine, cocaine, and Ecstasy? An example of the former mechanism is found with benzodiazepines. Some people who try to give them up after years of repeat prescriptions find that distressing symptoms persist for months or even years. This may be due to long-term changes in the cell membrane receptor complexes associated with the inhibitory neurotransmitter, gamma amino butyric acid (GABA). Dependency could then be explained as a manifestation of the need for a drug simply to restore normal physiological harmony. Both this concept, and the inherent deficit model, suggest that the logical response to addiction is long-term replacement therapy.

A fascinating discovery of the 1980s was the identification of a brain pathway concerned with the mediation and experience of pleasure and the drive to seek novel experiences. Pleasurable activities are associated with dopamine release in the meso-cortico-limbic system originating deep within the roots of the brain and projecting widely through a group of cell bodies called *nucleus accumbens* to brain areas concerned with emotion, reward, motivation, pain interpretation, memory, and reasoning. This is the ventral-tegmental dopaminergic system (VTDS). If a tiny electrode is implanted into the VTDS of a laboratory animal which is then given the opportunity to stimulate itself electrically by repeatedly pressing a bar, it will choose to do this to the exclusion of primary drives such as eating, mating, or sleeping. The animal will press the bar hundreds of times to achieve a single stimulus and, given free access, is likely to go on doing so until exhaustion or even death supervenes. Most drugs capable of producing addiction stimulate dopamine release within this pathway. This excessive dopamine signalling may induce plastic changes in the brain, strengthening neural connections underlying the association of drug use with reward and thereby enhancing the neurological mechanisms of addiction behaviour. This could account for the persisting extreme sensitivity of an abstinent addict to drug-related cues in the environment.

Paradoxically, the surge of dopamine signalling in VTDS is relatively modest following heroin, one of the most reinforcing of all drugs. This suggests that it may only be a correlate for a more subtle impact of dopamine within a specific sub-structure (such as the shell of nucleus accumbens). Dopamine signalling has also been found to be associated with the 'wanting' element of recreational drug use as distinct from the euphoria or reward.

An interesting phenomenon that can be explained by the existence of a pleasure pathway is called priming. Exposure to a small dose of an addictive substance can spark off a full relapse into addiction in abstinent subjects, an observation that formed a major plank in the emergence of a disease model for alcoholism in the 1930s. Priming can be demonstrated in previously addicted but currently drug-free animals trained to bar-press for reward. A small micro-injection of morphine delivered into the VTDS will immediately reinstate compulsive bar-pressing to obtain cocaine. The theory is that anything which tickles the pleasure pathway will spark off a 'positive appetitive state' with subsequent drug-seeking behaviours. It does not have to be a dose of the favoured drug; anything which twitches VTDS will do. This mechanism raises the possibility that everyday drugs such as caffeine and nicotine may be capable of instigating this process. Coffee or tobacco could then be unrecognized factors in inducing relapse in abstinent heroin or cocaine addicts. Recent work suggests that the priming effect in the VTDS can also be induced by environmental cues associated in the addict's mind with previous drug use.

The role of the VTDS can only offer a partial explanation of addictive behaviour in humans, most of whom do not respond to cocaine in the same way as experimental animals. Most reasonably well-adjusted individuals who snort cocaine a few times do not go on to sacrifice everything to the drug. The ability to think abstractly, to weigh up cost–benefit, to defer reward, and to place social obligations above the satiation of basic appetites usually provides an effective counterbalance against primitive messages from the pleasure pathway. It is also now apparent that VTDS is not the only brain system underpinning addictive syndromes. Information processing, learning, memory, planning, and inhibitory control are all highly relevant, and recent research has focused on the role of prefrontal and cingulate cortex, amygdala, hippocampus and orbito-frontal cortex. Extended periods of drug use may lead to structural changes (plasticity) in the brain which impair behavioural control and diminish the pleasure of alternative pursuits. A recent brain imaging study in alcoholics showed that a smaller amygdala was associated with increased craving and consumption and a greater likelihood of relapse following detoxification. Other work showed that abnormalities in the anterior frontal-subcortical region were also associated with relapse in alcoholics undergoing treatment.

Reinforcing effects of benzodiazepines may be partly mediated via opioid receptors, but another route to reward is by the relief of unpleasant stimuli such as fear or stress. Benzodiazepines antagonize the effects of corticotrophin-releasing hormone and thereby down-regulate the hypothalamo-pituitary-adrenocortical axis, and also modulate stress-mediating neurotransmitters such as neuropeptide Y and cholecystokinin. Drugs which neutralize punishment (depression, fear, pain, anxiety) can be as addictive as those which magnify pleasure.

Another relevant variable is the way the body transports and breaks down drugs, and there are important discreancies between individuals in the balance of metabolites emanating from the liver and other disposal mechanisms. This can explain the wide differences in addiction-liability to alcohol. If a person is physiologically programmed to produce lots of acetaldehyde (an unpleasantly toxic metabolite) but less good at completing the next stage in the metabolic process, the unpleasant symptoms which result will make alcohol consumption unrewarding. In contrast, an unusually efficient metabolism might necessitate a large intake simply to achieve comparable inebriation to less well-endowed companions. The enzyme systems that drive these metabolic processes are genetically determined, so patterns of response tend to be consistent within families.

Uterine exposure to psychoactive drugs as a result of maternal consumption may affect that individual's response to these drugs as an adolescent or adult and perhaps increase the risk of dependence. This association has been demonstrated for both alcohol and tobacco, but it is very difficult to separate congenital causation from a subsequent conditioning effect as a result of observed parental behaviour.

Psychological processes

Psychological models can be subdivided into psychoanalytic, behavioural, cognitive, and personality theories.

Psychoanalytical explanations vary according to the particular school of thought – Freudian, Jungian, Kleinian, and so forth. Put simply, the basic concept is that observed behaviour is the result of an interaction between external events and repressed or unconscious mental processes of which the subject remains unaware. The key task is to explore and interpret these internal processes, and merely tinkering with the addictive behaviour is seen as a waste of time. Even if you succeed in getting rid of it, the argument goes, the internal unconscious conflicts remain and will re-manifest in due course either in the form of relapse or by the appearance of some other 'neurotic' activity (symptom substitution). There are various more specific explanations of addiction. Some analysts believe that addicts are regressing to unfulfilled phases of psychosexual development. Others refer to defects in personality structure such as a poorly developed 'super-ego' or retention of 'infantile thought processing'. Subjects may be in the grip of 'narcissistic rage'. In treatment it may be relevant to search for evidence of some failure of natural satiation in early childhood, of oral fixation, or anal regression. The drug user may be seen as 'fundamentally suicidal'. Attempts have been made to explain why particular individuals are drawn to particular drugs. Heroin users, for example, may experience '. . . *a need for the ego to control feelings of rage and aggression, emotions that relate to the anal stage of psychosexual development*'. The 'weak ego structure' of such an individual leads them to seek quiet and lonely lives, hence the attraction to narcotics. Psychoanalytic concepts such as denial and rationalization provide an explanation for the persistence and dominance of maladaptive beliefs in spite of tangible evidence to the contrary, and destructive behaviours with serious negative consequences to the individual.

There was a time when such ideas underpinned the treatment philosophy of many drug and alcohol units, but this is no longer the case. Abstract hypotheses like these do not lend themselves to scientific testing, and even analysts from within the same theoretical school often come up with completely different interpretations of the same observed phenomena. Psychodynamic treatments of addiction have not proved particularly successful, and they are very time-consuming. The psychodynamic approach can sometimes seem patronizing and judgemental. Since it hinges on the ability of some external 'expert' to understand and interpret the hidden meaning of the various behaviours and feelings, it can also have the effect of increasing the addict's sense of helplessness and passivity.

Behavioural models are based upon various forms of learning theory. Classical conditioning is familiar through the efforts of Pavlov and his dogs. When a hungry dog is exposed to food (unconditioned stimulus) it salivates (unconditioned response). If a bell (conditioned stimulus) is rung on a number of occasions at about the same time the food is presented, after a number of exposures the dog will salivate on hearing the bell (conditioned response) even when the food is omitted. By the same process, elements of a drug user's environment (cues) become linked to highs and lows of the drug experience. A cue which has become a conditioned stimulus for euphoria may spark off positive memories of drug use leading to craving, whilst one which induces the symptoms of withdrawal will lead to drug-seeking behaviour to alleviate the misery.

Many injecting drug users find that the process of injecting itself becomes highly rewarding to the extent that they sometimes inject themselves with water or other inert substances between 'live' hits. This can be explained on the basis of classical conditioning, which also suggests a specific treatment (cue exposure and response prevention—see Chapter 14).

'Instrumental' or 'operant' conditioning is induced according to the outcome of the behaviour. Activities which have a pleasant outcome or take away an unpleasant experience like depression or fear, are reinforcing and likely to be repeated.

A third form of conditioning is vicarious learning, through contemplation of what happens to others. This 'modelling' can take place after observing the behaviour of family or friends, or activities portrayed in the media. Analysis of the effect of advertising confirms that compelling images such as the 'Marlboro man' do actually succeed in associating, in this case, the act of smoking with feeling tough, fearless, and independent. Repeatedly seeing the heroes (or anti-heroes) of films puffing contendedly on cigarettes or gulping whisky has a measurably reinforcing effect on viewers of all ages.

There are many experimental models by which the reinforcing properties of different drugs can be compared and quantified. A rat or monkey can be trained to press a bar to obtain a reward, and the number of times it is prepared to do so is a measure of the reinforcing power of that particular reward. If the reward is a small amount of amphetamine, cocaine, or heroin, a monkey will press the bar persistently to obtain a single dose. Alcohol, barbiturates, and benzodiazepines are also active in this model, but induce lower rates of bar-pressing. By comparing the number of bar presses with the results obtained from standard rewards such as access to food or water, the findings can be calibrated to the real world.

The way in which the reward is presented is also influential, the most reinforcing pattern being intermittent and random rather than a predictable one-to-one with the activity. This is what makes slot machines so addictive, so no surprise that these mechanical pickpockets were invented by a psychologist.

Psychological mechanisms may play a central role even in outcomes which appear at first sight overwhelmingly biological. An example is the phenomenon of tolerance. Regular, repeated exposure to many drugs leads to increasing resistance to some or all of their effects. Larger doses are required to achieve the same result, and the individual can eventually tolerate doses that would be highly toxic to an inexperienced user. Pharmacological explanations for this include the way the body is metabolizing the drug, changes in the number or sensitivity of receptors, and homeostatic responses from oppositional brain systems. A simple experiment illustrates that there is more to this than basic physiology. An animal exposed to gradually increasing doses of morphine in a completely consistent environment will eventually develop tolerance to huge doses as expected. If it is then moved to an unfamiliar place and given exactly the same dose, it will keel over and die of overdose as if it were a drug-naive animal. Similarly, addicted rats which have been withdrawn from opiates become re-addicted much more quickly in the cage associated with the previous addiction. These observations show that what the animal has learnt to expect powerfully shapes what actually happens.

Cognitive theories focus on the way people interpret and account for their experiences in life. Emotions are seen as the logical outcome of particular patterns of thinking. Key thoughts are usually so fleeting and familiar that the subject is completely unaware of them and the profound effect they are having in shaping her view of the world and herself. Cognitive therapists aim to uncover these 'automatic' thoughts, then collaborate with the subject to explore how true or useful they are.

To illustrate this with an example, a student suffered frequent, inexplicable bouts of gloominess which he self-medicated with cannabis. The cannabis was interfering with his ability to study and satisfy his tutors, so he sought help. Asked for the most recent example of these attacks, he described being gripped by one on the way to the clinic. Going back over the journey in his mind, he was able to pinpoint the onset of the mood at a particular place on the street, then remembered that at about the same moment he had nodded to a passing acquaintance without receiving any acknowledgement. Asked to imagine himself back there and examine the thoughts going through his head at that moment, he came up with the following sequence: 'He's ignoring me; he thinks I'm pathetic; he obviously doesn't like me; who the hell does like me?; I *am* pathetic; nobody likes me; I'm always going to be lonely'. If this interpretation was true depression would certainly be a logical outcome, but is it really the most likely explanation? Perhaps the fellow simply didn't see him. Repetitive undermining thought sequences often stem from deep-seated negative beliefs the individual has about himself. Ways in which the cognitive therapist gets to grips with these are described in Chapter 14.

The way people explain what has happened in the past also shapes their expectations for the future. These explanations or 'attributions' can be categorized as internal or external, stable or unstable, specific or general. Individuals tend to be consistent in their 'attributional style', and this has a profound effect on self-concept and confidence. Imagine three people who have all failed a maths exam. One is miserable, one is unmoved, the third is delighted. How is one to account for such different reactions to the same event? The first person thinks he failed because he is stupid. This attribution is internal, stable (he will still be stupid tomorrow and next year), and general (it has implications beyond the boundaries of the current event). No wonder he is miserable. The second person blames the examiner for setting such poorly worded, inappropriate questions (external, stable, specific); the result has little bearing on his ability or future. The third believes that he is destined to be a great painter (internal, stable, general) and that maths is a complete waste of his time; this result will finally convince his parents that a career in engineering, though secure, is not for him. Most 'normally' functioning individuals adopt a 'self-serving attributional bias' most of the time, giving themselves the credit when things are working out well but blaming external agencies (luck, the Government, God's will) when they are not.

A self-defeating attributional style can lie at the heart of the helplessness expressed by many drug-dependent people. Telling myself 'I've got a disease, it's not my fault, there's nothing I can do about it' is likely to be a self-fulfilling prophesy in that it gives me licence to sit back and wait for someone else to come along with a magic pill or some other passive cure. The subtle, undeclared advantages of continuing an apparently self-destructive behaviour are sometimes overlooked in the face of disadvantages which seem horrific to the observer but, perhaps contrary to what he says, have little genuine impact upon the subject. How desirable, all things considered, the addict *really* regards a particular outcome, such as abstinence, is not always easy to ascertain for patient or therapist, and will obviously influence the likelihood of reaching an outcome that may be more attractive to therapist, employer, or spouse than the 'addict' himself.

To illustrate this, consider the case of a journalist whose addiction to heroin has cost him his job and marriage, and who now presents at a drug unit with a large abscess on his leg from a dirty injection. He begs to be admitted for detoxification and rehabilitation, explaining that at last he has reached rock bottom and is absolutely determined to achieve abstinence. Five days in and through the worst, he suddenly announces he can't take any more and discharges himself. Within half an hour of leaving the ward, he has scored a gram of heroin and is 'on the nod' in a lavatory at the bus depot. The medical team, the wife, and the employer scratch their heads and wonder at the mystery of addiction.

The difficulty is that all these people are looking at the 'problem' from a completely different perspective to the 'addict'. They think of the pain and fear of illness, the loneliness and squalor of life in a bedsit away from the family home, the waste of a promising career. The 'addict' knows that heroin will kill the pain and take away all thought of illness. Long-term risk is trumped by immediate reward, be it ever so slight and fleeting. Family life carries a ton of responsibility and frustration as well as reward and satisfaction. Being in the office at 8.00 a.m. every morning, meeting impossible deadlines, running on the treadmill. Nobody expects a junkie to be tidy and polite, confident and cheery in the face of hassle or boredom, considerate and unselfish. How easy it is to compress all these obstacles and worries into just one question: where's my next fix coming from? It's only when this last dilemma can no longer be answered, when the energy and deviousness to survive at the coal-face of addiction have ebbed away, that the addict throws himself temporarily on the mercies of the 'caring' professions.

Self-efficacy and self-esteem are two other concepts with relevance to addiction. The former is the degree to which a person believes she possesses the skills necessary to achieve a desired outcome. Many distressed addicts can accept that giving up would be a good idea but do not believe that they could tolerate detoxification, manage their emotions without the drug cocoon, or resist temptation to use again if they did achieve abstinence. Self-esteem is the sense of contentment and self-acceptance that stems from a person's judgement of her own worth. People arrive at this by self-appraisal in a number of areas: perceived competence and ability to persevere in valued tasks; an estimation of worthiness and significance in comparison with others; perceived attractiveness to, and approval by, other people; the ability to like oneself in the absence of support from others, or in the face of active criticism and disapproval; and an idea of the value of existence in general. Many therapists in the drug and alcohol field regard low self-esteem as an important causative or maintaining factor, and essential to target in some way during treatment. If you don't like yourself, why should you care what happens in the future?

Personality theories—A clearly defined 'addictive personality' has little scientific credence, but certain personality traits (which may be genetically determined) may well increase the risk of compulsive or dependent drug use. These include a consistent tendency to impulsive behaviour, a low tolerance for frustration, insecurity and a low sense of self-worth, chronic ('trait') anxiety, and a persistent feeling of alienation from family and peers. Individuals diagnosed with anti-social personality disorder have a much increased prevalence of substance dependence. However, cause and effect are difficult to disentangle. When confronted with an addict of ten years' standing with a maladaptive or unpleasant personality, could this simply be the effect of all that drug use rather than its cause?

In studies of normally functioning adolescents, the only trait which is consistently associated with an increased likelihood of experimenting with drugs is 'sensation seeking' or risk taking. Children who climb highest in a tree, ride their bike the fastest down a hill, or swim the furthest out to sea are also the most likely to try whatever drugs are going.

Attempts have been made to pigeon-hole drug users according to some particular trait or motivation. One classification separates them into pleasure seekers, conformists (responding to peer pressure), experimenters, and self-therapists. Intuitively, it is the latter group that will be more vulnerable to dependent use. As remarked elsewhere, the more a drug is able to offer a particular individual, the more it overcomes or camouflages a deficit or weakness, the harder it will be to relinquish. Shyness, low self-esteem, poor self-confidence, boredom, fear, anger, loneliness—it is hard to go back to all that once you have found a way to push it out of sight. The more 'normal' a population exposed to a drug, the less will be the casualty rate in terms of dependent use. In the 1980s cocaine epidemic in the US, the proportion of individuals who became compulsive users was estimated at between 10% and 15%, a figure similar to that found with alcohol. In the population attending an average drug dependency unit the proportion would be much higher. This may be explicable in terms of the higher prevalence of psychological disorder or maladaptive personality traits in this latter group, or in more sociological terms.

Socio-cultural influences

Despite the power of individual neurobiology and personality structures, a person's attitudes and behaviour are profoundly influenced by the family, the peer group, and the rules and mores of society at large.

The family, circle of friends and neighbourhood networks are crucial in both starting and maintaining social drug use. Attitudes and expectations will have been absorbed ahead of exposure. Initiation, whether it is a first diluted glass of wine at the family supper table, a cigarette behind the bike shed, or the first toke off a spliff, will characteristically take place in a context of rules and rituals. First use of an illicit drug is almost always sourced from within the immediate family or social circle. Patterns of drug use are powerfully modulated by membership within such groups. For example, in the US alcoholism is much commoner than average amongst Irish-Americans and extremely uncommon in Jewish communities.

Becoming delinquent is not only a matter of consciously rejecting one lifestyle but gradually learning an alternative which seems to deliver better results, particularly in the short term. Excessive or destructive drug use within deviant subgroups in any society may simply be consistent with the other illegal or antisocial activities which the group adopts. The junkie lifestyle, despite its obvious disadvantages and risks, in many ways fulfils the role of a club with its rituals and camaraderie, and for some people may be the very first time they experience a degree of social support. In that context, overcoming addiction would have the major disadvantage of expulsion from that particular club.

A clear example of socio-cultural influences on drug use can be found among American GIs who used heroin whilst on active service in Vietnam. There were a number of environmental reasons that encouraged the use of the drug: the normal cultural and moral restraints were absent; familiar close interpersonal relationships were disrupted; the surroundings were alien, hostile, and frightening; high purity heroin was cheap and easily accessible; and the immediate peer group regarded heroin use as socially acceptable and even desirable. Heroin use became highly prevalent, often involving very large daily doses. However, most of these individuals did not use it on leave in the US, or when their tour of duty finished. Amongst those that became physically and psychologically dependent in Vietnam, only 20% ever used heroin in the US: their 'addiction' seemingly evaporated as soon as the supporting sociological parameters were removed.

Compulsive, self-destructive drug use is much more prevalent among subgroups in society that are poor and deprived. Such individuals will have had little prospect of adequate education or material advance, disrupted or abusive families, daily exposure to deviant or criminal behaviour, and poor access to leisure facilities.

Anomie (Greek for 'absence of law') was a term used by the sociologist Émile Durkheim to describe a state in which cohesion within society has been weakened to the point that individuals begin to pursue their own goals with little concern for the common good. At times, this state of affairs can almost seem to become consistent with government policy. It certainly appeared that way in the UK and US of the 1980s, the decade of the yuppie and the flaunting of new-found wealth. Margaret Thatcher's famous quote *'there is no such thing as society'* has been much misunderstood but to many it has become a literal personal philosophy. The early years of the 21st century brought a resurgence of blatant consumerism, but for many sections of society such a lifestyle remains unattainable for reasons of opportunity or personal attributes. A person in that situation has only three alternatives: lower her aspirations, and settle for a mundane job with a modest lifestyle; rebel, and become a criminal or revolutionary; or retreat, perhaps by numbing herself out with drugs.

Issues of personal morality

Writers such as the psychologist Stanton Peele and the psychiatrist Sally Satel have argued controversially that the addiction treatment industry has consistently failed to acknowledge or confront the moral and emotional infirmity at the heart of addictive behaviour. They do not accept that some drugs are too rewarding to resist and that addiction may strike anyone. The low prevalence of alcoholism amongst Jews mentioned above is not the result of some quirk of biology or personality: it is because Jews disapprove of drunken behaviour and ostracize those who indulge in it. In the face of this strong motivational pressure, a member of the Jewish community exerts personal control over intake despite the neuropharmacological power of the drug.

It is necessary to work at becoming addicted to a drug over many weeks, which suggests that the individual is making a positive choice. Many who become addicted display a range of other antisocial or destructive behaviours which are linked by the individual's propensity to put self-gratification ahead of other priorities or responsibilities to others. Becoming involved in deviant social groups is also a matter of choice for which the individual must accept responsibility. A politically correct reluctance to criticize bad behaviour removes the powerful restraining effect of guilt or shame which might otherwise inhibit further deterioration. Nor is it possible to argue that the intense psychoactive effects or come-down from the drugs eliminate the possibility of free choice. Sally Satel has pointed out that in the long intervals between cocaine binges or heroin scores addicts are constantly making decisions about lifestyle issues or every day tasks. Although nobody would say it is easy, it is not constitutionally impossible for such a person to take the decision to enrol in a self-help programme, or decide that it's more important to pick up your child from school than go out and score.

Abstinence from addictive behaviour is achieved far more frequently by naturalistic means than as a result of therapy. Alcohol and drug abuse diminish with age, driven by changes in personal aspirations, attitudes and expectations. Such a change of perspective may be brought about by circumstances much removed from 'hitting bottom', often quite a minor event at a key moment is sufficient to achieve this. A journalist who had been a heroin addict explained in a BBC interview: *'My experience was you know I had plenty of things that from the outside you'd say this guy should stop. Several times I overdosed, ended up in hospital. I got hepatitis C. I had trouble with the police. In the end it was something kind of internal in me. I just had one of those epiphanies and I saw myself through the eyes of my children actually looking at me—me standing there looking like a lunatic—and I saw myself as they saw me. I had a moment of clarity, I suppose'.*

Conclusion

The nature of addiction remains controversial, and the degree of autonomy and free choice that a person in its grip can be expected to demonstrate is argued about fiercely. Some experts and specialists will strongly espouse just one of the four domains summarized above, but it seems more likely that all play a part to a variable degree for different individuals. Perhaps the most important conclusion is that addiction should not be regarded as a walled-off, stand-alone, cross-sectional 'condition'. Rather, it is a dynamic state of mind and pattern of behaviour maintained by a volatile balance of drives stemming from the individual, whose particular genes and neuropharmacology, attitudes, values, and patterns of learned behaviour interacts with the social and physical environment.

Some individuals, for internal and/or external reasons, are more vulnerable to becoming addicted than others, but in prospective studies of large groups of adolescents it has proved very difficult to pick out the ones most at risk with any accuracy. Once dependency is established, there is no external 'cure'. Addicts have choices and must take responsibility for their actions but, as we have seen, there are powerful physical, psychological, and social forces at work which can make behaviour change very difficult. Nevertheless, most people find their own way out of addiction. Treatment can only succeed if it takes place as a collaborative venture, with the 'addict' encouraged to be the prime mover.

Selected references

Babor, T. F., Cooney, N. L., Lauerman, R. J. (1987). The dependence syndrome concept as a psychological theory of relapse behaviour: an empirical evaluation of alcoholic and opiate addicts. *British Journal of Addiction*, **82**, 393–405.

Childress, A. R., McLellan, A. T., O'Brien, C. P. (1986). Conditioned responses in a methadone population: a comparison of laboratory, clinic, and natural settings. *Journal of Substance Abuse Treatment*, **3**, 173–9.

Daglish M. R. C., Williams T. M., Wilson S. J. et al. (2008). Brain dopamine response in human opioid addiction. *British Journal of Psychiatry* **193**, 65–72.

Dimond, S. J. (1980). Consciousness. In: *Neuropsychology: a textbook of systems and psychological functions of the human brain* (ed. S. J. Dimond). Butterworths, London.

Epping-Jordan, M. P., Watkins, S. S., Koob, G. F., Markou, A. (1998). Dramatic decreases in brain reward function during nicotine withdrawal. *Nature*, **393**, 76–9.

Glassman, A. H., Koob, G. F. (1996). Psychoactive smoke. *Nature*, **379**, 677–8.

Gossop, M. (1976). Drug dependence and self-esteem. *International Journal of the Addictions*, **11**, 741–53.

Hyman, S. E., (2007). The neurobiology of addiction: implications for voluntary control of behaviour. *Am J Bioeth*, **7**, 8–11.

Joslyn, G., Brush, G., Robertson, M. (2008). Chromosome 15q25.1 genetic markers associated with level of response to alcohol in humans. *Proc Nat Acad Sci USA*, **105**, 20368–73.

Kalivas, P. W., Volkow, N. D. (2005). The neural basis of addiction: a pathology of motivation and choice. *Am J Psych*, **162**, 1403–13.

Lart, R. (1992). Changing images of the addict and addiction. *International Journal of Drug Policy*, **3**, 118–25.

Legarda, J. J., Bradley, B. P., Sartory, G. (1987). Subjective and psychophysiological effects of drug-related cues in drug users. *Journal of Psychophysiology*, **4**, 393–400.

Le Moal M., Koob G. F. (2007). Drug addiction: pathways to the disease and pathophysiological perspectives. *European Neuropsychopharmacology* **17**, 377–393.

McAuliffe, W. E., Rohman, M., Felman, B., Launer, E. K. (1985). The role of euphoric effects in the opiate addictions of heroin addicts, medical patients, and impaired health professionals. *Journal of Drug Issues*, **Spring**, 203–24.

Peele S. (1987). A moral vision of addiction: how people's values determine whether they become and remain addicts. *Journal of Drug Issues* **17**, 187–215.

Pidoplichko, V. I., DeBiasi, M., Williams, J. T., Dani, J. A. (1997). Nicotine activates and desensitizes midbrain dopamine neurons. *Nature*, **390**, 401–4.

Room, R. (1989). Drugs, consciousness, and self-control: popular and medical conceptions. *International Review of Psychiatry*, **1**, 63–70.

Satel S., Lilienfeld S. (2007). Medical misnomer: addiction isn't a brain disease, Congress. Slate, Medical Examiner: http://www.slate.com/id/2171131/.

Saunders, B., Allsop, S. (1987). Relapse: a psychological perspective. *British Journal of Addiction*, **82**, 417–29.

Stelten, B. M. L., Nobless, L. H. M., Ackermans, L. et al. (2008). The neurosurgical treatment of addiction. *Neurosurg Focus*, **25**, 1–5.

Stewart, J., de Wit, H., and Eikelboom, R. (1984). Role of unconditioned and conditioned drug effects in the self-administration of opiates and stimulants. *Psychological Review*, **91**, 251–68.

Volkow N. D., Wang G. J., Telang F. et al. (2006). Cocaine cues and dopamine in the dorsal striatum: mechanism of craving in cocaine addiction. *Journal of Neuroscience* **26**, 6583–8.

West, R. (1989). The psychological basis of addiction. *International Review of Psychiatry*, **1**, 71–80.

Wikler, A., Pescor, F. T. (1967). Classical conditioning of a morphine abstinence phenomenon, reinforcement of opioid-drinking behaviour, and 'relapse' in morphine-addicted rats. *Psychopharmacologia*, **10**, 255–84.

Wilson, G. T. (1987). Cognitive processes in addiction. *British Journal of Addiction*, **82**, 343–53.

Wise, R. A. (1988). The neurobiology of craving: implications for the understanding and treatment of addiction. *Journal of Abnormal Psychology*, **97**, 118–32.

Chapter 14

Helping problem drug users

The essential first step towards obtaining help with a drug-related problem (throughout this chapter 'drug' will include alcohol and tobacco) is to recognize that one exists. The affected person is often the last to realize or admit that things are getting out of hand, and it falls to friends or family to bring it to his or her attention. This may be the result of 'defence mechanisms', those unconscious mental devices we all use to fend off unwelcome thoughts or inner conflicts, or simply because it isn't the user that has the problem; doing badly at school or acting like a jackass at home are, in an immediate sense, problems for teachers and family rather than the rascal himself.

On the other hand, it is always possible that concerned onlookers are making a value judgement and regarding drug use in itself as inherently problematic. Whilst it is true that any flirtation with a legal or illegal recreational drug has the potential to become problematic, it is far from inevitable that this will come about. Many people, both adolescent and adult, are able to keep their lives under control even while using drugs quite regularly, and don't seem any the worse for the experience.

Drugs and young people

Regular use of any drug, including tobacco and alcohol, is likely to be counterproductive for younger teenagers who are still developing physically and emotionally. They are more vulnerable to physical and psychological unwanted or toxic effects, and drug use with the rituals that surround it can disrupt the relationships, education, activities, and interests which are most likely to lead to a happy and productive adult life.

Some young people are particularly susceptible to excessive drug use. Examples include those whose parents misuse alcohol or other drugs, the homeless and those 'in care', regular truants from school, those involved in crime and prostitution, and those with physical disability or learning difficulties.

There are a number of pointers which may suggest to parents that their child is developing a problem related to drug use. An altered pattern of sleeping may become evident, with the child active later into the night and showing a greater than usual reluctance to respond to the alarm clock. A previously healthy appetite may fade with resulting weight loss, or alternatively mounds of food are devoured. A previously placid person may become moody or unpredictable, or a live-wire appear lethargic and torpid. Concentration span or memory may be diminished. The child may seem suspicious or secretive, irritable or restless, or pale, tired, and apathetic. Favourite hobbies and interests get abandoned, friendship patterns change.

These rather non-specific clues would carry much more weight if there were also reports of declining school performance, or the person had actually been seen to be clumsy of demeanour and slurred of speech. The obvious clinching factor would be the discovery of drug paraphernalia around the house, such as hidden alcohol, peculiar-looking cigarette ends, powder or plant material in twists of paper or small plastic bags, tablets, or capsules. Regular solvent inhalers often leave a conspicuous trail: pungent smells from the bedroom or on the breath; plastic bags, cans, bottles, and rags in waste-paper baskets; spill marks on clothes or bedding, faded sleeves from surreptitious sniffing; spots or sores round the nose and mouth, cracked and dry lips, chronic cough and cold.

Discovery of needles, syringes, or ampoules would indicate that problems had progressed into a different league.

How should a parent or guardian react to evidence suggestive of drug use? The most important thing is not to *over*-react, and there are several reasons for this. Firstly, many of the earlier pointers are part and parcel of ordinary adolescence and may have nothing whatsoever to do with drugs. But even if they do, it is essential not to make matters worse by going off at the deep end and further alienating the child. There are also some immediate physical risks in winding up the emotional tone in someone who is currently intoxicated. A surge of anxiety, fear, or anger can prove fatal to a glue-sniffer because of the effect on the heart, and could provoke a panic attack or worse in someone deep into an LSD trip.

So first, remain calm by keeping things in perspective. Remember that your offspring is by no means unique since many of his or her peers will have tried an illegal drug before leaving school, and that the chances of emerging unscathed are very high. The most constructive approach is to be prepared to listen to what the child says, understand the worries and conflicts he or she is facing, and help to find practical solutions to problems. Gaining the confidence of the child, improving communication, and restoring trust will enable the parent to find out the true extent of the drug use, and develop the sort of collaborative approach that will be most likely to establish more constructive priorities.

To change direction, a person needs to see the prospects of clear benefits resulting from that change. Threats or punishment produce only short-term, superficial responses. Factual information should flow both ways since many teenagers know a lot more about street drugs than their parents or teachers (and doctors). The most important task is to provide the information most relevant to immediate life-goals, and instigate honest discussion. For example, horror stories about cannabis causing lung cancer or mental illness at some point in the future will have little impact on school students, but the fact that it can threaten an exam outcome or selection for the football team is more likely to capture their attention.

Once this collaborative approach is established, the practical steps taken depend on the scale of the problem. There may be health issues which necessitate a check-up from the family doctor. Broadly, the aim is to boost the young person's confidence and self-esteem by giving a sympathetic ear, good advice, and practical support, whilst avoiding wading in and taking control. Getting the person to keep a diary can be a useful way of estimating progress, and it also serves to sharpen the insight of the diary-keeper. Self-monitoring of this sort has been shown to be therapeutic as well as informative in people with out-of-control binge-eating and other counter-productive habits. Various practical ways of solving a particular problem can be discussed and perhaps written down for retention and review but the responsibility for carrying these through should always remain with the young person so that the sense of personal control and self-determination is fostered.

Parents faced with adolescent drug use should be prepared to examine their own conduct and relationships for the source of their child's troubles. It may even be necessary to examine the rest of the family's use of drugs to determine whether the 'do as I say, not as I do' factor might have got a bit out of hand. A father who regularly enjoys a bar-crawl with his buddies or a valium-popping mother are hardly in a strong position to castigate a son or daughter caught in possession of a few dodgy tablets or an 8th of hash.

Information, advice, and ways of accessing help can be obtained via the internet (e.g. http://ncadi.samhsa.gov/ in the US or http://www.nhs.uk/Livewell/drugs/Pages/Drugtreatment.aspx in the UK) or through local resources such as the family doctor or voluntary agencies. Counselling, self-help groups, training and support for families, mediation, and crisis support teams are normally available in most developed countries. For more serious problems, similar strategies for detoxification, rehabilitation, and relapse prevention will be required as for adults.

The UK organization SCODA identified 10 key principles for drug interventions aimed at young people. The approach has to reflect issues such as legal competence, age appropriateness, and particular confidentiality requirements. The welfare of the child supercedes the interests of the adults concerned, and the views of the young person must be heard and supported whenever possible. Parental responsibility must be factored in, and there must be careful coordination between the various authorities and organizations involved which must combine to produce a holistic approach. The services must be attractive, accessible, and safe for young people, with a comprehensive scope and operating according to principles of good practice with evidence-based techniques. Unfortunately, such an ideal is rarely available under current funding constraints.

Ideally, each larger town or city should have an informal walk-in centre where a young person can get confidential advice and information, counselling, or referral to relevant services. Outreach work, with streetwise individuals mingling with drug users in their natural habitat giving non-judgemental support and advice, is an important component. Such workers are often highly effective at spreading the health protection message to individuals leading risky lifestyles who are not in contact with services, and who have scant regard for the advice of professionals or official pronouncements.

In the case of volatile substance abuse (VSA), early intervention organized by the family doctor with a focus on practical problem solving and dealing with any family or social difficulties is often effective. If VSA has been regular or heavy a careful neurological examination is essential, and counselling and support from specialist services will probably be required. Information and advice on how to access this can be obtained online: http://www.re-solv.org/ in the UK and http://www.inhalants.drugabuse.gov/ in the US.

Psychological treatments—general principles

Psychological interventions are central to the management of all drug-related problems. A wide range of techniques has been applied over the decades, but evidence of effectiveness for many is limited.

The cornerstone approach is counselling. A good counsellor will be an excellent listener, and the sort of person who is able to build up trust and rapport with their clients. Having clarified what the person wishes to achieve, the aim will be to guide her towards realistic goals, then advise, educate, problem solve, and support. Central to the process is the establishment of a confidence-enhancing and supportive personal interaction, collaborating with the client without compromising his or her autonomy. The effectiveness of counselling depends more on the personal attributes of the counsellor than the details of technique. Many of these are inherent rather than taught: natural warmth and empathy, patience, confidence and inner strength, and communication skills. The sort of concrete benefits demonstrated include reductions in prescribed and illicit drug use, arrests, and convictions. Clients maintained on substitute medication (e.g. methadone) achieve better results if they also receive regular counselling.

A very influential paper from the 1980s separated drug users into four categories. A 'pre-contemplator' is someone happily puffing away at their cigarettes or shooting up their heroin without any thought or concern about possible consequences. A 'contemplator' has begun to think now and again that it would be good to cut down, experiences the occasional twinge of guilt or anxiety whilst consuming, and dreads coming across an article about lung cancer or HIV in the newspaper (it *could* happen to me!). A person who is taking practical steps towards giving up has reached the stage of 'active change', whilst someone who is abstinent and struggling to stay that way is at the level of 'relapse prevention'. The point of this classification is to emphasize that the therapeutic intervention must be appropriate to the stage the person has reached. There is no future in attempting to persuade pre-contemplators to give up; the aim should be to nudge them up to the next stage, to get them to begin the process of weighing up the pros and cons of the habit.

More specialized psychological treatments are of proven worth in the treatment of anxiety and depression, but are also effectively deployed against drug-related problems where resources permit this. Many therapists now rely heavily on the principles of cognitive behavioural therapy (CBT). Unlike many psychological treatments, its efficacy is supported by results of carefully controlled clinical trials. The underlying principle of CBT is to uncover self-defeating patterns of thinking which, it is argued, lie at the heart of depression, anxiety, and guilt. Instead of relying on subjective opinions of either therapist or client, behavioural experiments are devised to test out these opinions empirically. For a simple example, imagine a person who concedes that his heroin use has become rather more regular recently, but says that this is not a matter for concern because he could give it up any time he wished. The therapist disagrees. Instead of arguing about what is, at this stage, just a matter of opinion, she suggests a little trial: 'Just out of interest, why not see if you can manage without a hit until the day after tomorrow'. The outcome of this experiment will be useful whichever way it goes. Success would result in a psychological boost to the client, whilst failure might bring home an important insight to build upon. The therapist will also be interested in analysing with the client the rules by which he governs his life—the 'shoulds, musts, and oughts'—attitudes and beliefs, habits and rituals, in order to reflect with him on which are helpful and life-enhancing and which are not.

'Motivational interviewing' became fashionable in the 1990s and remains an important and effective technique. It is based on an attitude towards the client which is fundamentally different from the traditional, paternalistic view of old. Individuals are expected to take full responsibility for actions and their consequences, encouraged in the belief that they have the power to shape their own destiny, and helped in developing the skills and confidence to achieve personal goals. 'Denial', that great let-out clause for unsuccessful therapy, is seen not as an immovable character trait, but rather as a product of a confronting client-therapist interaction without genuine rapport. The therapist tries in various ways to raise the client's self-esteem and confidence, in the expectation that this improved internal concept will become more and more incompatible with self-damaging behaviour. The therapist then collaborates with the client to resolve this 'cognitive dissonance' by positive changes in behaviour. Strategies drawn from CBT are used to challenge assumptions and experiment with new solutions.

Symptoms of anxiety or depression are common in dependent drug users presenting to health services, but usually clear up spontaneously when the problems related to the addiction are sorted out. A small proportion turn out to have a genuine depressive illness, and these are amenable in the usual way to antidepressant medicines or psychological treatments such as CBT.

Relapse, prevention and rehabilitation

Relapse prevention is all about planning ahead so as to foresee high-risk situations, and understanding how subtle lifestyle decisions may bring these about. An example would be an abstinent alcoholic deciding to keep a bottle in the house just in case an old drinking companion should call round. Risky situations, such as returning to old haunts or friendships, are either avoided or confronted with rehearsed coping responses. Coping is generally more desirable than avoiding since, if successful, it will lead to an increase in self-confidence and self-esteem, making future relapse less likely. The converse is also true, so the choice between avoidance and control is a tactical one.

The therapist will be aware that a small lapse may induce what is known as the 'abstinence violation effect'—'that's it, I've had a hit, all that effort's been a complete waste of time, I'll always be a junkie, might as well go the whole hog'—at which point a single lapse turns into full-scale relapse. Some even plan a 'controlled lapse' with the client so these feelings can be explored with greater realism.

The basic planks of relapse prevention consist of predicting likely high-risk situations and planning in advance how to deal with them, increasing drug-free social contacts and avoiding the drug culture or favourite drinking haunts, reinforcing the negative memories of drug use as opposed to the positive, providing continuing support and help with problem solving, and perhaps urging membership of a self-help group. Sometimes, pharmacological treatment may have a place (see below).

The common causes of relapse include low mood, feeling physically unwell or suffering drawn-out withdrawal symptoms, experiencing powerful craving, falling out with families or partners, and pressure from other drug users or former drinking buddies. A less obvious danger is feeling good: 'Life's so great I must snort a line to make it perfect!' Some people come a cropper when they decide to test their personal resolve, confident that enough time has passed to have cracked the problem.

For many people who have become seriously drug dependent, some sort of post-detoxification rehabilitation is essential if abstinence is to be maintained. Non-residential programmes usually consist of long-term counselling, individual or group psychotherapy of one sort or another, family or marital therapy, or more pragmatic approaches like help in moving to another district or finding work.

Residential rehabilitation often takes place in units practising the so-called 'Minnesota Method', or in therapeutic communities of one sort or another. The Minnesota Method is a rather ill-defined, individually tailored package applied over a fixed time-span, usually between four and six weeks. It relies heavily on the AA 12-step approach (see below), with a tightly structured time-table including education, individual and group therapy sessions, skills training, confidence building, and attention to physical health. Families may be involved in the process. After completing the programme, there is an expectation that most clients would continue to attend AA or NA meetings regularly, or move into a hostel or some other sheltered environment.

Therapeutic communities aim to provide a safe, drug-free environment in which maladaptive ways of coping with life's challenges can be confronted by the peer group, and new ways explored. The organization of such communities varies from place to place, and it makes sense for an interested person to shop around in order to find a regime which seems acceptable. Most programmes last many months, and often involve long periods in which contact with family and friends is discouraged or banned. This sort of arrangement may not be appropriate or desirable for someone who retains a degree of social structure, such as an intact family or regular employment. In certain circumstances, the courts are prepared to consider placement in a suitable community as an alternative to a prison sentence.

Many therapeutic communities operate as 'concept houses'. This idea originated in 1959 with the Synanon organization of California. Daily life is highly structured with inmates organized in a formal hierarchy based on seniority and progress through the system. Staff are generally recovered addicts or, more correctly, 'addicts who are not using at the moment' since this is not seen as a condition which can be cured, only put into remission. The aim is to provide a surrogate family in which a global change in life-view can be nurtured. All behaviour and interactions are closely scrutinized by other residents and subject to peer review through regular 'encounter' groups. These potentially harrowing and confrontational sessions may sometimes go on for hours. Individuals are brought face to face with their behaviour or personal foibles in a very direct way and exposed to a particularly vigorous form of peer pressure. Privileges and responsibilities have to be earned, and a system of rewards and punishment is stringently applied. To get into such a community, a number of hurdles must first be cleared, for example becoming drug-free and getting through a detailed assessment procedure. New admissions are accorded low status, and may be given a range of menial and unpleasant tasks in the service of the community. Shame, guilt, and public humiliation are sometimes used to enforce conformity. Serious transgression of the rules can result in expulsion and immediate cessation of all access to community members. If a person stays the distance, profound changes for the better are claimed but concrete research evidence to prove this is lacking. Reintegration into the outside world after a long stay in a community of this sort can prove problematic.

Self-help groups

Self-help groups are made up of people with a common difficulty who meet regularly to provide mutual support, encouragement, and advice. Through regular attendance, people struggling to attain or retain abstinence may find the resolve to do so. Many find that self-help groups give a sense of purpose and belonging, and provide a credible abstinence role-model for those who have got used to thinking that this is beyond their reach.

Most are organized on the basis of principles first formulated by Alcoholics Anonymous (AA), which was founded in the 1930s. Members meet regularly, and anyone who is an ex-user or has a desire to abstain is welcome to attend. Complete honesty is expected, and new attenders may be allocated an experienced 'sponsor' to whom they can turn for advice or support. At the heart of the meetings is the 'twelve steps philosophy' which requires each member:

(1) to admit to powerlessness over his addiction, and concede that life has become unmanageable;

(2) to believe that a power greater than himself could restore him to sanity;

(3) to undertake to turn his will and life over to God 'as he understands Him';

(4) to make a 'searching and fearless moral inventory' of himself;

(5) to admit to God, himself, and to another human being the exact nature of his wrongs;

(6) to be entirely ready to have God remove all these defects of character;

(7) to 'humbly ask Him to remove his shortcomings';

(8) to make a list of all the persons he has harmed, and be willing to make amends to them all;

(9) to make direct amends to such people whenever possible, except when to do so would injure them or others;

(10) to continue to take personal inventory, and when wrong promptly admit it;

(11) to seek through prayer and meditation to improve conscious contact with God, 'praying only for knowledge of His will for us and the power to carry that out';

(12) having had a spiritual awakening as a result of these steps, to try to carry this message to other addicts and practise these principles in all his affairs.

Recognizing that the religious orientation would not appeal to everybody, it is stressed that the way of attaining the spiritual dimension which is central to the process is left entirely to the individual to determine. A humanistic orientation would be equally acceptable. Members are accustomed to concentrating on 'one day at a time' rather than trying to envisage a life without drugs stretching ahead interminably. This results in the rewards and satisfaction of success being experienced immediately rather than at some indeterminate point in the future.

Many offshoots have subsequently appeared. Narcotics Anonymous (NA) was established in the 1950s, and there are now groups aimed at stimulant users, gamblers, and 'overeaters'. Groups also exist for young people (Alateen), and families and partners (Al-Anon and Nar-Anon). AA and NA groups are accessible in almost all locations in the US and UK, and according to Reuters around five million people in the US attend regularly.

Despite their apparent effectiveness for many, AA and NA are not without their critics. Objective evidence that the 12-step approach significantly enhances the likelihood of abstinence in comparison with natural remission or other interventions is lacking. The emphasis on the disease model of alcoholism (and other addictions) is controversial, and rules out controlled consumption as an alternative to complete abstinence. Some find the group ethos dogmatic and more like a religious ritual than a scientifically-based undertaking, and are concerned that dependence upon the group is encouraged at the expense of personal autonomy and responsibility.

Specific strategies for smokers

The need for smoking cessation interventions is pressing given that only 5% of smokers quit spontaneously each year despite the fact that three-quarters say they would like to stop and a third will have made at least one serious but unsuccessful attempt to quit within the past twelve months.

Brief interventions by a doctor or other professional consisting of health education, practical advice about problem solving, and provision of leaflets, can increase the natural quit rate by about 2% but is likely to be effective only for light smokers. Abrupt withdrawal offers better prospects for success than attempts at gradually cutting down. Regular sessions to provide continuing support and encouragement will enhance this effect. It will often be helpful to ask the smoker to make a list of the benefits and cost savings of giving up, set a firm date, involve friends and family in the decision, change routines to avoid environmental cues associated with a habitual cigarette, and remain vigilant and plan ahead for high-risk situations for relapse. It is important to address secondary issues such as unwanted weight gain, or the role of alcohol or caffeine in cementing the habit or bringing about relapse. Risk factors for relapse (such as a smoking spouse) must be identified and coping strategies worked out in advance. Self-help leaflets and hypnosis have some research support, and acupuncture is sometimes helpful.

Regular smokers are likely to experience physical dependence, which is signalled by lighting up the first cigarette soon after waking, preoccupation and craving when circumstances preclude smoking, continuing to smoke even when unwell, and smoking very regularly throughout the day no matter how inconvenient this may be. For such individuals, a pharmacological component alongside the psychological intervention may be needed.

Nicotine replacement therapy (NRT) is available in the form of chewing gum, skin patches, lozenges, nasal spray or 'inhalator'. The gum delivers 2–4 mg per stick, and is usually taken for around three months after quitting then gradually withdrawn. It relies on absorption through the lining of the mouth, which is impeded in acidic conditions caused, for example, by coffee or Coca-Cola. Patches come in varying strengths, and to start with a delivery of 22 mg each 24 hours is usual. After a month or so, a patch delivering 14 mg daily is substituted, then 7 mg a month after that. These substitutes are of proven value in reducing anxiety and depression, craving, irritability, and poor concentration. They are less successful in combating insomnia and weight gain. Fear of the latter is a major barrier to giving up for many people, especially women. Very few adverse effects have been reported, especially in the case of gum. Patches sometimes cause rashes, nausea, insomnia, or vivid dreams. In association with other strategies, trials indicate that NRT can push the quit rate 8–10% above spontaneous rates.

A vaccine is in development which would cause the generation of antibodies to nicotine which could persist in the bloodstream for an extended period. When tobacco smoke is inhaled passively or the ex-smoker has a brief lapse, the antibodies would bind with the absorbed nicotine and slow or prevent its entry into the brain. By this means the vaccine could provide protection against re-addiction.

Bupropion (also known as amfebutamone) is an antidepressant which acts by enhancing CNS signalling of dopamine and noradrenaline. It also inhibits the nicotinergic acetylcholine receptors and for this reason has been used widely alongside behavioural smoking cessation programmes. It is started a couple of weeks before the cessation date and continued for two or three months thereafter. In clinical trials it reduced craving and withdrawal symptoms and improved abstinence rates 10% more than placebo. It carries the risk of inducing seizures and should be avoided by anyone with a history of epilepsy. Bupropion can also cause psychiatric symptoms and is therefore contraindicated in those with pre-existing mental health problems. Nortriptyline is another antidepressant which has in the past been used to reduce craving.

Varenicline (Champix/Chantix) is a partial agonist at the α4β2 neuronal nicotinic acetylcholine receptor (AChR) which was first licenced in 2006 and has since been prescribed to several million smokers. It is used in the same way as bupropion to reduce craving and withdrawal, and clinical trials suggest it is significantly more effective. By blocking the binding of nicotine to the AChR it reduces the rewarding effects of smoking. Unfortunately it also carries a risk of inducing agitation, depression, and suicidal ideas or behaviour. In 2008 the US Food and Drug Administration (FDA) issued a warning of the risk of suicide, aggressive or erratic behaviour, or other psychiatric symptoms in people taking the drug. This led the Federal Aviation Administration to ban the use of varenicline by pilots and air-traffic controllers.

Clinical trials have suggested that the cannabinoid CB_1 receptor antagonist rimonabant may significantly increase the chances of quitting and may also prevent weight gain in ex-smokers. However, at the time of writing the drug is under a cloud because of a high incidence of psychiatric adverse effects. Because of these concerns FDA declined to licence the drug in the US for its primary anti-obesity indication, and in October 2008 the European Medicines Agency followed suit.

Specific strategies for drinkers

No opportunities should be lost to uncover asymptomatic heavy drinkers through routine screening of accessible populations such as visitors to family doctors and hospital in-patients. This consists of taking the opportunity of an unrelated consultation to ask about alcohol (and smoking) habits and checking for signs and symptoms of related disorders, handing out questionnaires to vulnerable populations, or including a liver function test or other relevant measure when blood is taken for other reasons.

At-risk individuals identified in this way are often responsive to brief interventions from family doctors or practice nurses, with reduction of intake averaging around 24% in most studies. These reductions are associated with reduced absenteeism from work, and even mortality. A typical intervention consists of giving clear information about risks, firm advice to cut down or abstain, a request to keep a drinking diary (to boost insight), and a self-help booklet.

The evidence in support of more specialized treatments targeted on people who have already developed alcohol-related problems is less convincing, but alcoholics in treatment generally drink less than those untreated. Intensive (and expensive) in-patient regimes are not demonstrably more effective than out-patient or community work.

For those who have become physically dependent, abrupt withdrawal carries some risk and may require medical support. For milder cases of the shakes and agitation, a long-acting benzodiazepine such as diazepam tapered off over a week or so plus some vitamin supplements will be all that is required. Full-blown delirium tremens ('the DTs') is potentially life-threatening and should be treated in hospital. Sedation, intravenous fluids, electrolytes, carbohydrates and thiamine (to prevent brain damage with severe, permanent memory loss), and skilled nursing are likely to be required.

Behavioural treatments (assertiveness and social-skills training, contracting, deconditioning, outcome reinforcement, relapse prevention) work better than insight-oriented therapy (e.g. psychoanalysis). 'Controlled drinking' rather than abstinence can be a realistic goal, especially in younger, socially stable, less physically dependent people, and women seem to do better at this than men. Marital therapy may be appropriate, and attendance at Alcoholics Anonymous also helps some people. Whatever the form of treatment, long-term, low-intensity interventions usually achieve better results than intensive, short-term measures.

'Dual diagnosis', the coexistence of mental illness with addiction, requires a specialized approach but symptoms of anxiety and depression which very frequently accompany alcoholism usually clear up spontaneously once the addiction is brought under control.

Disulfiram (Antabuse) and calcium carbimide have been used for many years to prevent relapse in abstinent alcoholics. They work by inhibiting the enzyme aldehyde dehydrogenase, which results in a rapid build-up of toxic acetaldehyde in the blood if the subject drinks. Severe vomiting and diarrhoea, and potentially dangerous increases in blood pressure, then ensue. Adverse effects of these drugs are quite unpleasant, so it is hardly surprising that compliance is usually poor and the evidence for their usefulness less than compelling.

Naltrexone, an opioid antagonist, attracted interest in the early 1990s in this context because alcohol had been shown to stimulate certain opioid receptors in the brain. Research conducted over the past two decades suggests that abstinent alcoholics given naltrexone take longer to relapse and drink less if they do relapse than people given placebo. Alcoholics with a family history of alcoholism may be more likely to benefit. Overall, efficacy levels are quite modest and the drug can cause gastrointestinal and psychiatric adverse effects. An injectable depot formulation is available to improve compliance for long-term maintenance.

Acamprosate has also been available for more than two decades in Europe and is also now approved in the US. It seems to work by inhibiting excitatory brain neurotransmitters whilst mimicking the effects of the inhibitory neuro-transmitter GABA. Like naltrexone its overall efficacy in clinical trials is less than spectacular, though it may be marginally better at producing initial absti-nence. However in one large US study with a head-to-head comparison it appeared significantly inferior to both naltrexone and cognitive therapy.

The anti-convulsant gabapentin has been found to reduce consumption and craving in dependent subjects. In those who have achieved abstinence it can reduce the likelihood and delay the onset of relapse. Mode of action remains uncertain, but gabapentin resembles GABA structurally and mimics its effects in the brain. Enhancing GABA signalling in the amygdala may be a key mecha-nism. Topiramate, another anti-convulsant, reduced the rewarding effects of alcohol and improved drinking outcomes in a recent clinical trial, presumably by a similar mechanism. It also reduced the risk of alcohol-induced cardiovas-cular and liver disease.

Two other drugs are undergoing preliminary assessment. The atypical anti-psychotic aripiprazole increased the sedative effects and decreased eupho-ria following alcohol in an exploratory trial. LY686017, which blocks the neurokinin-1 brain receptor, may reduce alcohol craving and improve well-being during abstinence.

When liver disease is established drugs such as naltrexone are contra-indicated because they may aggravate the condition. In these circumstances the anti-spasticity drug baclofen has the advantage of minimal liver metabo-lism and has been shown to improve abstinence rates and reduce craving.

Most people dependent on alcohol are also troubled by insomnia. The anti-depressant trazodone is frequently used off-label to treat this but though effective as a hypnotic it may actually worsen abstinence outcome.

Specific strategies for opioid users

A vigorous approach is justified since treatment is highly cost-effective: UK research shows that for every £1 spent more than £9 is saved in health and crime costs.

The threat of a world-wide HIV epidemic in the 1980s and more recently the rampant spread of hepatitis C has transformed the political and clinical response to injecting drug use. A 'harm reduction philosophy' is now a central strategy in many countries. Instead of focusing only on individuals wishing to become abstinent the aim is to establish contact with as wide a range as possible, including those intending to go on using for the foreseeable future.

Having made contact the minimal requirement in the 'treatment hierarchy' is risk reduction. This involves giving advice about safer sex and injecting, including instructions on how to clean used equipment effectively if fresh 'works' are unavailable. It may be possible to provide basic health care and help with housing, child care, or legal issues. Many people present with problems partly related to drug use but partly related also to the ubiquitous difficulties of homelessness, poverty, and a life without prospects or hope. Such individuals can benefit greatly from practical help, even if they are initially reluctant to confront their drug dependence.

The hierarchical approach does not imply defeatism. It will often be possible to substitute oral drug use for injecting, stabilize the lifestyle to the point that detoxification becomes feasible and desirable, then go on to arrange rehabilitation or strategies to prevent relapse. The harm-reduction approach sets a more practical perspective, in that limiting the spread of infectious diseases and the burden of criminal activity generated by drug addiction is arguably of greater importance to society at large than inducing abstinence in a subgroup of addicts. Ignoring chaotic drug users has in the past cost the taxpayer huge sums in hospital bills, prison and probation costs, street crime, and the break-up of families. A lack of drug services can have frightening consequences. In Edinburgh, for example, a culture developed among drug users in which the sharing of injecting equipment was routine. The HIV infection rate in a sample of these people in 1987 was 52%. Twenty per cent had shared needles with users in other parts of the country. A disaster of this sort has sombre implications for the population at large. In this same city, screening people aged between 20 and 30 attending a particular family health practice revealed an HIV positivity rate of one in 14 men and one in 28 women.

Needles, syringes, and condoms should be made easily available (on an exchange basis for injecting equipment to encourage safe disposal) free of charge from street agencies and elsewhere because of the individual and public health benefits that can result from such simple harm-reduction measures.

The savings in medical and social expenditure from preventing a single case of AIDS would support one of these agencies for a whole year. Three quarters of attenders at needle-exchange clinics have no other contact with services, so this represents a unique opportunity to provide health education, explore ambivalence about drug use, and initiate motivational input to an otherwise invisible group. Although most attenders know something about HIV and hepatitis around a third continue sharing needles or syringes, and only a minority regularly use a condom. Easy availability of needles and syringes has not been shown to result in an increase in injecting drug use, though this needs careful monitoring. Needle exchange schemes are now available in 24 European member states but in the US availability is limited to a few hundred centres nationwide because schemes are not allowed to receive federal funding.

Assessment of a new patient will include a physical examination and relevant biochemical investigations. Vaccination should be offered to injectors who test negative for hepatitis B. HIV testing, with counselling before and after the test, should be on offer. Recent drug consumption can be confirmed or monitored by urine or blood testing.

Pregnant users should be given accurate information about drugs being taken, attention to general health and emotional well-being, and support in establishing a more stable lifestyle. Some drugs, including barbiturates, cocaine, and amphetamine, have been linked with direct damage to the foetus. If the mother feels she simply cannot give up, or has a physical dependency, the best option is to wean her away from street drugs with a substitute prescription whilst avoiding withdrawal symptoms which may bring on premature labour.

Detoxification

For those wishing to become abstinent medical help with detoxification may be required. This is usually the case when alcohol (see above), tranquillizers, or opiates have been taken in sufficient quantity and regularity to induce physical dependence. Benzodiazepine detoxification is usually best carried out at home. If the individual is dependent on a short-acting compound such as temazepam, withdrawal symptoms are often made more tolerable by transferring to an equivalent dose of a longer-acting drug such as diazepam before beginning the reduction. Reasons for choosing hospital detoxification would include a history of serious complications during previous detoxifications or coexisting medical or psychiatric problems.

Opiate detoxification is usually unpleasant and feared disproportionately by addicts, but it is not dangerous to those in reasonable health and so can usually be undertaken out of hospital. Sometimes all that is needed is brief symptomatic treatment from the family doctor with lofexidine, diphenoxylate, hyoscine, metaclopramide, or benzodiazepines, or a reducing dose of a prescription opioid over a few days.

Unfortunately, a steady reduction of methadone or some other opioid over days, weeks, or months in the community, or symptomatic treatment of withdrawal symptoms as described above has a low success rate. Only one in five on average will successfully resist the temptation to revert to the black market. An alternative, when resources permit, is a residential methadone withdrawal regime which will have a much higher immediate success rate. Many will relapse shortly after discharge, though, because withdrawal symptoms are usually at their height towards the end of the procedure and immediately thereafter. Patients must be warned of this and given regular support in these early days of abstinence.

An alternative detoxification method is the clonidine-naltrexone technique. Clonidine specifically antagonizes many of the withdrawal symptoms while naltrexone speeds up the withdrawal process, possibly by displacing the opioid from receptors in the brain. Apart from the advantage of a briefer hospital stay of seven to 10 days, quicker if necessary, persistent withdrawal symptoms may be less prominent. Lofexidine is a more expensive alternative to clonidine and better tolerated by some patients, but both may cause fainting due to lowered blood pressure.

The chances of remaining abstinent following detoxification are marginally improved by long term maintenance on the opioid antagonist naltrexone. Compliance is a major difficulty, so sustained injections or implants may enhance efficacy.

'Cue exposure and response prevention' may help people with an addiction to the act of injecting itself ('needle fixation'). This consists of exposing the client to a 'cue', such as a loaded syringe, without allowing him to inject. The resulting intense agitation and craving gradually subsides over an hour or so, and the patient is kept in contact with the cue until this is complete. If repeated at regular intervals the subject's response to the cue diminishes ('habituates') or disappears completely.

Detoxification on its own has no influence on longer-term outcome. It is only useful if it forms part of some more general treatment plan.

Substitute or long-term prescribing

For those not yet ready to abstain from opioids, some form of substitute prescribing may be indicated. Addiction specialists vary widely in their attitude to this. Some regard it as colluding with dependency and akin to handing out money to compulsive gamblers, and will not contemplate it under any circumstances.

Others go to the opposite extreme and think that heroin and cocaine for injection, smoking, or snorting should be readily available to addicts in order to prize them away from the black market and undermine the profits of criminals. A middle position would be that substitute prescribing can bring stability to selected individuals but that if employed indiscriminately it may encourage or worsen addiction and swell the black market, as happened in the late 1960s.

Methadone remains the most widely used substitute opioid. Unlike heroin, it is effective by mouth and a single dose goes on working for 24 hours, permitting a simple routine which encourages a more stable lifestyle. It is just as addictive as heroin itself and produces a withdrawal syndrome of equal severity. It is in no sense a cure, merely an effective palliative. Methadone is itself easily and cheaply available on the black market

Providing methadone to someone not genuinely addicted to opioids would be to create a new addict. It is therefore essential to confirm opioid dependence by observing the patient actively withdrawing before prescribing. The correct dose is arrived at by titrating against visible withdrawal effects and increasing the dose on a daily basis as required. Once stabilization has been achieved the methadone is either reduced and stopped according to a negotiated time-scale, or continued long term at the same level.

Clinical trials show that methadone maintenance patients are more likely to remain in treatment and use less street drugs than those in drug-free programmes or on long-term naltrexone. Other benefits include lower levels of drug dealing and criminality, improved physical and mental health, more stability in family life, and lower rates of unemployment. Arguments against maintenance are that it is social manipulation rather than treatment, that it colludes with dependency, and that methadone is harder to come off than heroin. Apart from the risk of overdose methadone is generally well tolerated. Recently, several unexplained cases of sudden cardiac arrest in methadone maintenance patients have been published. It remains to be seen if a causative role emerges.

In a few countries (not including the US) a small number of selected addicts receive injectable prescriptions of methadone or pharmaceutical heroin, usually when oral methadone has proved unsuccessful in achieving stabilization. The aim is to create a therapeutic relationship with the more chaotic users and help them sever links with the black market. This remains a controversial practice. At the time of writing controlled clinical trials are in progress in the UK, the Netherlands, Germany, and Switzerland, and preliminary feedback suggests that heroin prescription is associated with better retention and less black market drug use than either oral or intravenous methadone. However, the prevalence of adverse events may be higher in both injectable groups.

The results of a clinical trial in the 1970s illustrates the difficulty in defining a successful outcome in such trials. Opiate addicts seeking injectable heroin were randomly allocated to receive either oral methadone or IV heroin and followed up for a year whether or not they remained in the trial. Three-quarters of the heroin group remained in treatment for the year of study but, of course, all were continuing to inject. Twelve per cent of this group regularly sold some of their script into the black market. In the methadone group, 12% left the trial immediately on learning that heroin was not available to them, and after a year only 29% of the original sample remained in treatment. However, 40% of those who had quit the trial had given up illegal drugs. Overall, the two groups ended up with similar rates of illicit drug use, time spent in the drug culture, unemployment, criminality, and poor general health, but this equivalence concealed a polarization effect in the methadone group; some did unusually well in terms of illicit drug use, crime, and so forth, but a similar proportion fared very badly. So which is the better result? Only a politician can decide!

Buprenorphine, a partial μ-opioid agonist with a long duration of action, is an alternative to methadone for long-term maintenance. Initially marketed as an analgesic, its use as a substitute opioid in addiction was pioneered in France and Australia, and it is now licenced for this purpose in over 30 countries including the US where it is in a lower controlled drug schedule than methadone. This means it can be prescribed from office-based practices as well as in a hospital setting or methadone clinics. Clinical trials suggest that it has equivalent efficacy and adverse event profile to methadone, but as a partial agonist it should theoretically be safer in overdose and have less abuse potential. It may also be easier to come off, and so could have particular merit for younger subjects with a shorter addiction history. Recently a formulation which combines buprenorphine with naloxone has become available. Naloxone is an opioid antagonist effective only by injection so that in normal oral use it has no effect. If the formulation is injected, however, it will antagonise the euphoric effect of buprenorphine.

Contingency management is becoming fashionable in maintenance programmes. Incentives such as shopping vouchers or allowing take-home doses of methadone are given to participants who have negative urine screens or achieve some other goal such as employment.

Specific strategies for amphetamine and cocaine users

Abstinence following regular, heavy use of stimulants (or hallucinogens) does not cause a physical withdrawal syndrome and so will not require medical help. However, the psychological effects and craving will likely be intense, so skilled psychological support may be needed along with short-term symptomatic prescribing for anxiety or insomnia.

Long-term management of stimulant dependency hinges around the psychological principles summarized above. In the US, a protocol-based programme incorporating drug education and monitoring and drawing on established techniques from individual, group and family therapies alongside attendance at self-help groups has been created. Several studies have produced evidence that use of this so-called Matrix Model can produce significant reductions in drug and alcohol use, improvements in mental health and reduced levels of risky sexual behaviour.

Several medicines have been used in an attempt to ameliorate the intense craving often associated with quitting stimulants, but there is little research evidence in support. Disulfiram is thought to reverse the brain dopamine deficiency which can result from chronic stimulant use by preventing the conversion of dopamine to noradrenaline. Significantly more cocaine addicts achieved a drug free urine following disulfiram than following placebo. Preliminary evidence suggests it might also be useful for methamphetamine addicts. Naltrexone was found to reduce craving for amphetamine in a small pilot trial. Several antidepressants have been tried with no success, and other drugs currently under investigation include baclofen, vigabatrin, flumazenil, gabapentin, hydroxyzine, aripiprazole, and bupropion.

Based on a similar theoretical base as described above for nicotine, there are hopes of developing a cocaine vaccine to generate antibodies that would combine with cocaine in the bloodstream and prevent its entry into the brain. Preliminary trials suggest that the vaccine is safe and well tolerated, and is associated with reduced use of cocaine.

For stimulant users who are unwilling to quit, the prescribing of substitute stimulants such as amphetamine or cocaine is even more controversial than opioid maintenance. It has been tried on a relatively small scale in centres in the UK, Australia, Canada, and the US. As yet there is no research evidence to justify it, but anecdotal reports suggest it can stabilize the lives and improve the physical and mental health of carefully selected subjects.

Specific strategies for cannabis smokers

Abrupt cannabis withdrawal may be associated with sleep disturbance, emotional lability, reduced appetite, sweating, shaking, and stomach cramps lasting a few days and for which brief symptomatic treatment may be indicated. In severe cases a reducing course over a week or so of the oral cannabinoid dronabinol (or nabilone in countries where this is not licenced) may prove helpful.

There is no agreed strategy for rehabilitation and relapse prevention for cannabis dependency. Most research into this has been conducted in the US and Australia where it is the most frequent drug requiring treatment (as is also the case in Africa). Some other countries (e.g. France) have now set up specialized services for cannabis users, but the best approach is according to the principles of psychological treatments summarized above.

One current line of research is exploring whether an inhibitor of the enzyme catechol-o-methyl-transferase (COMT) might reduce cannabis craving. COMT breaks down dopamine, so inhibiting it may produce a 'natural high' which could take the place of marijuana smoking.

Selected references

Academic ED SBIRT Research Collaborative (2007). The impact of screening, brief intervention and referral for treatment on emergency department patients' alcohol use. *Annals of Emergency Medicine* 50, 699–710.

Addolorato G., Leggio L., Ferrulli A. et al. (2007). Effectiveness and safety of baclofen for maintenance of alcohol abstinence in alcohol-dependent patients with liver cirrhosis: randomised, double blind, controlled trial. *Lancet* 370, 1915–22.

Aubin H. J., Bobak A., Britton J. R. et al. (2008). Varenicline versus transdermal nicotine patch for smoking cessation: results from a randomised open label trial. *Thorax* 63, 717–24.

Bennett, T., Wright, R. (1986). The impact of prescribing on the crimes of opioid users. *British Journal of Addiction*, 81, 265–73.

Boothby L., Doering P. L. (2007). Buprenorphine for the treatment of opioid dependence. *American Journal of Health-System Pharmacy,* 64, 266–72.

Bradley, B. P., Phillips, G., Green, L., Gossop, M. (1989). Circumstances surrounding the initial lapse to opiate use following detoxification. *British Journal of Psychiatry*, 154, 354–9.

Brettle, R. P., Bisset, K., Burns, S., Davidson, J., Davidson, S. J., Gray, J. M. N., *et al.* (1987). Human immunodeficiency virus and drug misuse: the Edinburgh experience. *British Medical Journal*, 295, 421–4.

Cahill K., Ussher M. (2007). Cannabinoid type 1 receptor antagonists (rimonabant) for smoking cessation. *Cochrane Database Systematic Review 2007* Oct 17(4)CD005353.

Charney, D. S., Heringer, G. R., Kleber, H. D. (1986). Combined use of clonidine and naltrexone as a rapid, safe, and effective treatment of abrupt withdrawal from methadone. *American Journal of Psychiatry*, 143, 831–7.

Chugh S. S., Socoteanu C., Reinier K. et al. (2008). A community-based evaluation of sudden death associated with therapeutic levels of methadone. *American Journal of Medicine,* 121, 66–71.

Ciraulo D. A., Dong Q., Silverman B. L. et al. (2008). Early treatment response in alcohol dependence with extended-release naltrexone. *Journal of Clinical Psychiatry*, 69, 190–5.

Drugscope and Drugs Prevention Advisory Service (2002).*Assessing local need: planning services for young people.* Home Office, London.

Drummond, D. C. (1997). Alcohol interventions: do the best things come in small packages? *Addiction*, **92**, 375–9.

Ernst D. B., Pettinati H. M., Weiss R. D. et al. (2008). An intervention for treating alcohol dependence: relating elements of Medical Management to patient outcomes with implications for primary care. *Annals of Family Medicine*, **6**, 435–40.

Fischer B., Oviedo-Joekes E., Blanken P. et al. (2007). Heroin-assisted treatment (HAT) a decade later: a brief update on science and politics. *Journal of Urban Health*, **84**, 552–62.

Friedmann P. D., Rose J.S., Swift R. et al. (2008). Trazodone for sleep disturbance after alcohol detoxification: a double-blind, placebo-controlled trial. *Alcohol Clinical & Experimental Research*, **32**, 1652–60.

Fudala P. J., Bridge T. P., Herbert S. et al. (2003). Office-based treatment of opiate addiction with a sublingual tablet formulation of buprenorphine and naloxone. *New England Journal of Medicine*, **349**, 949–58.

Furiera F. A., Nakamuria-Palacios E. M. (2007). Gabapentin reduces alcohol consumption and craving: a randomised, double-blind, placeob-controlled trial. *Journal of Clinical Psychiatry*, **68**, 1691–700.

George G. T., Gilman J., Hersh J. et al. (2008). Neurokinin 1 receptor antagonism as a possible therapy for alcoholism. *Science*, **319**, 1536–9.

Gorelick D. A., Gardner E. L., Xi Z. X. (2004). Agents in development for the management of cocaine abuse. *Drugs*, **64**, 1457–73.

Gossop, M. (1978). A review of the evidence for methadone maintenance as a treatment for narcotic addiction. *Lancet*, **1**, 812–15.

Gossop, M., Green, L., Phillips, G., Bradley, B. (1989). Lapse, relapse, and survival among opiate addicts after treatment – a prospective follow-up study. *British Journal of Psychiatry*, **154**, 348–53.

Gossop, M., Griffiths, P., Bradley, B., Strang, J. (1989). Opiate withdrawal symptoms in response to 10-day and 21-day methadone withdrawal programmes.*British Journal of Psychiatry*, **154**, 360–3.

Hajek, P., West, R. (1998). Treating nicotine dependence: the case for specialist smokers' clinics. *Addiction*, **93**, 637–40.

Hartnoll, L., Mitcheson, M. C., Battersby, A., Brown, G., Ellis, M., Fleming, P., et al. (1980). Evaluation of heroin maintenance in controlled trial. *Archives of General Psychiatry*, **37**, 877–84.

Hayes J. T., Ebbert J. O. (2008). Varenicline for tobacco dependence. *New England Journal of Medicine*, **359**, 2018–24.

Hughes, J. R. et al. (1996). Practice guidelines for the treatment of patients with nicotine dependence. *American Journal of Psychiatry*, **153**, 1–31.

Jansson L. M., Choo R., Velez M. L. et al. (2008). Methadone maintenance and breastfeeding in the neonatal period. *Pediatrics*, **121**, 106–14.

Jayaram-Lindstrom N., Hammarburg A., Beck O. et al. (2008). Naltrexone for the treatment of amphetamine dependence: a randomised, placebo-controlled trial. *American Journal of Psychiatry*, **165**, 1442–8.

Joe, G. W., Simpson, D. D. (1975). Retention in treatment of drug abusers: 1971–72 DARP admissions. *American Journal of Drug and Alcohol Abuse*, **2**, 63–71.

Joe, G. W., Simpson, D. D., Broome, K. M. (1998). Effects of readiness for drug abuse treatment on client retention and assessment of process. *Addiction*, **93**, 1177–90.

Johnson B. A., Rosenthal N., Capece J. A. (2007). Topiramate for treating alcohol dependence: a randomised controlled trial. *JAMA,* **298**, 1641–51.

Judson, B. A., Goldstein, A. (1982). Prediction of long-term outcome for heroin addicts admitted to a methadone maintenance program. *Drug and Alcohol Dependence*, **10**, 383–91.

Kleber, H. D. (1989). Treatment of drug dependence: what works. *International Review of Psychiatry*, **1**, 81–100.

Kranzler H. R., Covault J., Pierucci-Lagha A. et al. (2008). Effects of aripiprazole on subjective and physiological responses to alcohol. *Alcohol Clinical & Experimental Research,* **32**, 573–9.

Kreek, M. J. (1979). Methadone in treatment: physiological and pharmacological issues. In: *Handbook on drug abuse* (ed. R. L. Dupont, A. Goldstein, and J. O'Donnell), pp. 57–86, N.I.D.A., Washington.

Lee N. K., Rawson R. A. (2008). A systematic review of cognitive and behavioural therapies for methamphetamine dependence. *Drug & Alcohol Reviews*, **27**, 309–17.

Luty J., Carnwath T. (2008). Specialised alcohol treatment services are a luxury the NHS cannot afford. *British Journal of Psychiatry*, **192**, 245–7.

McCrady, B. S., Langenbucher, J. W. (1996). Alcohol treatment and health care system reform. *Archives of General Psychiatry*, **53**, 737–46.

McLellan, A. T. Luborsky, L., Woody, G. E., O'Brien, C. P., Druley, K. A. (1982). Is treatment for substance abuse effective? *Journal of the American Medical Association*, **247**, 1423–8.

McLellan, A. T., Luborsky, L., O'Brien, W. G. E., Druley, K. A. (1983). Predicting response to alcohol and drug abuse treatments. *Archives of General Psychiatry*, **40**, 620–5.

McLellan, A. T., Woody, G. E., Luborsky, L., Geohl, L. (1988). Is the counsellor an 'active ingredient' in substance abuse rehabilitation? (An examination of treatment success among four counsellors.) *Journal of Nervous and Mental Disease*, **176**, 423–30.

McSweeney T, Turnbull PJ, Hough M (2008). *Tackling drug markets and distribution networks in the UK* UK Drug Policy Commission www.ukdpc.org.uk/reports.shtml.

Maddux, J. F., Desmond, D. P. (1982). Residence relocation inhibits opioid dependence. *Archives of General Psychiatry*, **39**, 1313–17.

Marks, I. (1990). Behavioural (non-chemical) addictions. *British Journal of Addiction*, **85**, 1389–94.

Marks, J. (1987). State-rationed drugs. *Druglink*, **2**, 14.

Marlatt, G. A., George, W. H. (1984). Relapse prevention: introduction and overview of the model. *British Journal of Addiction*, **79**, 261–73.

Marsch, L. A. (1998). The efficacy of methadone maintenance interventions in reducing illicit opiate use, HIV risk behaviour, and criminality: a meta-analysis. *Addiction*, **88**, 515–32.

Mason B. J., Goodman A. M., Chabac S., Lehert P. (2006). Effect of oral acamprosate on abstinence in patients with alcohol dependence in a double-blind, placebo controlled trial: the role of patient motivation. *Journal of Psychiatric Research*, **40**, 383–93.

Miller, W. R. (1983). Motivational interviewing with problem drinkers. *Behavioural Psychotherapy*, **11**, 147–72.

Mintzer I. L., Eisenberg M., Terra M. et al. (2007). Treating opioid addiction with buprenorphine-naloxone in community-based primary care settings. *Annals of Family Medicine*, **5**, 146–50.

Moore T.J., Cohen M. R., Furberg C. D. (2008). *Strong safety signal seen for new varenicline risks*. Report prepared for the Institute for Safe Medication Practices http://www.ismp. org/docs/vareniclineStudy.asp.

National Institute for Health and Clinical Excellence (2007). *Drug misuse: psychosocial interventions and opiate detoxification*. NICE Clinical Guidelines 51 and 52; NICE, London.

Ngo H. T., Tait R. J., Hulse G. K. (2008). Comparing drug-related hospital morbidity following heroin dependence treatment with methadone maintenance or naltrexone implantation. *Archives of General Psychiatry*, **65**, 457–65.

Orson F. M., Kinsey B. M., Singh R. A. et al. (2008). Substance abuse vaccines. *Annals of the New York Academy of Sciences*, **1141**, 257–69.

Perneger, T. V., Giner, F., del Rio, M., Mino, A. (1998). Randomised trial of heroin maintenance programme for addicts who fail in conventional drug treatments. *British Medical Journal*, **317**, 13–18.

Polkinghorne, J. (1996). *Task force to review services for drug misusers: a final report*. Department of Health Publications, London.

Prochaska, J. O., DiClemente, C. C. (1983). Stages and processes of self-change of smoking: toward an integrative model of change. *Journal of Consulting and Clinical Psychology*, **51**, 390–5.

Rathod, N. (1987). Substitution is not a solution. *Druglink*, **2**, 16.

Riley, D. (1987). The management of the pregnant drug addict. *Bulletin of the Royal College of Psychiatrist*, **11**, 362–5.

Roberto M., Gilpin N. W., O'Dell L. E. et al. (2008). Cellular and behavioural interactions of gabapentin with alcohol dependence. *Journal of Neuroscience*, **28**, 5762–71.

Robertson, J. R., Bucknall, A. B. V., Welsby, P. D., Roberts, J. J. K., Inglis, J. M., Peutherer, J. F. *et al.* (1986). Epidemic of AIDS-related virus infection among intravenous drug abusers. *British Medical Journal*, **292**, 527–9.

Robson, P. (1992). Opiate misusers: are treatments effective? In: *Practical problems in clinical psychiatry* (ed. K. Hawton and P. Cowen). Oxford University Press, Oxford.

Rounsaville, B. J., Glazer, W., Wiber, C. H., Weissman, M. M., Kleber, H. D. (1983). Short-term interpersonal psychotherapy in methadone-maintained opiate addicts. *Archives of General Psychiatry*, **40**, 629–36.

Russell, M. A., Stapleton, J. A., Jackson, P. H., Hajek, P., Belcher, M. (1987). District programme to reduce smoking: effect of clinic-supported brief intervention by general practitioners. *British Medical Journal*, **295**, 1240–4.

Schottenfeld R. S., Chawarski M. C., Mazlan M. (2008). Maintenance treatment with buprenorphine and naltrexone for heroin dependence in Malaysia: a randomised, double-blind, placebo-controlled trial. *Lancet*, **371**, 2192–200.

Schuckit, M. A. (1996). Recent developments in the pharmacotherapy of alcohol dependence. *Journal of Consulting and Clinical Psychology*, **64**, 669–76.

Simpson, D. (1979). The relation of time spent in drug-abuse treatment to post-treatment outcome. *American Journal of Psychiatry*, **136**, 1449–53.

Skidmore, C.A., Robertson, J. R., Roberts, J. J. K. (1989). Changes in HIV risk-taking behaviour in intravenous drug users: a second follow-up. *British Journal of Addiction*, **84**, 695–6.

Stewart, J., de Wit, H., Eikelboom, R. (1984). Role of unconditioned and conditioned drug effects in the self-administration of opiates and stimulants. *Psychological Review*, **91**, 251–68.

Strang, J. (1987). The prescribing debate. *Druglink*, **2**(4), 10–12.

Stimson, G. V., Alldritt, I. J., Dolan, K. A., Donoghue, M. C., Lart, R. A. (1988). *Injecting equipment exchange schemes: final report*. Monitoring Research Group, Sociology Department, Goldsmiths' College, London SE14 6NW.

Swift, W., Williams, G., Neill, O., Grenyer, B. (1990). The prevalence of minor psychopathology in opioid users seeking treatment. *British Journal of Addiction*, **85**, 629–34.

Volkow N. D., Li T-K. (2005). Drugs and alcohol: treating and preventing abuse, addiction and their medical consequences. *Pharmacology & Therapeutics*, **108**, 3–17.

Wolk, J., Wodak, A., Guinan, J. J., Macaskill, P., Simpson, J. M. (1990). The effect of a needle and syringe exchange on a methadone maintenance unit. *British Journal of Addiction*, **85**, 1445–50.

Woody, G. E., Luborsky, L., McLellan, A. T., O'Brien, C. P., Beek, A. T., Blaine, J., et al. (1983). Psychotherapy for opiate addicts – does it help? *Archives of General Psychiatry*, **40**, 639–45.

Woody G. E., Poole S. A., Subramanian G. et al. (2008). Extended versus short-term buprenorphine-naloxone for treatment of opioid-addicted youth: a randomised trial. *JAMA*, **300**, 2003–11.

Wrase J., Makris N., Braus D. F. et al. (2008). Amygdala volume associated with alcohol abuse relapse and craving. *American Journal of Psychiatry*, **165**, 1179–84.

Chapter 15

International drug policy—is it working?

Invited Contributors: Robert L. DuPont and Ethan Nadelmann

How are drugs controlled?

The 182 current signatory nations to the Single Convention on Narcotic Drugs (1961), the Convention on Psychotropic Substances (1971), and the Convention against Illicit Traffic in Narcotic Drugs and Psychotropic Substances (1988) are required to 'limit to medical and scientific purposes the cultivation, production, manufacture, export, import, distribution of, trade in, use, and possession of [certain] drugs'. Draconian enforcement of controls is imposed because of the grave public health, social, and economic risks the drugs are said to pose.

The main policy-making organization for international drug control is the Commission on Narcotic Drugs which has delegates from the member states of the United Nations (UN), along with representation from all non-UN signatories to the 1961 Convention. The Commission receives information and recommendations from interested organizations, and instigates surveys and research. Its role is to devise and monitor strategies for control of drug abuse and to advise governments on appropriate systems of legal restraint. The International Narcotics Control Board (INCB) is responsible for implementing the Conventions and monitoring compliance on a global basis. It appraises the legitimacy of scientific or medical uses of controlled drugs and oversees safeguards to prevent diversion into the illicit market. INCB provides regular reports on trends in drug consumption and trafficking, sales of precursor chemicals, and policy issues within individual nations. The United Nations Office on Drugs and Crime coordinates international drug control. Based in Vienna with satellite offices around the world, it was created in 2002 to improve the capacity of the UN to tackle '. . . *the interrelated issues of drug control, crime prevention and international terrorism in all its forms'.*

This system has many critics, not least from within the European Parliament. There have been calls for repeal on the grounds that despite the huge resources which have been applied '. . . *production and consumption of, and trafficking in, prohibited substances have increased exponentially over the past 30 years, representing what can only be described as a failure . . .*'. It was argued that the Conventions themselves had greatly enhanced the disastrous economic impact of the illegal drug trade and the resulting erosion of '. . . *the health, freedom and life of individuals*'. In practice, repeal seems almost impossible since the Conventions have no termination clause and as long as a single signatory persists would remain in effect. However, there is scope for individual nations to make their own interpretations of particular clauses or even to 'denounce' (withdraw) from the Conventions overall or selected components. Although this has never yet happened, it would, for example, be feasible for an individual nation to use denouncement and reaccession with a reservation to decriminalize cannabis yet retain membership of the Conventions.

Signatory nations are required to introduce legislation to implement the Conventions. Regulation in the UK is through the Misuse of Drugs Act (1971) and Regulations (2001). The former divides drugs into three classes according to perceived potential for causing harm, and defines penalties for offenders. Currently more than 300 drugs fall into Class A including heroin and the stronger opioids (including opium, dextromoramide, dipipanone, fentanyl, levomethorphan, levomoramide, methadone, morphine, pethidine), Ecstasy, LSD and other hallucinogens including magic mushrooms, cocaine powder and crack, methamphetamine, and other amphetamines when prepared for injection. Maximum penalty for using Class A drugs is seven years in prison and/or a fine, and life imprisonment for dealing. Class B consists mainly of barbiturates and similar compounds, the weaker opioids, amphetamine and dexamphetamine, and methylphenidate. Cannabis was restored to Class B in January 2009 against the advice of the government's own expert advisers. Class C contains benzodiazepines, ketamine, and gamma-hydroxybutyrate.

The Misuse of Drugs Regulations allocates drugs into five schedules which define how they must be stored, prescribed, and documented. Schedule 1 is for substances possessing no recognized application in conventional medical practice, such as coca leaf, opium, cannabis, and LSD. Doctors cannot prescribe these, and a special licence from the Home Office is required for use in research. Schedule 2 contains those drugs with high abuse potential but also recognized therapeutic utility, including opioids, dexamphetamine, and cocaine. Schedule 3 is for drugs known to be abused, but to a lesser degree than those in the previous category, including barbiturate-like sedatives and sleeping pills, temazepam, and a motley range of slimming tablets and milder painkillers. Schedule 4 entails only a modest level of control and includes the rest of the benzodiazepines, and Schedule 5 is reserved for concoctions which contain tiny amounts of substances from higher up the scale.

In the US compliance with the Conventions is achieved by the Comprehensive Drug Abuse Prevention and Control Act (1970), otherwise known as Controlled Substances Act (CSA). Controlled drugs are assigned to one of five Schedules according to perceived potential for abuse and/or dependence, and medical utility. Schedule 1 contains those with high abuse potential and no recognized medical utility including numerous opioids including heroin, the hallucinogens, and certain CNS stimulants and depressants. Schedules II–IV have medical utility and decreasing potential for abuse. Schedule II drugs are only available by prescription and their use is rigorously monitored by the Drug Enforcement Administration.

Other countries vary in their interpretation and implementation of the Conventions, and none more contrastingly than Sweden and the Netherlands.

Sweden has a long-standing temperance tradition. It has a state monopoly on sale of alcohol and the world's most generous social welfare system. Illegal drug use was virtually unknown before the 1960s, although the legal use of amphetamines as slimming agents and stimulants was widespread from the late 1930s. Sweden's initial response to an emerging illegal market was quite liberal and based upon harm reduction, but research of questionable quality conducted by a police doctor (Nils Bejerot) appeared to show that this was aggravating an intravenous drug epidemic. As a result, from the late 1970s a notably restrictive policy has been instituted. Drugs are seen as a major threat to social stability and the stated goal is a drug-free society. Marijuana is rigorously suppressed because it is seen as likely to lead to 'harder' drug use and a life of addiction. Although the aim is to rehabilitate rather than punish the user, harm reduction has largely been replaced by an abstinence orientation, coerced if necessary. Drug education programmes begin early in all schools, urine and drug screening are widely practiced to detect and deter users.

There appears to be widespread support for these policies within the media and general population even though there is little scientific evidence to support their efficacy. Amphetamine remains the main problem drug with heroin next, and as everywhere else in the world cannabis is the most widely used illegal drug. In retrospect it is difficult to see a convincing correlation between state interventions and drug prevalence. In the 1990s problem drug use rose sharply in comparison with the pattern elsewhere in Europe alongside falls in black market prices for heroin, amphetamine, and cocaine, but the new millenium has seen a sharp downturn. Throughout these oscillations the restrictive policies have remained unchanged.

In contrast, harm reduction has remained the central plank in the drug policy of the Netherlands for more than three decades. Whilst still aiming to minimize supply and remain in step with other European countries, the Dutch have placed less emphasis on punishing personal possession and use. The police cooperate with a declared wish to keep addicts integrated in society rather than force them underground. There is a belief that the effects of repressive drug policy are often confused in the public mind with the effects of drugs themselves. The misuse of drugs is seen as '. . . *a matter of social well-being and public health rather than as a problem for the police and the courts*'.

A fundamental practical distinction in the Dutch approach is the differentiation of 'drugs presenting unacceptable risks' from 'hemp products'. In 1976, a formal policy of non-enforcement was adopted whereby possession or trade in small amounts of cannabis would no longer be prosecuted, though such activity remained technically illegal. The reason given for this *de facto* decriminalization was to '. . . *avoid a situation in which consumers of cannabis suffer more damage from the criminal proceedings than from the drug itself*'. Currently, up to 5 grams per transaction can be purchased from 'brown' coffee shops, and possession of up to 30 grams is permitted. Retail outlets are supposed to limit their stock to 500 grams, minimum age for purchase is 18, alcohol sale is banned, and no advertising is allowed. Hard drugs are rigorously suppressed in these outlets. However, since the police continue to prosecute those dealing in larger amounts legitimate businessmen were and remain excluded from wholesale supply, leaving the field open to criminal entrepreneurs. This approach has not been popular with European neighbours, who have labelled Holland a 'narco-state'. One spin-off, desirable or not depending on your point of view, is that quality control has improved considerably as a result of customer discrimination; home-produced Dutch cannabis is reckoned by some to be the best in the world.

Public opinion, interestingly, is often at odds with government policy: there is generally a more repressive attitude to drugs among the Dutch than, for example, in Southern France where the law against personal use is rigorously enforced. The effect of depenalization on cannabis consumption has been analyzed by MacCoun and Reuter (1997). Between 1976 and 1983, it resulted in '*little if any effect on levels of use*' but between 1984 and 1996 prevalence of cannabis use 'increased sharply', particularly among young people aged between 18 and 20. Interpretation of this is complicated by the fact that prevalence rates increased equally rapidly in countries with total prohibition between 1992 and 1996. Currently, prevalence and price of cannabis are very similar in comparable Dutch and US cities, such as Amsterdam and San Francisco, where average age of first use is almost identical (16.95 and 16.43 years respectively). There is some evidence that the Dutch are having success in separating 'hard' and 'soft' drugs, since the prevalence of addiction to opioids and stimulants is much lower than that in France, UK, Italy, Spain, Switzerland, and the US.

The balance of the research evidence indicates that decriminalization of cannabis in the Netherlands did not significantly increase consumption, a finding that has been replicated in certain US and Australian States, Italy, and Spain. On the other hand, the current lifetime prevalence of cannabis smoking among students in Sweden is 7% compared to 28% in Holland (average for Europe = 21%) whilst figures for amphetamines, LSD, Ecstasy, sedatives, and inhalants are broadly similar. If this is the effect of a more restrictive policy on cannabis, why hasn't it worked for the US or UK? The answer must surely be that drug consumption in any particular country is determined by a multitude of individual, cultural, and logistic variables, many of which are poorly defined and understood. It appears that drug policy may exert only a limited impact within this hierarchy.

Strategies aimed at reducing smoking

The goals of most countries' tobacco policy are to reduce initiation by young people, to help smokers to quit, and to limit the damage and nuisance of passive smoking by restricting ignition in public places. Despite earning nearly £8,000 million last year in tobacco taxes, the UK government spent only £64 million on education programmes and helping people quit, and this discrepancy holds true for many developed countries. Meanwhile, despite bans on most forms of tobacco advertising, the tobacco industry continues to spend billions of dollars on cigarette promotion world wide. In the US, State programmes for control and prevention declined by 20% between 2002 and 2006, whilst over the same period the industry doubled its marketing expenditure (including discounting strategies) to over $13 billion. There is solid evidence of a link between advertising and prevalence of smoking by young people, and partial bans simply result in a switch to new media. Countries such as Norway and Sweden which have imposed a total ban on advertising have seen sharp falls in consumption. Calling in 2008 for a total world-wide ban, the World Health Organization points out that 95% of the global population is currently exposed to some form of promotion. For example, an international survey of adolescents found that more than half reported seeing billboard adverts for cigarettes within the previous month. The internet, magazines, music, and sports events continue to be favourite conduits to recruit new young smokers.

Health education campaigns in schools and through the media seem intuitively worthwhile, although there is little evidence that they influence behaviour very much. Packet warnings are reported to have stimulated a quit attempt by a substantial minority of smokers, especially following recent increases in size. 'Quit clinics' and self-help clubs are useful, and increased funding to improve access would be helpful. The age of legal purchase of tobacco should be at least 18, but probably would have little effect on access. Banning cigarette machines would have a major impact in the view of most experts, but only Britain is actively considering this at present. In December 2008, the open display of tobacco products was banned in British shops. Many countries have instigated bans on smoking in bars, restaurants, and other public places. Not only does this prevent passive smoking, it has also been shown to reduce average levels of consumption.

Tobacco is what is known as an 'elastic' commodity—if you make it more expensive, less people use it and those that do use it less. In both the UK and US, periodic boosts in the tax on cigarettes have been linked with downturns in consumption.

Strategies aimed at reducing drinking

Since most people use alcohol in an appropriate and life-enhancing way, most policy makers have as their target the reduction of high-risk drinking rather than all drinking. Alcohol, like tobacco, is an elastic commodity so increasing price through taxation undoubtedly reduces overall consumption, which in turn correlates with the prevalence of alcohol-related damage. The price of alcohol in real terms has fallen steadily over the past twenty years in most countries. On the other hand, many people find it hard to accept that what is for the majority a harmless pleasure should be manipulated excessively in this way, and it does produce sharp contrasts between prices in neighbouring countries which encourages smuggling and a black economy. Financial deterrence may be less influential for the heaviest dependent drinkers who are most at risk.

Limitations imposed upon advertising and promotion are undoubtedly effective. Life skills training in schools, educating the public about safe levels of drinking, encouraging employers and educators to instigate clear workplace policies on alcohol, restricting the number of licensed premises and points of sale, banning sale of alcohol to minors, and targeting drunk drivers are effective strategies adopted in most countries. Random, high-profile, roadside breath tests greatly enhance the impact of the latter. There is a strong argument for instituting lower or even zero blood alcohol limits for younger drivers. Compulsory rehabilitation programmes for drunk drivers have a modest effect in preventing reoffending.

Labelling drink containers with the alcohol content empowers the drinker to behave sensibly, and the production and promotion of low-alcohol beverages is to be encouraged. Putting pressure on retailers or bartenders not to supply more alcohol to people who are already drunk by holding them liable for damage caused by their customers is becoming more common in some countries. Warning labels drawing attention to the risks of drunk driving or drinking in pregnancy have been shown to stick in the mind, but whether they actually cause people to behave more prudently has yet to be demonstrated.

Current policy approaches to illegal drugs

The response of most countries to illegal drugs has centred on three aims: to reduce the supply of drugs, to stifle demand for them, and to provide treatment for those who develop drug-related problems. Since the US is so influential in shaping strategy elsewhere in the world, its policy will be described as a representative model.

The US regards the global industry in illegal drugs as a major threat to its national security. According to the National Drug Control Strategy 2008 Report this challenge is being met by a determination to '. . . *reduce the flow of illicit drugs into the United States; disrupt and dismantle major drug trafficking organizations; strengthen the democratic and law enforcement institutions of partner nations threatened by illegal drugs; and reduce the underlying financial and other support that drug trafficking provides to international terrorist organizations*'. A large-scale training programme is aimed at improving the detection by local law enforcement officials of bulk drug supplies as they are transported around the country. Clamping down on drug-related crime, street level dealing, and anti-social behaviour at the local level is a high priority. Targeting domestic marijuana production resulted in the destruction of nearly seven million plants in 2007. Tracking sale and transport of chemical precursors is an important strategy in combating stimulant and other synthetic drugs, and in conjunction with the UN this has been extended into countries with significant production or transit capacity. In cooperation with Mexico there is an unprecedented effort to stem the flow of marijuana, heroin, cocaine, and methamphetamine across the border between the two countries, the prinicipal access route to the US. An estimated $20 billion in cash annually flows the other way across this border, and along with other drug-trafficking assets is an important target for seizure. In Afghanistan the counternarcotics and counter-insurgency tactics are familiar to anyone that reads a newspaper, whilst the US has been collaborating with the Government of Colombia since 2000 on aerial eradication of coca, targeting jungle laboratories, and establishing better control of the extensive coastline. Prescription drug abuse has become a major concern, and alongside an educational campaign several online pharmacies have been successfully prosecuted.

Reducing demand begins with education programmes for children and parents, with a strong message that young people should not use drugs. Local drug challenges are tackled through the federally funded Drug Free Communities Support Program, and national media campaigns have been launched by organizations such as the Partnership for a Drug-free America. More controversially, and currently unacceptable in some countries, a policy of random drug testing in schools, the armed forces, and many workplaces has been instituted.

The US has many federally funded services and programmes targeting the needs of problem drug users, and the National Institute on Drug Abuse funds tens of millions of dollars worth of research every year. Addiction is regarded as a treatable disease afflicting up to one in ten adults, and since the vast majority of these do not see themselves as having a problem widespread screening and brief treatment programmes have been initiated in family medical practices, colleges, and universities. More physicians and other health workers are being trained to detect and manage problem drug users. Drug problems are particularly prevalent amongst prisoners, so providing treatment facilities during and after incarceration has received greater prioritisation. For non-violent offenders drug treatment courts have been shown to lower reconviction rates and improve treatment outcomes.

The US has been slow to incorporate a harm-reduction approach (see Chapter 14) which remains an extremely controversial topic amongst the nation's drug experts. This philosophy has been well established in Britain and many other countries since the mid-1980s when it was fuelled by the well-founded fear of an HIV epidemic among injecting drug users. UK government-funded research has shown that every £1 spent on harm reduction measures such as walk-in clinics, needle exchange schemes, and methadone/buprenorphine maintenance programmes results in more than £9 saved in health and crime costs.

The war on drugs

Drug prohibition requires the suppression of unauthorized cultivation, manufacture, transport across national frontiers, marketing, and personal use of controlled substances. This is the 'war on drugs', a concept spearheaded by the US in the early 1970s and subsequently adopted with varying degrees of enthusiasm in most countries round the world. It is an expensive undertaking, with a global cost around $100 billion annually. The UK is committed to this approach, and suppression of drug supply and criminal justice implementation now costs the British taxpayer almost £5 billion annually.

Is this money well spent? If the yardstick is price, availability and purity of street drugs, the answer would have to be 'no'. Despite heroic expenditure on enforcement over three decades, the real price of street drugs has fallen steadily while access, especially for young people, remains easy. Average purity of heroin and cocaine has remained constant or increased. Drug seizures go up steeply every year, but clearly represent the tip of an iceberg. In a 2008 report, the independent UK Drug Policy Commission found that '*Drug trafficking is considered to be the most profitable sector of transnational criminality and to pose the single greatest organised crime threat to the UK*'. The UK still has the highest prevalence of problem drug use in Europe. The report reviewed evidence that vast profits have motivated resilience and adaptability in the dealing and distribution networks despite the extensive resources deployed against them. Large seizures or the breaking up of a particular criminal grouping produces only a temporary disruption, quickly replaced by other sources of supply or fresh criminal 'faces'. Asset recovery and prevention of money laundering has achieved only marginal success, despite being a major priority. Successes may have unintended consequences. In Australia, a reduction in the availability of cannabis on one occasion was mirrored by an increased availability of amphetamine. Temporary shortages of heroin on American streets have stimulated the development of 'designer' drugs, often of horrifying toxicity. Nature, and the drugs black market, abhor a vaccum. Noting a dearth of evidence-based interventions, the report draws attention to '. . . *the need to establish the long-term effectiveness, cost-effectiveness and value for money offered by key components of previous and current drug strategies—and in particular of drug law enforcement*'.

Far from being discouraged by such evidence as has convinced many observers that the war on drugs can never be won, its proponents remain firmly committed to the cause and tend to regard critics as defeatists. Baruch Spinoza (1632–77) held that excessive legal controls are more likely to arouse vices than reform them. Does an emphasis on external regulation undermine processes of self-regulation that contain the pursuit of other pleasurable activities within reasonable limits?

A whole industry has grown up around the treatment and control of drug use and any number of experts with varying levels of vested interest are on hand to contribute a range of conflicting opinions. There is a reluctance amongst politicians to enter into serious debate about the merits of current policies because there are few votes in it and a risk of being labelled in the media as defeatist, naive, or unsound.

Two invited appraisals of present and future US drug policy

1. Robert L DuPont, M.D.—President, Institute for Behavior and Health, Inc.

"Although the 'war' over the future of drug policy, like drug use itself, has ancient roots, it is strikingly new. The world's old drug problems generally involved single drugs consumed by relatively ineffective routes of administration and they usually involved small segments of the population. Prior to the 20th century, drug policy generally permitted open markets for drugs of abuse.

The world's modern drug epidemic, started in the 1960s in the United States, has now spread throughout the world. Today's drug scene involves a myriad of different drugs taken by highly potent routes of administration—especially smoking and intravenous injection. It includes entire national populations with the initial focus on risk-taking youth. The modern illegal drug epidemic is as new as the computer. The new drug policy, reflecting this new reality of drug use, is a restrictive policy limiting the use of the illegal drugs.

In the late 1960s the unprecedented rise in the use of illegal drugs showed that the early efforts at a restrictive drug policy, which had been successful for six decades, was no longer adequate. By the early 1970s a new national drug abuse prevention strategy, again backed by strong bipartisan support, balanced earlier law enforcement efforts with a massive investment in drug abuse treatment and greatly expanded anti-drug law enforcement. This new policy has had significant, but incomplete success. A decade of rapidly escalating rates of illegal drug use peaked in 1979 with 14.1% of persons aged 12 or older having used an illicit drug in the past month. This number was cut in half by 1992, with 6.7% reporting current drug use. By 2007 the number increased slightly to 8%.[1] In 1979 25 million Americans were current users of illegal drugs. Since that time the US population has grown by 37% but the number of illegal drug users has fallen to 20 million.

---

[1] Substance Abuse and Mental Health Services Administration, Office of Applied Studies (2008). *Results from the 2007 National Survey on Drug Use and Health: National Findings* (NSDUH Series H-34, DHHS Publication No. SMA 08-4343). Rockville, MD.

From 1977 to the early 1990s a powerful grass-roots community movement, known as the Parents Movement, inspired American drug policy. Focusing on the negative health effects of marijuana, the most widely used illegal drug and usually the gateway drug for all other illegal drug use, the Parents Movement shifted the focus of drug policy from an initial timid policy of containment to an active commitment to drug-free goals. This bottom-up movement, started by parents in Atlanta, Georgia, was strongly supported in the final years of the Carter administration. It was picked up and greatly expanded in 1981 by Nancy Reagan as 'Just Say No'.

The results of this effort were spectacular. Drug use trends that appeared to be moving strongly in only one direction—up—suddenly turned even more steeply down as the number of current users of illegal drugs fell to 14 million in 1992. The pro-drug movement which had been prominent in the early 1970s was far less visible during those 14 years. However, since 1992 the movement to tolerate illegal drug use, having seized the flag of 'harm reduction', fuelled a modest up-tick in the number of illegal drug users although in the past decade there has been a return to a downward trend, especially for youth.

It is useful to consider the nation's experience with the two most widely used drugs – which are legal for adults but not children—nicotine and alcohol. In contrast to today's 20 million users of all of the hundreds of illegal drugs combined, most of which are more reinforcing than either alcohol or tobacco, there are 71 million tobacco smokers (28.6%) and 127 million alcohol drinkers (51.1%) in the United States. Reflecting these much higher levels of use, each of these two common drugs produce social costs for the nation that dwarf the costs of all the illegal drugs combined, including all of the criminal justice system costs of enforcing the current restrictive policy on illegal drug use and sale.

These facts are important when contemplating future drug prevention policies, especially more permissive policies toward the currently illegal drugs, precisely because the strident critiques of the century-long and still-evolving restrictive drug policies often claim that the war on drugs has failed. It is bizarre that the anti-drug efforts of the past four decades have been declared to have failed when the rates of illegal drug use have fallen significantly since 1979 and when the societal costs of both nicotine and alcohol vastly exceed all of the costs of illegal drug use. Would it be considered wise to stop the war on cancer or the war on poverty because those dreadful problems have not been entirely eliminated in a few decades?

There are two recurrent arguments against current drug prevention policies. First, there is a striking mismatch between the amount of effort devoted to criticism of current policies and the amount of effort devoted to the proposed changes to those polices. The objections to current policy begin by mocking the goal of 'prohibition' which is invariably compared to alcohol prohibition. The claim is often explicit, but always implicit, that it is the illegal status of drugs that creates the 'drug problem'.

Second, the common criticism of current American drug policy starts with a full-scale assault on 'prohibition' only to end with a list of tepid proposals which not only do not match the scale of the critique but which are all but irrelevant to the total costs of drug use or drug law enforcement. This mismatch is not accidental. It reflects the inherent problems with most criticisms of current drug policies.

Let's look at the first problem: the focus on the failures of current policy which dominate these arguments. They are based on easily recognized false assumptions. For starters, the claim is made that the drug problem exists because the drugs are illegal. Here is a fact that refutes this argument, an argument that is so often repeated it has become a cliché: the fastest growing segment of the drug problem in the United States today is the nonmedical use of prescription drugs, especially opioid pain medicines. In 2002 the number of new users of prescription pain killers passed the number of new marijuana users for the first time. This pattern has continued every year since.[2] These prescription drugs produce terrible social costs even though the mafia is nowhere to be seen. If a legal supply of drugs would reduce our social burden from the currently illegal drug, why are prescription pain killers so widely used nonmedically and why are they causing so many deaths?

The second problem with the current avalanche of criticism of American drug policy is the emptiness of the proposals the critics make for new drug policies. The top agenda item of the critics of today's drug policies is to legalize 'medical marijuana' for just about anyone to use for just about anything. In the same vein these critics want to legalize heroin to treat pain and to use LSD and other hallucinogens in the treatment of many illnesses from depression to drug addiction. They want to give needles to intravenous drug users to reduce the spread of HIV-AIDS. They want farmers to grow hemp. They want to make sure that the criminal justice system does not enforce the drug-free status of people arrested for crimes including, but not limited to, drug sales. That's their agenda.

Why is there such a dramatic mismatch between the criticisms leveled against current drug policies in the US on the one hand, and the proposed remedies on the other hand? The problem exists because the only answer that fits their

---

[2] Substance Abuse and Mental Health Services Administration, Office of Applied Studies (2008). *Results from the 2007 National Survey on Drug Use and Health: National Findings* (NSDUH Series H-34, DHHS Publication No. SMA 08-4343). Rockville, MD.

criticism is to legalize not just marijuana but all of the currently illegal drugs. Such a policy would require providing all drugs to all would-be users, regardless of age or any other factors. Anything less than access on the level of soft drinks today would not eliminate the illegal market for these drugs. The existence of a robust illegal drug market is the fundamental source of the criticism of current policies—which are labeled 'prohibition' to disparage them.

The call for a 'regulated' market in the currently illegal drugs is an illusion. How effectively do the current regulated markets for tobacco and alcohol limit the use of these drugs within the society? If regulation of additional drugs from marijuana to heroin and from cocaine to methamphetamine were to involve much tighter restrictions than now apply to tobacco and alcohol, the illegal drug market would eagerly meet the frustrated demand. Since flat-out legalization is a non-starter practically, the critics trim their proposals to the puny ideas they now promote.

As for the libertarian ideal of making all of the currently illegal drugs available in a free market for everyone on the assumption that drug use is a purely personal decision, the facts speak for themselves: drug use affects everyone around the user. Worse yet, when drug users get into trouble, as they commonly do, there is an irresistible public responsibility to help them including, but not limited to, drug abuse treatment.

One aspect of the criticism of current drug policies I enthusiastically endorse: Today the cost of illegal drug use in the US is far too high. New policies are needed to reduce illegal drug use and the societal burdens imposed by this use. More effective demand reduction is the key to improving national drug policies in the future. Think about a policy that relies only on law enforcement efforts that are aimed at reducing the supply of illegal drugs. If this policy were fully successful, without a similarly successful reduction in the demand for drugs, the price of illegal drugs would escalate creating additional incentive for the sophisticated and resourceful globalized drug suppliers. In other words, without demand reduction, supply reduction is a doomed strategy since it has within it the seeds of its own failure. Every one of the common proposals to 'reform' the current drug prevention policies, most of which are now labeled 'harm reduction', will increase the demand for, and use of, the currently illegal drugs.

Only reducing the demand for drugs will improve the effectiveness of America's current drug policy. Here are five new ideas—all furthering restrictive drug policies and all aiming for drug-free goals—that will reduce the demand for illegal drugs:

1. Reduce drugged driving which is now causing deaths and injuries on the nation's roads on the scale of the better known problem of drunk driving.

This is the best new idea to reduce the prevalence of illegal drug use in the country and to improve highway safety.

2. Promote non-punitive random student drug testing in the nation's schools to discourage drug use among teenagers, the age when almost all drug use begins. These programmes give young people another good reason not to use drugs. In addition, if students do use drugs these programmes provide an opportunity for families, schools, and communities to help the students get and stay drug free. This is the best new idea to reduce the onset of drug use.

3. Reduce prescription drug abuse by promoting abuse resistant formulations and by educating patients and physicians about the unique risks associated with prescribed controlled substances, and about their responsibilities when using these often useful but widely abused medicines

4. Improve treatment of drug abuse by encouraging long-term care with rigorous monitoring for continued drug use that is linked to meaningful consequences for the return to drug use. This will help stop the revolving door of today's treatment which wastes a large part of the money spent on treatment.

5. Improve the performance of the criminal justice system by promoting enforced abstinence among the five million convicted criminals now on supervised release in communities throughout the nation.

A national drug policy that accepts illegal drug use encourages the growth of illegal drug use, and the costs resulting from that use. Tossing out the bipartisan, balanced drug prevention policies of today in favour of surrendering to illegal drug use would be a tragedy."

2. Ethan Nadelmann, Ph.D.—Founder and Executive Director, Drug Policy Alliance

Is US drug policy a model for success?

"Looking to the United States as a role model for how to deal with drugs is like looking to apartheid South Africa for how to deal with race, or to Russia and China for lessons in human rights. The United States ranks first in the world in per capita incarceration, with less than 5% of the world's population but almost 25% of the world's incarcerated population. The number of people locked up for drug law violations has increased from roughly 50,000 in 1980 to almost 500,000 today; that's more than all of western Europe locks up for all offences. Hundreds of thousands more are incarcerated for other 'drug-related violations' including parole and probation violations involving 'dirty urines', petty crimes to support drug habits, and violent conflicts associated with the illegality of the drug trade. Millions of US citizens now have a felony record for a drug law violation, thereby rendering them second class citizens given the breadth of sanctions applied to former felons, often for life. The total cost to taxpayers of relying so heavily on the criminal justice system to deal with particular drugs approaches $50 billion in direct costs as well as possibly greater amounts in indirect costs.

Rates of illicit drug use in the US are roughly equivalent to rates in other advanced industrialized nations. What matters far more than rates of drug use, however, are the harms associated with drug misuse. While most other advanced industrialized nations implemented syringe exchange programmes and other harm reduction initiatives to reduce HIV/AIDS in the 1980s and 1990s, the United States largely rejected such policies, effectively opting to allow tens of thousands of people to die of the deadly disease. Political resistance to such programmes remains strong even today, notwithstanding the overwhelming scientific consensus regarding their effectiveness. Meanwhile, drug overdose fatalities have increased dramatically since the 1980s; by 2005 accidental overdose was second only to motor-vehicle crashes as a cause of death from unintentional injury in the United States. Once again, ideological and political resistance hobbles efforts to respond effectively.

Is supply reduction the best solution?

About 40% of Americans believe that supply reduction—i.e., stopping drugs at the border and reducing drug production abroad—is the best way to contain the illegal drug problem in the United States. That's unfortunate. The carrot and stick of crop substitution and eradication have been tried and failed—with rare exceptions—for half a century. They can work in targeted locales but inevitably result in simply shifting production from one place to another: opium production moves from Thailand to Burma, or from Afghanistan to Pakistan; coca production moves from Bolivia and Peru to Colombia; and cannabis production moves from Colombia and Mexico to the United States and Canada. The State Department estimates that total coca production in Latin America in 2005 was basically the same as in 1992—about 200,000 hectares—with only modest variation in the interim years. Opium flourishes today in Afghanistan, as it once did in Burma, Thailand, and Pakistan, and will somewhere else in years to come. And no one even pretends anymore that cannabis can be controlled.

The best thing to be said for an emphasis on supply reduction is that it provides a rationale for wealthier nations to spend a little money on economic development in poorer countries. But mostly the carrot and stick wreak havoc among impoverished farmers without impacting overall global supply. The stick, often in the form of aerial spraying, wipes out illicit and licit crops alike, and can be hazardous to both human health and local environments. Some members of Congress, led by Congressman Mark Souder (Repub., Indiana) now advocate employing mycoherbicides, i.e., biological warfare. The carrot, on the other hand, is typically both late and inadequate. And perverse consequences often follow, such as the spread of HIV/AIDS and other drug abuse problems when shortages of opium push local consumers to switch to heroin.

Faith in supply reduction strategies persists mostly by ignoring the fact that the global markets in cannabis, coca, and opium products are essentially the same as other global commodities markets. If one source is compromised due to bad weather, rising costs of production or political difficulties, another emerges. And if by chance overall global supply is temporarily interrupted, consumers typically switch to alternative drugs, which may be more or less problematic.

What about reducing demand?

Demand reduction would seem to be the most sensible strategy; after all, if there were no demand for drugs, there would be no supply and hence no illicit markets, traffickers and so on. It's generally good when fewer people use drugs, especially those that are easily misused.

Too rigid a focus on reducing the number of drug users rather than the harmful consequences of drug misuse, however, can prove disastrous. In the United States, drug war proponents often point to the 50% drop in the number of illegal drug users during the 1980s as a success story. But that drop consisted mostly of fewer teens smoking marijuana and fewer yuppies snorting cocaine—even as cocaine became endemic in American cities, HIV/AIDS spread rapidly among drug users and their lovers and children, incarceration of drug law offenders quintupled, and government drug war expenditures increased from a few billion a year to tens of billions. If that counts as success, one wonders at the definition of failure!

Demand reduction efforts that rely on honest education and positive alternatives to drug use are good and important, but not when they devolve into 'zero tolerance' rhetoric and policies. The DARE programme in the United States, which sends police officers into classrooms to teach drug prevention, has been amply evaluated and consistently found to have no impact on adolescent drug misuse. The same is true of the National Youth Anti-Drug Media Campaign, for which the US Congress appropriated nearly $1 billion between 1998 and 2004, and of random drug testing of teenage students in schools, which the Bush administration aggressively promoted from 2001 to 2008. 'Zero tolerance' policies inevitably deter some people from using drugs, but also dramatically increase the harms to those who do.

How about harm reduction?

'The answer', to the extent one exists, is to focus on reducing problematic drug use as well as the harms of drug use among those who cannot or will not stop using drugs. There's virtually never been a drug free society in the history of human civilization, after all, and more psychoactive drugs are discovered and devised every year, both legally and illegally. The desire to alter one's state of consciousness, and to use psychoactive drugs to do so, is near universal—and mostly not a problem. What needs to be reduced is not so much drug use per se as the death, disease, crime and suffering associated with both drug misuse and failed prohibitionist policies. Harm reduction with respect to legal drugs means promoting responsible drinking and designated driver norms, and getting people who can't quit smoking to smoke less, and switch to nicotine patches, chewing gums, and smokeless tobacco. With respect to illegal drugs, it means reducing HIV/AIDS, hepatitis C, and other infectious diseases through needle exchange programs; reducing overdose fatalities by making the antidote, naloxone, readily available, opening safer injection sites, and changing the ways that police and others deal with OD's before they turn fatal; and allowing drug addicts to obtain their drugs legally in medically supervised facilities like the heroin prescription programmes and research trials found in Switzerland, Germany, Britain, the Netherlands, and Canada. And of course it means ensuring that a diversity of treatment and rehabilitation services and options are readily available to those in need. Many thousands of scholarly studies demonstrate that such strategies decrease drug-related harms without increasing drug use and are far more cost-effective than criminal justice strategies in reducing illicit drug use, crime, recidivism, and incarceration.

What about decriminalizing or legalizing some or all drugs?

Global drug prohibition is clearly a costly disaster. In 1998, the UN estimated the value of the global market in illicit drugs at $400 billion, or 7% of global trade. The extraordinary profits available to those willing to assume the risks enrich organized and unorganized criminals, corrupt politicians and governments, and terrorists and others involved in political violence. Many cities, states and even countries in Latin America, the Caribbean, and Asia are reminiscent of Chicago under Al Capone—times 50. Legalization would radically change all this for the better.

Legalization would also make some drugs less dangerous and make it easier to address addiction as a health issue. Joseph Westermeyer's classic article, 'The Pro-Heroin Effects of Anti-Opium Laws in Asia', documented how opium bans in Asia stimulated heroin production and use. Similarly, during alcohol Prohibition, beer was mostly displaced by hard liquor; no surprise given the ways in which Prohibition prioritizes the need to escape detection and dramatically increases transportation costs. And, more recently, modestly successful crackdowns on marijuana appear to have stimulated new production and trafficking of cocaine and methamphetamine. Legalization would probably have the opposite effect, favouring less potent and problematic drugs and means of ingestion. New HIV infections, Hepatitis C cases, and fatal overdoses would surely drop.

Some say legalization is immoral. That's nonsense, unless one believes there is some principled basis for discriminating against and among people based solely on what they put into their bodies, absent harm to others. Others say legalization would open the floodgates to huge increases in drug abuse. But they forget that we already live in a world in which psychoactive drugs of all sorts are readily available—and in which people too poor to buy drugs resort to sniffing gasoline, glue, and other industrial products, which can be more harmful than any drug.

The greatest downside to legalization may well be the fact that the legal markets would fall into the hands of the alcohol, tobacco, and pharmaceutical companies. That's preferable to the current situation, but obviously problematic given their track record to date. One can also envision regulatory systems far stricter than contemporary controls on alcohol and cigarettes that still allow adults legal access to their drugs of choice. The case for legalization is strongest with respect to marijuana given its relative safety compared to most other drugs, legal and illegal. In the United States, 40% of Americans believe that marijuana should be taxed, controlled, and regulated more or less like alcohol. It's possible that the medical cannabis dispensaries operating throughout California, and beginning to pop up elsewhere, may evolve into outlets for non-medical consumers, not unlike the coffeeshops in The Netherlands.

What should be the priorities for US drug policy over the next decade?

The election of Barack Obama and the Democratic gains in the Congress and state governments bode well for drug policy reform. The priorities are clear: first and foremost, reducing the number of people unjustly and unnecessarily incarcerated for non-violent drug law violations; and second, incorporating harm reduction principles and objectives fully into US drug policies. That means dramatically expanding access to treatment and rehabilitation for people struggling with addiction, eliminating unreasonable discriminations against people with drug convictions and substance abuse problems, ensuring that the most effective, and cost-effective, steps are taken to reduce overdose fatalities as well as new HIV and Hepatitis C infections, and pushing aside ideological barriers to scientific inquiry and policy debate. The fiscal crisis offers a silver lining insofar as the United States can no longer afford the luxury of its prejudices in dealing with illegal drugs."

UK drug policy: is a more radical approach needed?

The consumption of psychoactive drugs by a substantial proportion of the population is here to stay. The past is the best guide to the future, and there has never been a tribe, race, or society which has not resorted to mind-altering drugs. All drugs carry risks, but most people who are adequately informed will avoid riskier options and modulate their intake of selected substances. That is why individuals with drug-related problems make up a small proportion of the overall population. This is not to minimize the enormous suffering and harm to society of drug abuse and addiction, but it does highlight the need for nationwide, well designed, accurate, and continuing drug education pro-grammes to support the natural inclination to self preservation.

Drug education for young people must be evidence-based, accurate, and credible, otherwise it can actually be counter-productive. Moralizing, propa-gandizing, or shock tactics such as the 'reefer madness' campaign of the 1950s, the 'heroin screws you up' adverts of the 1980s, and the Leah Betts Ecstasy warning posters all had the opposite effect to that desired on the target audience. If an exaggerated or distorted account of the risks of drugs familiar to the audience is given, overall credibility will be lost. The current legal clas-sification of some drugs also causes credibility problems since, according to an evidence-based appraisal of overall harm (Nutt et al. 2007), alcohol and tobacco outrank cannabis and ten other illegal drugs, including the Class A LSD and Ecstasy.

Tackling social conditions which foster self-destructive indulgence in alcohol and drugs receives insufficient attention. Improving the prospects for economically deprived families to achieve a better lifestyle beyond the benefits culture, rehabilitating decayed inner-city environments, and providing con-structive and enjoyable sports and leisure activities for urban youth are essen-tial if we are serious about reducing problem drug use. Chronic boredom, discomfort, or despair are powerful drivers for oblivion seekers.

The UK government's 2008 10-year drug strategy document reviews some undoubted successes and unveils constructive innovations aimed at education, demand reduction and treatment. There is a welcome focus on meeting the needs of families and communities, widening the prevention target beyond illegal drugs to incorporate tobacco and alcohol, and creating new incentives to move away from dependence into treatment, training and employment. The UK has always been in the forefront for evaluating new and radical ideas, such as the substitute prescribing of heroin to enhance harm reduction among opioid addicts.

Greater efforts should be made to reduce the unprecedented profitability of the drugs market for organized crime. One way to achieve this is to move further along the path of controlled availability of opioids and stimulants from doctors or other government administered sources with the involvement and support of other interested parties locally, particularly the police. A drug habit would become much cheaper even if the addict had to bear the cost of the drugs to the NHS, so that a deviant career would no longer be inevitable. Reintegration of the drug user into normal society would restore peer pressure as a potent restraint on behaviour. It is certainly possible that such 'normalization' initiatives might result in increased numbers of people using harder drugs, some of whom are bound to become dependent. Although an addiction to pharmaceutical drugs is much less dangerous to health and welfare than a street drug habit, it is still highly undesirable and poses risks to the individual and his or her social circle. For this reason, such initiatives could be organized as controlled trials in order that the effects can be monitored carefully by independent observers. This strategy has been criticized as colluding with dependence and encouraging a welfare mentality, and there is certainly weight in this argument. However, there are may historical examples of individuals who have led full and productive lives whilst maintained on pharmaceutical opioids, and recipients could be required to pay for their supply like any other commodity. Whether some increase in individual risk is a price worth paying for the benefits to society of undermining organized crime is a matter for public debate. Government-sponsored research of this sort would provide a more rational basis for answering this question than presently exists.

Every effort should be made to divert convicted drug misusers away from prison and into residential rehabilitation units. Many drug users continue to use drugs in prison and simply learn to be more deviant, while non-drug-using inmates are exposed to the temptation of taking up the habit to ease boredom or distress.

In her Foreword to the policy document, the Home Secretary writes: '*Through our new drug strategy, and the action that will flow from it, we will continue to send a clear message that drug use is unacceptable*'. Presumably she is not including alcohol (and tobacco?) within her definition of 'drug' in this edict, yet the expert review referred to above suggests that both are more harmful overall than several other drugs whose current use the law deems 'unacceptable'. In the case of alcohol, concern is focused on misuse rather than use: is it now the time to adopt a similar approach for drugs which are currently illegal?

Arguments for changes in the law do not in the least reflect a lack of concern about the undoubted risks that drugs pose. On the contrary, the unremitting economic and social burden of drug misuse and addiction in the face of all our best efforts to date demands a more radical response than simply doing more of the same. This is a timely consideration, since the UN is scheduled to conduct a strategic drug policy review in 2009.

The Misuse of Drugs Act (1971) requires revision to reflect a more evidence-based representation of relative potential for harm. A good example of the disparity between legal position and tabloid representation on the one hand and the scientific facts on the other is the case of Ecstasy. This came 18th out of 20 in terms of overall harm in the evidence-based ranking yet resides in Class A alongside heroin and cocaine. The dangers associated with the occasional use of pharmaceutically pure MDMA, though genuine and potentially tragic for a tiny proportion of users, must be kept in perspective. This risk is significantly increased when the drug is manufactured and supplied by a criminal, with all the possibilities of contamination and adulteration that this entails. Nevertheless, on the day that Leah Betts took her fatal Ecstasy tablet dozens of young people will have been crippled or killed as a result of alcohol-related trauma.

Injecting heroin or smoking crack is infinitely more dangerous and damaging than smoking cannabis, yet a disproportionate amount of police and customs time is focused on suppressing the latter. In 2006/7, there were 186,028 seizures of illegal drugs in England and Wales of which 140,406 consisted of cannabis in various forms. This amounted to 45.4 tons of herbal material or resin and 344,360 plants. More than 100,000 people received formal cautions or warnings for cannabis possession in that year. The discretionary nature of modern policing of cannabis possession risks uneven and arbitrary implementation of the law. The Government's decision to reclassify cannabis from Class C to B against the advice of its own experts flies in the face of logic, especially since cannabis use actually declined in the period following its down-regulation to Class C in 2004.

Decriminalizing cannabis would free up vast resources in money and police time which could be redeployed more appropriately, but what other reasons are there for taking this step? Despite global prohibition cannabis use is endemic in almost every country, and the illegal black market contributes massively to the profits of organized crime. Increased potency of some street cannabis is in part a by-product of its illegality: speed of production is a priority to minimize risk of detection and maximise profit, and the growing methods deployed to achieve this stimulate the plant to produce more of the main psychoactive component (THC). Millions of otherwise law abiding young people are criminalised every year, with potentially disastrous implications for their future employment and productivity. A government-controlled legal source of cannabis would ensure purity, inclusion of secondary and potentially protective components such as cannabidiol (see Chapter 5), and defined potency. This legal supply would produce healthy taxation revenue which would offset the costs of production. Like all drugs cannabis poses risks to the consumer, but an evidence-based analysis shows this to be less than alcohol or tobacco. Would legal availability in the absence of active promotion significantly increase the number of users? Such research as exists suggests not.

Changes in the international law pertaining to cannabis control are highly unlikely for the foreseeable future, so what modifications are feasible for individual nations such as the UK? In October 2008 the Beckley Foundation, an independent charitable trust, published the Global Cannabis Commission Report. This is an analysis of cannabis policy conducted by an international group of academics and public health experts. Following a review of available scientific data, the Commission found that enforcement efforts had done little to deter use and the probability of arrest for any single consumption is less than one in a thousand. However, the tiny minority who are convicted may be disproportionately damaged by loss of employment prospects or impairment of family and social integration. Current international treaties have impeded initiatives for reform, but the measures undertaken by the Dutch and others have mitigated to some extent some unwanted effects of prohibition. The Commission points out that prohibition rules out regulation, so there are '... *advantages for governments in moving toward a regime of regulated legal availability under strict controls, using the variety of mechanisms available to regulate a legal market, such as taxation, availability controls, minimum legal age for use and purchase, labeling and potency limits'*. However, and as pointed out by Robert DuPont above, a major risk of legalization would be commercial promotion leading to greatly increased levels of use and a repetition of the problems caused by alcohol and tobacco. Very tight market controls with particular attention to licencing and availability would be essential.

The Commission goes on to make several recommendations both within and beyond current international controls. Cannabis possession should not result in a criminal conviction (let alone imprisonment), and the police should give low priority to enforcement against cannabis use. Alternatives to fines such as referral to education or counselling should be considered. Driving a car after use should be treated in a similar way to alcohol. In the absence of changes to international policy, a country '... *can act on its own by denouncing the conventions and re-acceding with reservations, or by simply ignoring at least some provisions of the conventions. Any regime which makes cannabis legally available should involve state licensing or state operation of entities producing, wholesaleing and retailing the drug (as is true in many jurisdictions for alcoholic beverages). The state should, either directly or through regulation, control potency and quality, assure reasonably high prices and control access and availability in general and particularly to youth'.* Advertising and promotion should be banned, and the epidemiological effects closely monitored with revision an option if increased harm was evident. Such a step is by no means a novel suggestion. Many years ago Release, the respected London-based drugs and legal advice agency, called for the introduction of licensed premises such as cafes or clubs which could sell cannabis to members with strict monitoring of quality control and the normal regulations concerning trading standards and consumer protection.

There is scant political will for changes in UK drug policy at present, probably because it does not seem much of a vote winner, but such changes are clearly feasible even under the existing international controls. However, very careful consideration of the possible disadvantages pointed out above by Robert DuPont is essential. Avoiding commercialization should be possible in that very tight regulations could be initiated from the start, rather than post-hoc tinkering as with alcohol and tobacco. Peer pressure and self-regulation should not be underestimated as behavioural determinants: increasing social unacceptability of tobacco smoking in middle-class circles has greatly inhibited consumption in that segment of the population. Although an illegal market would still remain for underage users, there would be vastly increased resources to focus on this.

The momentum for change can only come from better informed and wider public discussion of the issues. As we contemplate the prospects of a lengthy recession and credit crunch, alongside eye-watering national debt and public sector liabilities throughout 2009 and beyond, UK taxpayers face a daunting future. In this context the war on drugs should not be exempt from a rigorous re-evaluation of its cost-effectiveness based on evidence rather than rhetoric, with consideration given to radical innovations beyond the current regime.

Selected references

Advisory Council on the Misuse of Drugs (2008). *Cannabis: classification and public health.* Home Office, London http://drugs.homeoffice.gov.uk/publication-search/acmd/acmd-cannabis-report-2008?view=Binary.

Advisory Council on Misuse of Drugs (1988). *AIDS and drug misuse.* DHSS, HMSO, London.

Alexander, B. K. (1990). Alternatives to the war on drugs. *Journal of Drug Issues,* **20**, 1–27.

Berridge, V. (1984). Drugs and social policy: the establishment of drug control in Britain 1900–1930. *British Journal of Addiction,* **79**, 17–29.

Berridge, V., Rawson, N. S. B. (1979). Opiate use and legislative control: a nineteenth-century case study. *Social Science and Medicine*, **13**, 351–63.

Clark, A. (1993). Adding up the pros and cons of legalization. *International Journal of Drug Policy*, **4**, 116–21.

Degenhardt L., Hall W. D., Roxburgh A. et al. (2007). UK classification of cannabis: is a change needed and why? (letter to the editor) *Lancet*, **370**, 1541

Degenhardt L., Chiu W.-T., Sampson N. et al. (2008). Towards a global view of alcohol, tobacco, cannabis, and cocaine use: findings from the WHO world mental health surveys. *PLoS Medicine*, **5**, e141, 0001–0015.

Drug Policy Alliance Network (2009). *Drug policy around the world: Sweden.* http://www.drugpolicy.org/global/drugpolicyby/westerneurop/sweden/.

Editorial (1987). Management of drug addicts: hostility, humanity, and pragmatism. *Lancet*, **May 9**, i, 1068–9.

Engelsman, E. L. (1989). Dutch policy on the management of drug-related problems. *British Journal of Addiction*, **84**, 211–18.

Engelsman, E. L. (1991). Drug misuse and the Dutch. *British Medical Journal*, **302**, 484–5.

Cappato M., Davis C., Cohn-Bendit D. M. et al. (2002). *Proposal for a recommendation on the reform of the Conventions on drugs.* European Parliament; http://www.europarl.europa.eu/sides/getDoc.do?pubRef=-//EP//NONSGML±MOTION±B5-2002-0541±0±DOC±WORD±V0//EN&language=EN.

Farrell, M., Strang, J. (1990). The lure of masterstrokes: drug legalization. *British Journal of Addiction*, **85**, 5–7.

Gerada, C., Orgel, M., Strang, J. (1992). Health clinics for problem drug misusers. *Health Trends*, **24**, 68–9.

Glanz, A. (1986). Findings of a national survey of the role of general practitioners in the treatment of opiate misuse: views on treatment. *British Medical Journal*, **293**, 543–5.

H.M. Government (2008). *Drugs: protecting families and communities. Action Plan 2008–2011.* Home Office, London. ISBN 978-1-84726-616-3.

Lemmens, P. H. H. M., Garretson, H. F. L. (1998). Unstable pragmatism: Dutch policy under national and international pressure. *Addiction*, **93**, 157–62.

MacCoun, R., Reuter, P. (1997). Interpreting Dutch cannabis policy: reasoning by analogy in the legalization debate. *Science*, **278** 47–52.

MacCoun, R., Reuter, P. (2001). Evaluating alternative cannabis regimes. *British Journal of Psychiatry*, **178**, 123–8.

Marks, J. (1985). Opium, the religion of the people. *Lancet*, **2**, 1439–40.

McSweeney, T., Turnbull, P. J., Hough, M. (2008). *Tackling drug markets and distribution networks in the UK.* UK Drug Policy Commission. www.ukdpc.org.uk/reports.shtml.

National Drug Intelligence Center (2008). *National Drug Threat Assessment (2008).* US Department of Justice; Johnstown, PA.

Nutt D., King L. A., Saulsbury W., Blakemore C. (2007). Development of a rational scale to assess the harm of drugs of potential misuse. *Lancet*, **369**, 1047–53.

Office of National Drug Control Policy (2009). *US National Drug Control Strategy 2008 Annual Report* http://www.whitehousedrugpolicy.gov/publications/policy/ndcs08/2008ndcs.pdf.

Plant, M., Single, E., Stockwell, T. (1997). *Alcohol: minimising the harm*. Free Association Books, London.

Potter D. (2009). Cannabis cultivation: link between illegal light and potency. *Personal Communication*.

Reinarman C., Cohen P. D. A., Kaal H. L. (2004). The limited relevance of drug policy: cannabis in Amsterdam and San Francisco. *American Journal of Public Health*, **94**, 836–42.

Reuter P., Stevens A. (2007). *An analysis of UK drug policy*. UK Drug Policy Commission; ISBN 978-1-906246-01-3.

Robson, P. (1992). Illegal drugs: time to change the law? *Oxford Medical School Gazette*, **43**, 20–3.

Roemer, R. (1991). Public health and the law. In: *Oxford textbook of public health*, Vol. 1. (Ed. W. W. Holland, G. Knox, R. Detels) Oxford University Press, Oxford.

Room R., Fischer B., Hall W. et al. (2008). *Cannabis policy: moving beyond stalemate*. The Global Cannabis Commission Report: Beckley Foundation, Oxford.

Ruttenber, A. J. (1991). Stalking the elusive designer drugs: techniques for monitoring new problems in drug abuse. *Journal of Addictive Diseases*, **11**, 71–7.

Smee, C., Parsonage, M., Anderson, R., Duckworth, S. (1992). The effect of tobacco advertising on tobacco consumption. *Health Trends*, **24**, 111–16.

Stevenson, R. (1991). The case for legalizing drugs. *Economic Affairs*, **11**, 14–17.

Smart, C. (1984). Social policy and drug addiction: a critical study of policy development. *British Journal of Addiction*, **79**, 31–9.

Strang, J., Ghodse, H., Johns, A. (1987). Responding flexibly but not gullibly to drug addiction. *British Medical Journal*, **295**, 1364.

Turnbull P. J., Hough M. (2008). *Tackling drug markets and distribution networks in the UK*. UK Drug Policy Commission Report; ISBN 978-1-906246-07-5.

UK Drug Policy Commission (2008). *Submission to the ACMD cannabis classification review 2008*. http://www.ukdpc.org.uk/resources/ACMD_Cannabis_Submission_Jan_2008.pdf.

United Nations Office on Drugs and Crime (2007). *Sweden's successful drug policy: a review of the evidence*. United Nations, Geneva: http://www.unodc.org/pdf/research/Swedish_drug_control.pdf.

van de Wijngaart, G. J. (1989). What lessons from the Dutch experience can be applied? *British Journal of Addiction*, **84**, 990–2.

Willis, J. H. (1987). Reflection [editorial]. *British Journal of Addictions*, **82**, 1181–2.

Bibliography and Reports

Books

Abadinski, H. (1989). *Drug abuse: an introduction.* Nelson-Hall, Chicago.

Braun, S. (1996). *Buzz: the science and lore of alcohol and caffeine.* Oxford University Press, Oxford.

Burroughs, W. (1996). *Junkie.* The Olympia Press, London.

CIBA Foundation Symposium 166 (1992). *Cocaine: scientific and social dimensions.* John Wiley & Sons, Chichester.

Cocteau, J. (1957). *Opium: diary of a cure.* Owen, London.

Crowley, A. (1922). *Diary of a drug fiend.* Collins, London.

Davies, J. B. (1992). *The myth of addiction.* Harwood Academic Publications Gmbh, Switzerland.

Galizio, M., Maisto, S. A. (ed.) (1985). *Determinants of substance abuse: biological, psychological, and environmental factors.* Plenum Press, New York and London.

Gerstein, D. R., Green, I. W. (ed.) (1993). *Preventing drug abuse: what do we know?* National Academic Press, Washington, DC.

Ghodse, H. (1989). *Drugs and addictive behaviour—a guide to treatment.* Blackwell, Oxford.

Gossop, M. (1987). *Living with drugs* (2nd edn). Wildwood House Ltd, Aldershot.

Grahame-Smith, D.G, Aronson, J.K (2002). *Oxford textbook of clinical pharmacology and drug therapy* (3rd edn). Oxford University Press, Oxford.

Grinspoon, L. (1975). *The speed culture.* Harvard University Press, Cambridge, MA.

Grinspoon, L. (1977). *Marihuana reconsidered* (2nd edn). Harvard University Press, Cambridge, MA.

Grinspoon, L., Bakalar, J. B. (1979). *Psychedelic drugs reconsidered.* Basic Books, New York.

Guy G.W., Whittle B.A., Robson P.J. (2004). *The medicinal use of cannabis and cannabinoids.* Pharmaceutical Press, London.

Hoffer, A., Osmond, H. (1967). *The hallucinogens.* Academic Press, New York.

Huxley, A. (1959). *The doors of perception and heaven and hell.* Penguin Books, Harmondsworth.

Iversen L (2008). *Speed, Ecstasy, Ritalin: the science of amphetamines.* Oxford University Press, Oxford.

Kerouac, J. (1976). *On the road.* Penguin Books, Harmondsworth.

Laurence, D. R., Bennett, P. N. (1992). *Clinical pharmacology* (7th edn). Churchill Livingstone, Edinburgh.

Laurie, P. (1967). *Drugs: medical, psychological, and social facts.* Penguin Books, Harmondsworth.

Leary, T. (1968). *The politics of Ecstasy.* G. P. Putnam, New York.

Lowinson, J. H., Ruiz, P., Millman, R. B., Langrod, J. G. (ed.) (1992). *Substance abuse*. Williams & Wilkins, Baltimore.

Miller, W. (ed.) (1985). *The addictive behaviours*. Pergamon, New York.

Orford, J. (1985). *Excessive appetites: a psychological view of addictions*. John Wiley & Sons, Chichester.

Plant, M., Plant, M. (1992). *Risk takers*. Routledge, London.

Plant, M., Single, E., Stockwell, T. (1997). *Alcohol: minimising the harm*. Free Association Books, London.

Russell, R. (1973). *Bird lives!* Quartet Books, London.

Shapiro, H. (1988). *Waiting for the man: the story of drugs and popular music*. Quartet Books, London.

Stockley, D. (1992). *Drug warning: an illustrated guide for parents, teachers, and employers* (2nd edn). Optima Books, London.

Szasz, T. S. (1985). *Ceremonial chemistry: the ritual persecution of drugs, addicts, and pushers*. (rev. edn). Learning Publications, Holmes Beach, Fl.

Szasz, T. S. (1992). *Our right to drugs: the case for a free market*. Praeger, New York.

Trocchi, A. (1966). *Cain's book*. Jupiter Books, Calder & Boyars Ltd, London.

Tyler, A. (1966). *Street drugs* (rev. edn). New English Library, London.

Watson, R. R. (ed.) (1990). *Drug and alcohol abuse prevention*. The Humana Press, Inc., New York.

Weil, A. (1973). *The natural mind*. Jonathan Cape, London.

Wolfe, T. (1969). *The electric kool-aid acid test*. Bantam Books, New York.

Reports

Action on Smoking and Health (1997). *Basic facts on smoking*. ASH, London.

Advisory Council on Misuse of Drugs (1988). *AIDS and drug misuse, Part 1*. HMSO, London.

Advisory Council on the Misuse of Drugs (2000). *Reducing drug related deaths*. The Stationery Office, London. ISBN 0 11 341239 8.

Advisory Council on Misuse of Drugs (2006). *Pathways to Problems: Hazardous use of tobacco, alcohol, and other drugs by young people in the UK and its implications for policy*. HMSO, London.

Chatlos, J. C. (1997). Substance use and abuse and the impact on academic difficulties. *Child and Adolescent Psychiatric Clinics of North America*, **6**, 545–68.

Department of Health (England) (2007). Drug misuse and dependence: UK guidelines on clinical management. London: Department of Health (England), the Scottish Government, Welsh Assembly Government and Northern Ireland Executive.

European Commission (2006). *Report: alcohol in Europe* http://ec.europa.eu/health-eu/news_alcoholineurope_en.htm.

European Monitoring Centre for Drugs and Drug Addiction (2007). *The State of the Drugs Problem in Europe*. Office for Official Publications of the Euroean Communities, Luxembourg.

European School Survey Project on Alcohol and Other Drugs (ESPAD) Report (2003). *Alcohol and other drug use among students in 35 European countries*. The Swedish Council for Information on alcohol and other drugs, CAN Council of Europe, Co-operation Group to Combat Drug Abuse and Illicit Trafficking in Drug (Pompidou Group).

European Monitoring Centre for Drugs and Drug Addiction (2007). *The state of the drug problem in Europe*. Luxembourg: Office for Official Publication of the European Communities.

Health Education Authority (1997). *Results of the 1995 National Drugs Campaign Survey*. HEA, London.

HM Government (2005). *Young people and drugs* DfES Publications, Nottingham.

Home Office Statistical Bulletin (2008). *Crime in England and Wales 2007/08*. Research & Statistics Directorate, London.

House of Lords Select Committee on Science and Technology (1998). *Cannabis: the Scientific and Medical evidence*. HL Paper 151. The Stationery Office, London.

International Centre for Drugs Policy (2008). *Drug-related deaths in the UK: Annual Report 2008*. National Programme on Substance Abuse Deaths, St George's, University of London.

International Narcotics Control Board (2008). *Report of the International Narcotics Control Board for 2007*. United Nations, Geneva.

National Treatment Agency for Substance Misuse (2007). *Reducing drug-related harm: an action plan*. Department of Health, London.

NHS Information Centre (2007). *Statistics on drug misuse: England 2007*. The Information Centre, Lifestyles Statistics.

NHS Information Centre (2008). *Drug use, smoking, and drinking among young people in England in 2007*. The Health and Social Care Information Centre. National Centre for Social Research, London.

Office of Population Censuses and Statistics (1996). *Living in Britain*. HMSO, London.

Reed E (2007). *Seizures of drugs in England and Wales, 2005*. Home Office Statistical Bulletin.

Royal College of Physicians (1992). *Smoking and the young*, RCP, London.

Royal Colleges of Physicians, Psychiatrists, and General Practitioners (1995). *Alcohol and the heart in perspective*. Report of a joint working group, Oxford.

Solowij, N., Lee, N. (1991). *Survey of Ecstasy (MDMA) users in Sydney*. Research Grant Report Series DAD 91–69. Drug and Alcohol Directorate, NSW health Department, Australia.

Substance Abuse and Mental Health Services Administration (2008). *Results from the 2007 National Survey on Drug Use and Health: National Findings*. (Office of Applied Studies, NSDUH Series H-34, DHHS Publication No. SMA 08-4343). Rockville, MD.

United Nations Office on Drugs and Crime (2008). *Annual Report 2008*. http://www.unodc.org/documents/about-unodc/AR08_WEB.pdf.

United Nations Office on Drugs and Crime (2008). *World Drug Report 2008*. United Nations Publication Sales No. E.08.X1.1 978-92-1-148229-4.

Wootton Committee (1968). *Cannabis: Report by the Advisory Committee on Drug Dependence*. HMSO, London.

Index